ILLUSTRATED PHYSIOLOGY

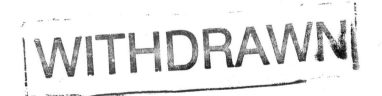

For Churchill Livingstone:

Publisher: Timothy Horne
Project Editor: Janice Urquhart
Indexer: Helen McKillop
Project Controller: Nancy Arnott
Design Direction: Jim Farley

ILLUSTRATED PHYSIOLOGY

B. R. Mackenna MB ChB PhD FRCP(Glasg)
Formerly Senior Lecturer, Institute of Physiology,
University of Glasgow, Glasgow, UK

R. Callander FFPh FMAA AIMBI
Formerly Director of Medical Illustration,
University of Glasgow, Glasgow, UK

SIXTH EDITION

CHURCHILL LIVINGSTONE
EDINBURGH LONDON NEW YORK PHILADELPHIA SAN FRANCISCO SYDNEY TORONTO 1997

CHURCHILL LIVINGSTONE
A Medical Division of Harcourt Brace and Company Limited

 is a registered trademark of Harcourt Brace and Company Limited

First edition 1963
   Italian translation 1966
Second edition 1970
   Danish translation 1973
Third edition 1975
   Japanese translation 1976
   Spanish translation 1981

Fourth edition 1983
   Reprinted 1984, 1986
Fifth edition 1990
   Reprinted 1991, 1992, 1995
Sixth edition 1997
   Reprinted 1998

Standard Edition ISBN 0-443-05060-0

International Student Edition ISBN 0-443-05779-6
   Reprinted 1997
   Reprinted 1998

British Library Cataloguing in Publication Data
A catalogue record for this book is available from the British
Library.

Library of Congress Cataloging in Publication Data
A catalog record for this book is available from the Library
of Congress.

Medical knowledge is constantly changing. As new information
becomes available, changes in treatment, procedures, equipment
and the use of drugs become necessary. The authors and the
publishers have, as far as it is possible, taken care to ensure that
the information given in this text is accurate and up to date.
However, readers are strongly advised to confirm that the
information, especially with regard to drug usage, complies with
current legislation and standards of practice.

The
publisher's
policy is to use
paper manufactured
from sustainable forests

Produced by Addison Wesley Longman China Limited, Hong Kong
NPCC/02

PREFACE TO THE SIXTH EDITION

We continue to be encouraged by the number of students who find Illustrated Physiology useful.

As the demands on students' time continue to increase, the use of a book with minimal text seems to be popular with many of them.

All the material has again been updated for this edition. For students lacking knowledge of chemistry or physics we have added pages on atomic and molecular structure with a special mention for DNA and RNA since it is clear that an understanding of genes and their role in body function is increasingly essential for all those who take an interest in advancements in medicine.

New material has been added about immunity, the alimentary system, the cardiovascular system, the autonomic nervous system and especially the renal system all of which are particularly important to medical students and health-care professionals. Difficult concepts such as the function of the loop of Henle, visual and muscle receptors and plasma clearance have been given additional coverage.

We are indebted to the following colleagues and friends in the Institute of Physiology for helpful discussion and suggestions: Ms Georgie Docherty, Dr H. Y. Elder, Dr M. Gladden, Dr D. J. Miller and Dr J. D. Morrison.

We should like to express our gratitude to our Project Editor, Janice Urquhart of Churchill Livingstone, Edinburgh for the efficient way she has guided the production of this edition of our book.

We hope that Illustrated Physiology will continue to be useful to nurses and other health-care workers and that many medical and dental students both undergraduate and postgraduate will find it a valuable aid to learning and revision.

1997

B. R. Mackenna
R. Callander

PREFACE TO THE FIRST EDITION

This book grew originally from the need to provide visual aids for the large number of students in this department who come to the study of human physiology with no background of mammalian anatomy and often without any conventional training in either the biological or the physical and chemical sciences. Such students include postgraduates studying for the Diploma or Degree in Education, undergraduates working for Degrees in Science, laboratory technicians taking courses for the Ordinary and High National Certificates in Biology, and the increasing number of medical auxiliaries (physiotherapists, occupational therapists, radiographers, cardiographers, dieticians, almoners and social workers) many of whom are required to study to quite advanced levels at least regional parts of the subject.

Many medical, dental and pharmacy students, as well as nurses in training, have been good enough to indicate that they too find diagrams which summarize the salient points of each topic valuable aids to learning or revision. It is our hope that some of these groups may find our book helpful.

Each page is complete in itself and has been designed to oppose its neighbour. It is hoped that this will facilitate the choice of those pages thought suitable for any one course while making it easy to omit those which are too detailed for immediate consideration.

A book of this sort is largely derivative and it is impossible to acknowledge our wider debt. We wish to record our gratitude, however, to Professor R. C. Garry for his generous permission to borrow freely from the large collection of teaching diagrams built up over the years by himself and his staff; to Dr H. S. D. Garven and Dr G. Leaf for permission to use some of their own teaching material; and to Messrs Ciba Pharmaceutical Products Inc. from whose fine book of Medical Illustrations by Dr Frank H. Netter the diagram of the Cranial Nerves has been modified.

We are indebted to the following colleagues and friends who read parts of the original draft and offered helpful criticism: Dr H. S. D. Garven, Dr J. S. Gillespie, Mr J. A. Gilmour, Dr M. Holmes, Dr B. R. Mackenna, Mr T. McClurg Anderson, Dr I. A. Boyd, Dr R. Y. Thomson, Dr J. B. deV. Weir.

We should like to express our gratitude to Mr Charles Macmillan and Mr James Parker of Messrs E. & S. Livingstone Ltd. for their unfailing courtesy and encouragement, and to Mrs Elizabeth Callander for help in preparing the index.

Ann B. McNaught
Robin Callander 1963

WHAT IS PHYSIOLOGY?

Physiology is the study of the function of living matter. Hence, there are many types of Physiology including Bacterial Physiology, Plant Physiology and **Human Physiology**.

To understand how human beings function it is necessary to appreciate that all living things are made of microscopic units of **protoplasm** called **cells**. There are some very simple living creatures which consist of just one cell, for example the **amoeba** which lives in pond water. These unicellular creatures demonstrate the structure of all animal cells and show the phenomena which distinguish living from non-living things. Hence we start with a brief look at such creatures.

The human being is made up of 75 trillion cells which are arranged in a variety of combinations and form various degrees of organized structure. Collections of cells with similar properties form **tissues** (e.g. muscular tissue, nervous tissue). Different tissues combine to form **organs** (e.g. kidneys, brain, heart). Organs are linked together to form **organ systems** (e.g. the heart and blood vessels form the cardiovascular system).

56% of the adult human body is fluid. Most is **inside** the cells (**intracellular fluid**). However about one third is **outside** the cells (**extracellular fluid**) and consists of the **plasma** of the blood which circulates in the cardiovascular system, plus the fluid which surrounds the cells (**intercellular** or **interstitial fluid**). Cells receive their nutrients from the interstitial fluid and as the nutrients are used up more must be brought to this surrounding fluid. Likewise the cells pass waste products to their bathing fluid and this waste must not be allowed to accumulate or it will poison the cells. In addition, the concentration of salts in the interstitial fluid must be kept constant for the cells to function normally.

The extracellular fluid was given the special name **the internal environment** of the body or the **milieu interieur** in the 19th century by the French physiologist Claude Bernard. Physiologists use the term **homeostasis** to mean maintenance of constant conditions in the internal environment.

Thus the main function of most of the tissues and organ systems of the human body is to maintain the constancy of the internal environment so that its cells can function normally. However, to do so the systems must be controlled and regulated. The nervous and hormonal systems are specialized for this regulatory function.

How cells function, how the tissues and organ systems maintain homeostasis and how the systems are regulated is basically what human physiology is about and that is what is illustrated in the following pages.

CONTENTS

CHAPTER 1

INTRODUCTION: ATOMS, ELEMENTS, CELLS, TISSUES AND SYSTEMS

ELEMENTS, ATOMS AND ISOTOPES

The chemical **ELEMENT** cannot be broken into simpler materials by chemical means. If two or more elements are combined they form a COMPOUND. The letter abbreviations by which elements are labelled are called CHEMICAL SYMBOLS and are derived from the first or first and second letters of the English or Latin names of the element. The commonest elements found in the body are C (carbon), H (hydrogen), N (nitrogen) and O (oxygen). See page 5.

Each element is made up of **ATOMS** which are composed of even smaller particles.

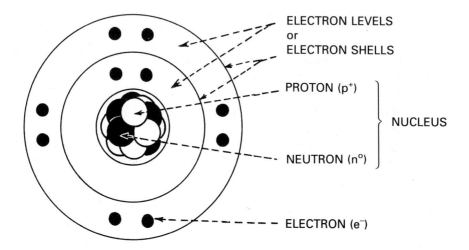

ELECTRON LEVELS
or
ELECTRON SHELLS

PROTON (p^+)

NUCLEUS

NEUTRON (n^o)

ELECTRON (e^-)

Positively charged PROTONS and uncharged NEUTRONS are located in the NUCLEUS. Negatively charged ELECTRONS are in constant motion round the nucleus in energy levels or electron shells (page 3).

The numbers of +ve protons and -ve electrons are equal, hence atoms are electrically neutral.

The unit of mass for atoms and their particles is the DALTON. A neutron has a mass of 1.008 daltons; a proton 1.007 daltons; an electron 0.0005 daltons, hence practically all the mass of an atom is in the nucleus.

The difference between one element and another is due to the difference in the number of PROTONS in their atoms. However, some atoms of the SAME element have different numbers of NEUTRONS. Those different atoms are called **ISOTOPES** of the element. All isotopes have the same chemical properties because the chemical properties of an element are determined by their ELECTRONS and all atoms of an element have the same number of electrons.

Certain isotopes, called RADIOACTIVE ISOTOPES, are unstable and emit various kinds of radiation viz. ALPHA (α) particles composed of two protons and two neutrons; BETA (β) particles composed of particles like electrons but can be either positively or negatively charged; GAMMA (γ) radiation, electromagnetic waves similar to very strong X-rays.

ELECTRONS; ATOMIC NUMBERS AND WEIGHTS; MASS NUMBERS

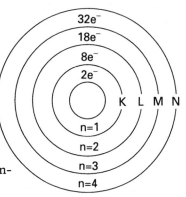

ELECTRONS possess different amounts of energy and are located in numbered ENERGY LEVELS. The lowest energy level (n = 1) can contain a maximum of 2 electrons. The second energy level (n = 2) can contain 8 electrons, the third (n =3) up to 18 electrons, and so on up to n = 7. Electron levels are sometimes called SHELLS and are labelled K,L,M,N, etc. To achieve stability, atoms either empty their outermost energy levels or fill it up to the maximum. In so doing they may give up, accept or share electrons with other atoms, whichever is easiest. The VALENCE (combining capacity) is the number of extra or deficient electrons inthe valence electron energy level (outermost).

ATOMIC STRUCTURE OF COMMON ELEMENTS

Atomic number = number of protons.

Mass number = number of protons + neutrons (mass numbers of only the commonest isotopes are given). Atomic weight = total mass of protons + neutrons + electrons.

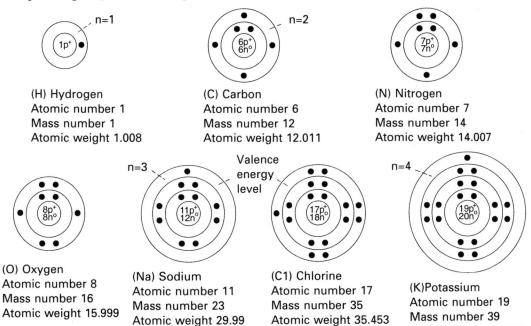

(H) Hydrogen
Atomic number 1
Mass number 1
Atomic weight 1.008

(C) Carbon
Atomic number 6
Mass number 12
Atomic weight 12.011

(N) Nitrogen
Atomic number 7
Mass number 14
Atomic weight 14.007

(O) Oxygen
Atomic number 8
Mass number 16
Atomic weight 15.999

(Na) Sodium
Atomic number 11
Mass number 23
Atomic weight 29.99

(C1) Chlorine
Atomic number 17
Mass number 35
Atomic weight 35.453

(K)Potassium
Atomic number 19
Mass number 39
Atomic weight 39.098

The valence electron energy levels of both sodium (n=3) and potassium (n=4) have only one electron. It is easier to get rid of one electron than to fill these outermost levels with electrons. The valence level of chlorine (n=3) is one short of stability, hence Na and K tend to combine with Cl in chemical reactions. When atoms combine in this way they form MOLECULES.

3

BONDS BETWEEN ATOMS

The outer electrons of one atom may interact with the outer electrons of other atoms, producing attractive forces or CHEMICAL BONDS: IONIC, COVALENT or HYDROGEN.

In **IONIC BONDS**, electrons are actually transferred from one atom to another. Such atoms or aggregates of atoms are then called IONS. The atom gaining an electron or electrons becomes negatively charged, called an ANION (more -ve electrons than +ve protons). The atom which loses electrons becomes positively charged, called a CATION (more +ve protons than -ve electrons).

Since oppositely charged particles attract one another, oppositely charged ions can be held together by this attraction to form electrically neutral ionic compounds. Such attractions are called ionic attractions or IONIC BONDS.

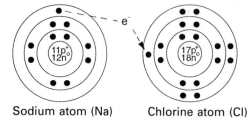

Sodium atom (Na)   Chlorine atom (Cl)

Sodium ion (Na$^+$) Chlorine ion (Cl$^-$)

Sodium chloride molecule (NaCl)

In **COVALENT BONDS**, atoms SHARE electrons in their outer energy level. This is very common.

In an H_2 molecule the two atoms share one pair of electrons which are most often in the region between the two nuclei. The attraction between the ELECTRONS in the middle and the PROTONS in the two nuclei holds the molecule strongly together. If

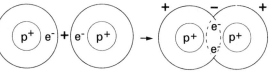

Hydrogen atoms   Hydrogen molecule

one pair of electrons are shared (e.g. H_2) a SINGLE covalent bond is formed. Two pairs shared (e.g. O_2) form a DOUBLE bond. Three pairs (e.g. N_2) a TRIPLE bond.

Shared electrons, attracted equally to both atoms, as with H_2, form

H_2O

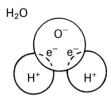

a NON-POLAR COVALENT BOND. However, if one atom attracts the shared electrons more strongly than the other, the bond is a POLAR COVALENT BOND and produces POLAR MOLECULES with positive and negative areas. Water is a polar molecule. Oxygen attracts the shared electrons more strongly and becomes somewhat negative. The hydrogen portions become somewhat positive. Polar bonds allow water to dissolve many molecules that are important to life.

HYDROGEN BONDS Oppositely charged regions of polar molecules can attract one another. Such a bond between hydrogen and e.g. oxygen or nitrogen is called a HYDROGEN BOND. These occur in water, proteins and other large molecules but are weak bonds (5% as strong as covalent bonds). However, large molecules may contain many H-bonds e.g. between bases in DNA and can thus give strength and three-dimensional shape to e.g proteins and nucleic acids.

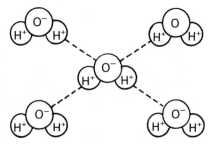

BASIC CONSTITUENTS OF PROTOPLASM

Protoplasm is made up of certain
ELEMENTS — present mainly in — **CHEMICAL COMBINATION**

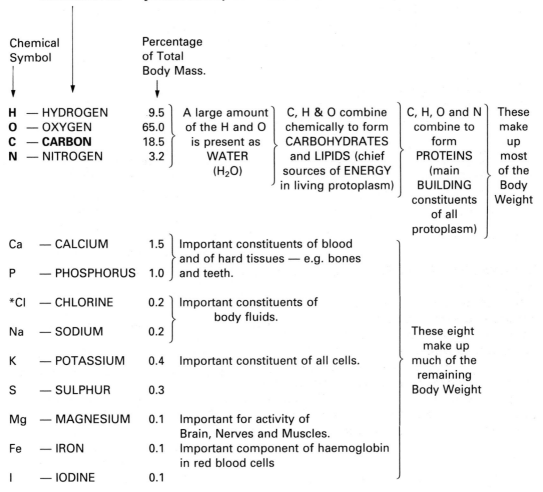

Chemical Symbol		Percentage of Total Body Mass.					
H — HYDROGEN		9.5	A large amount of the H and O is present as WATER (H_2O)	C, H & O combine chemically to form CARBOHYDRATES and LIPIDS (chief sources of ENERGY in living protoplasm)	C, H, O and N combine to form PROTEINS (main BUILDING constituents of all protoplasm)	These make up most of the Body Weight	
O — OXYGEN		65.0					
C — **CARBON**		18.5					
N — NITROGEN		3.2					
Ca — CALCIUM		1.5	Important constituents of blood and of hard tissues — e.g. bones and teeth.				
P — PHOSPHORUS		1.0					
*Cl — CHLORINE		0.2	Important constituents of body fluids.				
Na — SODIUM		0.2			These eight make up much of the remaining Body Weight		
K — POTASSIUM		0.4	Important constituent of all cells.				
S — SULPHUR		0.3					
Mg — MAGNESIUM		0.1	Important for activity of Brain, Nerves and Muscles.				
Fe — IRON		0.1	Important component of haemoglobin in red blood cells				
I — IODINE		0.1					

Trace elements make up the last few grams or so.

These include: Manganese, copper, zinc, cobalt, molybdenum, aluminium, chromium, silicon, fluorine, selenium, boron, strontium and vanadium.
NOTE: Many of these inorganic substances in the protoplasm are in chemical combination. Apart from water, the chief constituents are present as compounds of **carbon**, i.e. they are **organic substances**.

NB: Cl element is chlor**ine**; Salt, e.g. NaCl is chlor**ide**; Ion is chlor**ide** ion (Cl⁻).

THE AMOEBA

All living things are made of **protoplasm**. Protoplasm exists in microscopic units called **cells**. The **amoeba** (which lives in pond water) consists of just one cell but demonstrates the basic structure of all animal cells and shows the phenomena which distinguish living from non-living things.

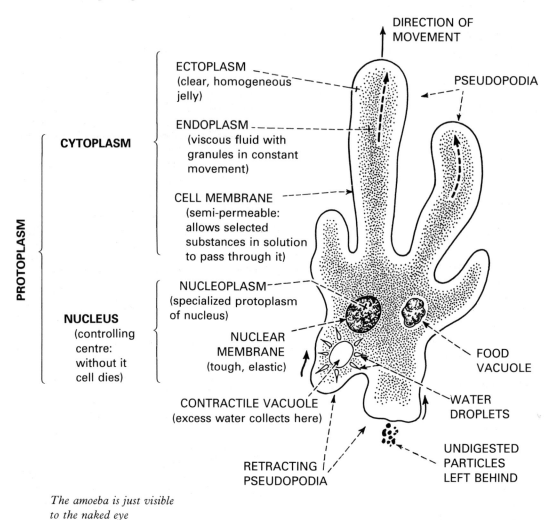

The amoeba is just visible to the naked eye

The constituents of all protoplasm are water, proteins, lipids, carbohydrates and electrolytes.

THE PHENOMENA WHICH CHARACTERIZE ALL LIVING THINGS ARE SHOWN BY THE AMOEBA

1 ORGANIZATION
Autoregulation —
inherent ability to control
all life processes.

2 IRRITABILITY
Ability to respond to
stimuli (from changes
in the environment).

3 CONTRACTILITY
Ability to move.

4 NUTRITION
Ability to ingest,
digest, absorb and
assimilate food.

5 METABOLISM AND GROWTH
Ability to liberate potential
energy of food and to convert
it into mechanical work
(*e.g. movement*) and to
rebuild simple absorbed
units into the complex
protoplasm of the living cell.

6 RESPIRATION
Ability to take in oxygen
for oxidation of food
with release of energy;
and to eliminate the
resulting carbon dioxide.

7 EXCRETION
Ability to eliminate
waste products of
metabolism.

8 REPRODUCTION
Ability to reproduce the
species.

PSEUDOPODIA FORMATION

Small elevation
arises on surface

Cytoplasm
streams
forward

forming
long
pseudopodium

2, 3

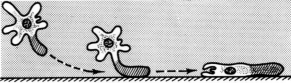

Free
floating

Contact
made

Crawling
along surface

Attracted by favourable stimuli.
Repelled by unfavourable stimuli.

FOOD VACUOLE FORMATION

INGESTION: *Amoeba flows round and engulfs*

food particle.

4

SECRETION of Enzymes
(organic catalysts)
which DIGEST (break
down) complex foods.

ABSORPTION &
UTILIZATION of
simple units by
the living cell

EXPULSION
of
undigested
particles.

RESPIRATION and EXCRETION

Oxygen
(in solution)

Carbon
Dioxide
(in solution)

6, 7

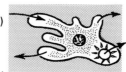

Waste Products
(in solution)

Water periodically
expelled at
surface

REPRODUCTION

Asexual in the amoeba
— by simple fission.

8

THE PARAMECIUM

The paramecium (another one-celled fresh water creature) shows:–
Modification and localization of structure for specialization and localization of certain functions

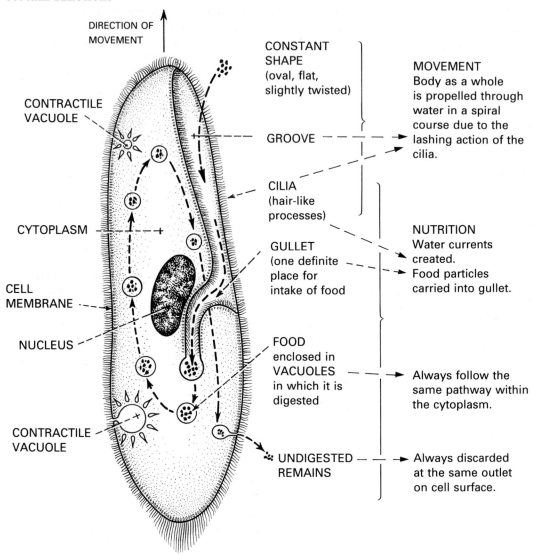

DIRECTION OF MOVEMENT

CONSTANT SHAPE (oval, flat, slightly twisted)

MOVEMENT
Body as a whole is propelled through water in a spiral course due to the lashing action of the cilia.

CONTRACTILE VACUOLE

GROOVE

CILIA (hair-like processes)

CYTOPLASM

GULLET (one definite place for intake of food

NUTRITION
Water currents created.
Food particles carried into gullet.

CELL MEMBRANE

NUCLEUS

FOOD enclosed in VACUOLES in which it is digested

Always follow the same pathway within the cytoplasm.

CONTRACTILE VACUOLE

UNDIGESTED REMAINS

Always discarded at the same outlet on cell surface.

The paramecium is just visible to the naked eye

Many other one-celled animals show elaborate organization and specialization.

THE CELL

The cell is the **structural** and **functional** unit of the many-celled animal. Higher animals, including man, are made up of millions of living cells which vary widely in structure and function but have certain features in common.

The cell contains an outer membrane, the **plasma (cell) membrane**, a nucleus (a spherical or oval organelle often near the centre) and cytoplasm, the region outside the nucleus, in which are cell **organelles** (little organs) suspended in a fluid, the cytosol, and **inclusion bodies** containing secretion and storage substances.

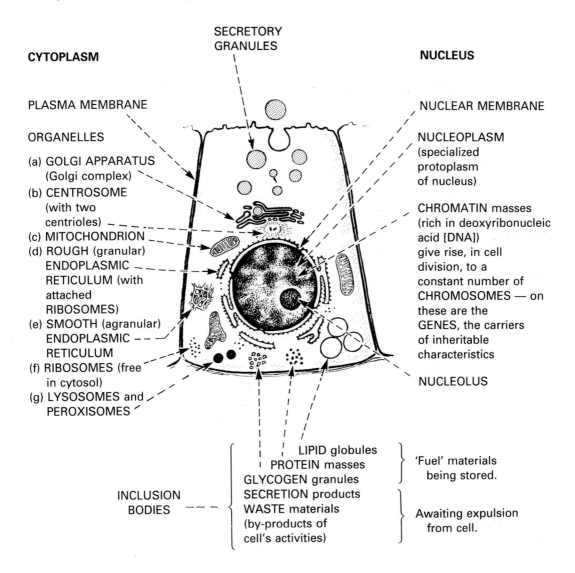

CYTOPLASM

SECRETORY GRANULES

PLASMA MEMBRANE

ORGANELLES

(a) GOLGI APPARATUS (Golgi complex)
(b) CENTROSOME (with two centrioles)
(c) MITOCHONDRION
(d) ROUGH (granular) ENDOPLASMIC RETICULUM (with attached RIBOSOMES)
(e) SMOOTH (agranular) ENDOPLASMIC RETICULUM
(f) RIBOSOMES (free in cytosol)
(g) LYSOSOMES and PEROXISOMES

NUCLEUS

NUCLEAR MEMBRANE

NUCLEOPLASM (specialized protoplasm of nucleus)

CHROMATIN masses (rich in deoxyribonucleic acid [DNA]) give rise, in cell division, to a constant number of CHROMOSOMES — on these are the GENES, the carriers of inheritable characteristics

NUCLEOLUS

INCLUSION BODIES

LIPID globules
PROTEIN masses
GLYCOGEN granules

'Fuel' materials being stored.

SECRETION products
WASTE materials (by-products of cell's activities)

Awaiting expulsion from cell.

FINE STRUCTURE OF CELLS

PLASMA MEMBRANE

The wall of the cell is the **plasma membrane** which controls the rate and type of ions and molecules passing into and out of the cell. It consists of two layers of **phospholipid** molecules interspersed with **protein** molecules.

Note the clothes-pin shape of the phospholipid molecules. The head is the phosphate portion — relatively soluble in water (polar, hydrophilic). The tails are the lipid — relatively insoluble (non-polar, hydrophobic) and they meet in the interior of the membrane. **Integral** proteins are embedded in the membrane: **peripheral** proteins are loosely bound to the inner or outer surface.

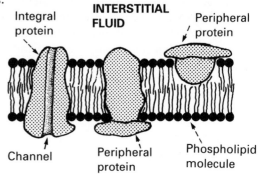

The proteins can function as:
(a) anchors for the cytoskeleton (internal network of protein rods supporting the cell's walls).   (b) carriers to transport substances across the membrane.   (c) channels for ions. Change in the shape of the protein can result in opening or closing of channel. (d) receptors, binding nerve transmitters and hormones which can initiate changes inside the cell.   (e) enzymes catalysing chemical reactions at the membrane surface.

NUCLEUS A nuclear envelope (or membrane), which is really two membranes separated by a space, surrounds the nucleus. At numerous points these membranes are joined, forming the rims of circular openings, the water filled nuclear pores, through which large molecules e.g. ribonucleic acid (RNA) can pass in and out of the nucleus.

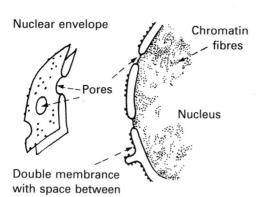

The nucleus is packed with fibres of chromatin which, when the cell divides, coils and shortens into 46 rod-shaped chromosomes. Chromatin fibres appear like 'beads on a string'. Each 'bead' has a central core of eight proteins called histones, around which are two coils of a double strand of deoxyribonucleic acid (DNA). The DNA also links the 'beads' together. Small segments of the DNA molecule are called genes. Each gene provides information required to determine a protein's amino acid sequence.

DNA molecules are too large to pass out of the nucleus. Hence part of the DNA molecule assembles (by a process called **transcription**) a nucleic acid which is smaller than DNA, called messenger ribonucleic acid (mRNA) which can pass into the cytoplasm. mRNA carries the code for polypeptide and protein assembly to the ribosomes. Amino acids are also carried to the ribosomes attached to other, smaller RNA molecules, called transfer RNA (tRNA). Polypeptides and proteins can then be assembled on the ribosomes from the amino acids according to the mRNA code (a process called **translation**).

ORGANELLES

NUCLEOLUS

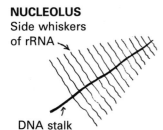

Side whiskers
of rRNA

DNA stalk

RIBOSOMES

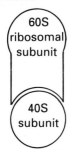

60S
ribosomal
subunit

40S
subunit

GOLGI APPARATUS

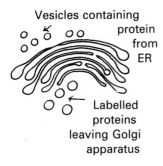

Vesicles containing
protein
from
ER

Labelled
proteins
leaving Golgi
apparatus

LYSOSOMES

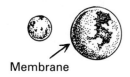

Membrane

PEROXISOMES

The **nucleolus** is a spherical body within the nucleus. It has no membrane and is **packed** with 'fern-like' structures, each consisting of a stalk of DNA and side whiskers of ribosomal ribonucleic acid (rRNA). The rRNA molecules are combined with protein to form subunits of ribosomes which pass into the cytoplasm where the subunits combine to form ribosomes.

Each **ribosome** consists of over 70 protein molecules and rRNA molecules, and is divided into two subunits called 40S and 60S on the basis of their sedimentation rates in a centrifuge. Some ribosomes are bound to a structure called **endoplasmic reticulum (ER)** and some are free in the cytosol. Ribosomes synthesize polypeptides and proteins from amino acids carried to the ribosomes by transfer RNA (tRNA) and assembled using instructions carried by mRNA molecules from genes in the nucleus. Proteins synthesized by endoplasmic reticulum ribosomes pass into the ER lumen then to the **Golgi apparatus** where they are processed as described below. Proteins manufactured by free ribosomes perform their functions in the cytosol.

The **Golgi apparatus** consists of a collection of membrane-enclosed sacs like 4–6 stacked saucers. Proteins from the endoplasmic reticulum have their structure altered here. This alteration is a kind of label which determines whether the protein will be (a) passed into **lysosomes** (see below), (b) stored in secretory granules or (c) inserted into the plasma membrane.

Lysosomes are large membrane-bound organelles of various sizes which act as intracellular scavengers. They contain digestive enzymes which digest e.g. bacteria, which have been engulfed by the cell, and cellular debris such as damaged organelles.

Peroxisomes are similar in structure to the lysosomes. They contain (a) enzymes which combine oxygen and hydrogen to form hydrogen peroxide (H_2O_2) and (b) and enzyme which converts H_2O_2 to water.

11

ORGANELLES

ENDOPLASMIC RETICULUM

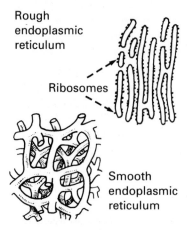

Rough endoplasmic reticulum

Ribosomes

Smooth endoplasmic reticulum

The endoplasmic reticulum is a network of interconnected tubular and flattened sac-like channels. The space between their walls is continuous with the space of the nuclear membrane and can thus transport substances from one part of the cell to another. One form of ER, **rough** or **granular** endoplasmic reticulum, has ribosomes attached to its outer surface and the other form, **smooth** or **agranular**, has no ribosomes. The spaces between both types are connected. Ribosomes on rough ER synthesize proteins while smooth ER is involved in carbohydrate metabolism. Specialized types of ER are present in some cells e.g. in skeletal muscle cells smooth ER stores calcium ions which are liberated to initiate contraction of muscle cells.

MITOCHONDRIA

Mitochondria are sausage or oval shaped organelles with a smooth outer membrane and an inner membrane which is folded to form shelves or **cristae** which extend into the internal space or **matrix**. The inner membrane is the power plant of the cell. Enzymes in the matrix function in association with oxidative enzymes on the cristae to convert the products of fat, protein and carbohydrate metabolism to carbon dioxide and water via the citric acid cycle (see p. 49). Energy is thus liberated and used to synthesize a high energy substance **adenosine triphosphate** (ATP). ATP is transported out of the mitochondria and diffuses throughout the cell to release its energy wherever it is required.

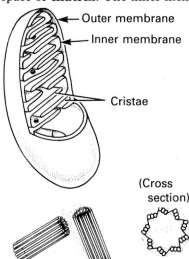

Outer membrane

Inner membrane

Cristae

(Cross section)

Centrioles

CENTROSOME

The centrosome consists of two rod-like structures called **centrioles** arranged at right angles to one another. It is concerned with the synthesis of microtubules, e.g. the spindle and aster microtubules present during cell division.

SECRETORY VESICLES

All secretory substances are formed by the endoplasmic reticulum — Golgi apparatus system. They are then released from the Golgi apparatus into the cytoplasm inside storage vesicles called **secretory vesicles** or **secretory granules**.

In addition to the above organelles the cytoplasm may contain any of a variety of rod-like filaments, microfilaments and microtubular structures, depending on the function of the cell.

CELL DIVISION (MITOSIS)

All cells arise from the division of pre-existing cells. In mitosis there is an exact *qualitative* division of the nucleus and a less exact *quantitative* division of the cytoplasm. The period of time between one mitosis and the next is called INTERPHASE.

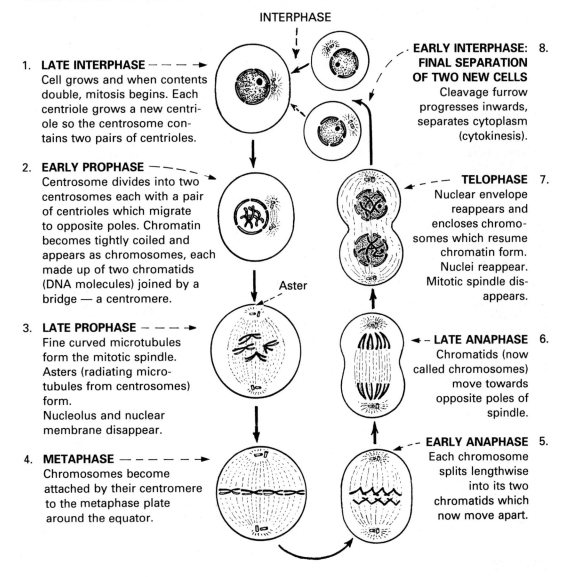

INTERPHASE

1. **LATE INTERPHASE** – – – ➤
Cell grows and when contents double, mitosis begins. Each centriole grows a new centriole so the centrosome contains two pairs of centrioles.

2. **EARLY PROPHASE** – – – –
Centrosome divides into two centrosomes each with a pair of centrioles which migrate to opposite poles. Chromatin becomes tightly coiled and appears as chromosomes, each made up of two chromatids (DNA molecules) joined by a bridge — a centromere.

Aster

3. **LATE PROPHASE** – – – ➤
Fine curved microtubules form the mitotic spindle. Asters (radiating microtubules from centrosomes) form.
Nucleolus and nuclear membrane disappear.

4. **METAPHASE** – – – – – ➤
Chromosomes become attached by their centromere to the metaphase plate around the equator.

EARLY INTERPHASE: 8.
FINAL SEPARATION OF TWO NEW CELLS
Cleavage furrow progresses inwards, separates cytoplasm (cytokinesis).

– – **TELOPHASE** 7.
Nuclear envelope reappears and encloses chromosomes which resume chromatin form. Nuclei reappear. Mitotic spindle disappears.

◄ – **LATE ANAPHASE** 6.
Chromatids (now called chromosomes) move towards opposite poles of spindle.

– – **EARLY ANAPHASE** 5.
Each chromosome splits lengthwise into its two chromatids which now move apart.

The longitudinal halving of chromosomes into two chromatids (DNA molecules) ensures that each new cell receives the same genes (hereditary factors) as the original cell.

The number of chromosomes is constant in any one species.

The cells of the human body (somatic cells) carry 23 pairs — i.e. 46 chromosomes.

For clarity only 4 chromosomes (2 pairs) are shown in these diagrams.

DIFFERENTIATION OF ANIMAL CELLS

Specialization distinguishes multicellular creatures from more primitive forms of life.

ONE-CELLED ORGANISMS — Capable of INDEPENDENT existence —
Undifferentiated ———— Show all activities or ----------**PHENOMENA of LIFE**
MANY-CELLED ANIMALS Cells COOPERATE for All cells retain powers of
well-being of whole body. ORGANIZATION
Differentiated ———— Groups of cells undergo IRRITABILITY
adaptations and sacrifice NUTRITION
some powers to fit them METABOLISM
for special duties. RESPIRATION
EXCRETION

MODIFICATION *for* SPECIALIZATION LOSS or REDUCTION
OF STRUCTURE *efficient* of FUNCTION ········ *with* ········ of VERSATILITY
e.g.

1. **SECRETORY CELL** -------- Highly developed powers Diminished powers of
of SECRETION CONTRACTION and
Cytoplasm Nucleus e.g. enzymes for REPRODUCTION
displaced chemical breakdown
to base by of foodstuffs.
Nucleus formed and
stored
secretion

2. **FAT CELL** ----------------- STORAGE of FAT Loss of powers of
Cytoplasm Cytoplasm CONTRACTION and
displaced SECRETION
by stored
Nucleus ----- fat

3. **MUSCLE CELL** ------------- Highly developed powers Diminished powers of
of CONTRACTILITY SECRETION and
Cytoplasm *Nucleus* REPRODUCTION
Elongated
cell body

4. **NERVE CELL** ------------ Highly developed powers Loss of powers of
Cytoplasm of IRRITABILITY REPRODUCTION

Cytoplasm (response to stimuli i.e. if nerve
drawn out and transmission of cell is destroyed
into long impulses over long no regeneration
Nucleus branching distances) is possible.
processes (If only axon is damaged,
x 500 it may grow a new axon.)

ORGANIZATION OF TISSUES

Cells which are alike are arranged together to form **tissues**. There are 4 main types of
tissue: 1. EPITHELIAL or LINING, 2. CONNECTIVE or SUPPORTING, 3.
MUSCULAR and 4. NERVOUS. These four join to form the organs of the body.

EPITHELIA

STRUCTURAL MODIFICATIONS   *SITE*   *SPECIALIZED
FUNCTIONS*

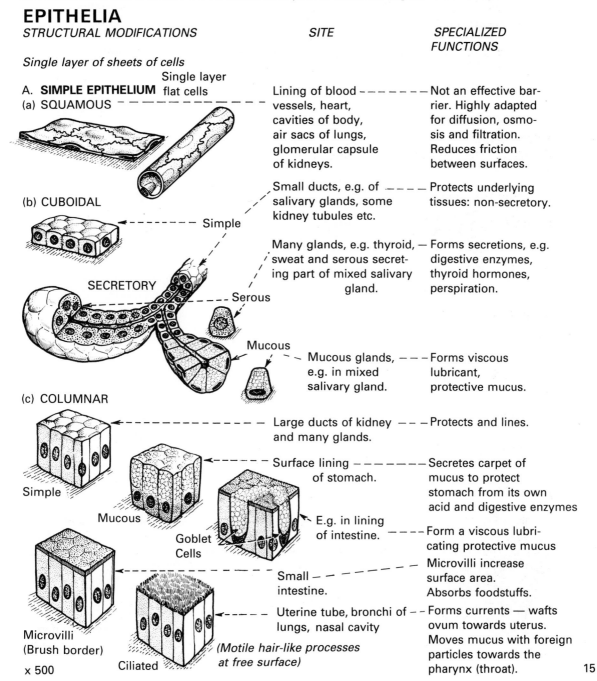

Single layer of sheets of cells

Single layer

A. **SIMPLE EPITHELIUM** flat cells

(a) SQUAMOUS

Lining of blood – – – – – – Not an effective bar-
vessels, heart, rier. Highly adapted
cavities of body, for diffusion, osmo-
air sacs of lungs, sis and filtration.
glomerular capsule Reduces friction
of kidneys. between surfaces.

(b) CUBOIDAL

Simple

Small ducts, e.g. of – – – – Protects underlying
salivary glands, some tissues: non-secretory.
kidney tubules etc.

SECRETORY

Serous

Many glands, e.g. thyroid, — Forms secretions, e.g.
sweat and serous secret- digestive enzymes,
ing part of mixed salivary thyroid hormones,
gland. perspiration.

Mucous

Mucous glands, – – – Forms viscous
e.g. in mixed lubricant,
salivary gland. protective mucus.

(c) COLUMNAR

Simple

Large ducts of kidney – – – Protects and lines.
and many glands.

Mucous

Surface lining – – – – – – Secretes carpet of
of stomach. mucus to protect
stomach from its own
acid and digestive enzymes

Goblet
Cells

E.g. in lining
of intestine. – – – – Form a viscous lubricating protective mucus

Microvilli
(Brush border)

Small – – – – Microvilli increase
intestine. surface area.
Absorbs foodstuffs.

Ciliated

Uterine tube, bronchi of – – Forms currents — wafts
lungs, nasal cavity ovum towards uterus.
Moves mucus with foreign
(Motile hair-like processes particles towards the
at free surface) pharynx (throat).

x 500

15

EPITHELIA

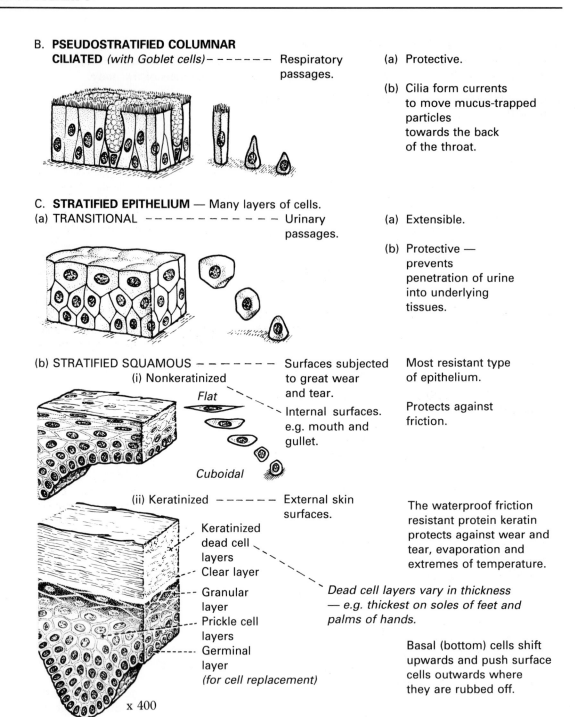

B. **PSEUDOSTRATIFIED COLUMNAR**
CILIATED *(with Goblet cells)*– – – – – – – Respiratory passages.

(a) Protective.

(b) Cilia form currents to move mucus-trapped particles towards the back of the throat.

C. **STRATIFIED EPITHELIUM** — Many layers of cells.
(a) TRANSITIONAL – – – – – – – – – – – Urinary passages.

(a) Extensible.

(b) Protective — prevents penetration of urine into underlying tissues.

(b) STRATIFIED SQUAMOUS – – – – – – –
    (i) Nonkeratinized

Flat

Surfaces subjected to great wear and tear.

Internal surfaces. e.g. mouth and gullet.

Most resistant type of epithelium.

Protects against friction.

Cuboidal

    (ii) Keratinized – – – – – – External skin surfaces.

Keratinized dead cell layers
Clear layer
Granular layer
Prickle cell layers
Germinal layer
(for cell replacement)

The waterproof friction resistant protein keratin protects against wear and tear, evaporation and extremes of temperature.

Dead cell layers vary in thickness — e.g. thickest on soles of feet and palms of hands.

Basal (bottom) cells shift upwards and push surface cells outwards where they are rubbed off.

x 400

Stratified cuboidal and stratified columnar epithelia are also found in the body but are uncommon.

CONNECTIVE TISSUES (CT)

STRUCTURAL MODIFICATIONS
Cells plus large amount of intercellular
matrix and extracellular elements.

SPECIALIZED FUNCTIONS
Form framework, connecting, supporting
and packing tissues of the body.

1. CELLS (floating free) in a FLUID MATRIX called PLASMA
   BLOOD

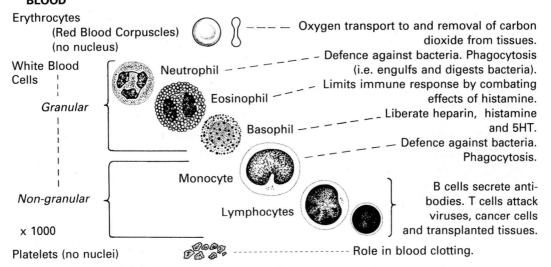

Erythrocytes
  (Red Blood Corpuscles)
  (no nucleus) — — — Oxygen transport to and removal of carbon
                      dioxide from tissues.

White Blood Cells

Granular

Neutrophil — — — Defence against bacteria. Phagocytosis
                  (i.e. engulfs and digests bacteria).

Eosinophil — — Limits immune response by combating
                effects of histamine.

Basophil — — — Liberate heparin, histamine
                and 5HT.

— — Defence against bacteria.
     Phagocytosis.

Monocyte

Non-granular

Lymphocytes

B cells secrete anti-
bodies. T cells attack
viruses, cancer cells
and transplanted tissues.

x 1000

Platelets (no nuclei) ---------- Role in blood clotting.

2. CELLS in SEMI-SOLID JELLY-LIKE MATRIX with fine fibrils.
   MESENCHYME

Mesenchymal cells
in semi-fluid
ground substance

Cytoplasm drawn
out to touch
neighbouring cells

Earliest type found in embryo.

From it other connective
tissues differentiate e.g.
bone, cartilage, blood
and fibres of connective
tissue.

3. CELLS in SEMI-SOLID MATRIX with fine network of
   extracellular RETICULAR FIBRES.
   RETICULAR

Reticular fibres — — — — — — — Form 3-dimensional 'net'.
                                  Framework of e.g. spleen,
                                  lymph nodes, bone marrow,
                                  liver, basement membrane.
                                  The glandular cells of these organs
                                  are anchored to the reticular framework.

Reticular
cells

x 500

Macrophages provide defence against microorganisms and are so important that they are often referred to collectively as the macrophage system (formerly called the reticuloendothelial system).

17

CONNECTIVE TISSUES (CT)

4. CELLS in SEMI-SOLID MATRIX with thicker collagenous and elastic fibres.

(a) LOOSE FIBROUS CT

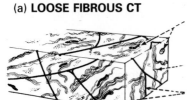

Fibroblasts (cells actively forming fibres)

Collagen fibres

Elastic fibres

Attaches skin to underlying tissue. 'Packing' tissue between organs: sheaths of muscles and nerves: surrounds and supports blood vessels. Contains large amount of tissue fluid.

(b) DENSE IRREGULAR CT

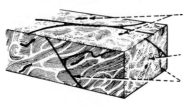

Fibrocytes (resting cells)

Collagen fibres

Elastic fibres

Like loose CT but with fewer cells and more collagen fibres which are randomly arranged.
Forms dermis of skin; fibrous capsules of liver, kidney, spleen etc.

(c) DENSE REGULAR CT

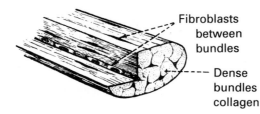

Fibroblasts between bundles

Dense bundles of collagen

Contains predominance of parallel bundles of collagenous fibres. The only cells are fibroblasts.
Forms tendons of muscles, ligaments of joints etc.

(d) ELASTIC CT

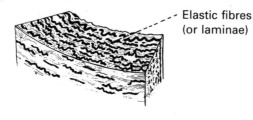

Elastic fibres (or laminae)

Strong extensible and flexible — e.g. in walls of blood vessels and air passages.

(e) ADIPOSE CT

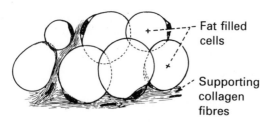

Fat filled cells

Supporting collagen fibres

Protective 'cushion' for organs. Insulating layer in skin. Storage of fat reserves

CONNECTIVE TISSUES (CT)

5. CELLS in SOLID ELASTIC MATRIX with fibres.
(a) HYALINE CARTILAGE

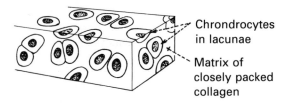

Chrondrocytes in lacunae

Matrix of closely packed collagen

Firm yet flexible. Forms embryonic skeleton, which is replaced by bone; also costal cartilages, rings of trachea and articular cartilages at ends of bones.

(b) WHITE FIBRO-CARTILAGE

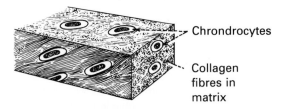

Chrondrocytes

Collagen fibres in matrix

Tough. Resistant to stretching. Slightly compressible. Acts as shock absorber between vertebrae — the intervertebral discs. Pubic symphysis.

(c) ELASTIC or YELLOW FIBRO-CARTILAGE

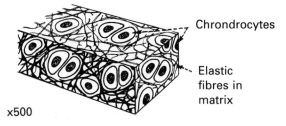

Chrondrocytes

Elastic fibres in matrix

More flexible, resilient — e.g. in larynx, external ear and the epiglottis.

x500

6. CELLS in SOLID RIGID MATRIX impregnated with mainly calcium salts reinforced with collagen fibres.

BONE

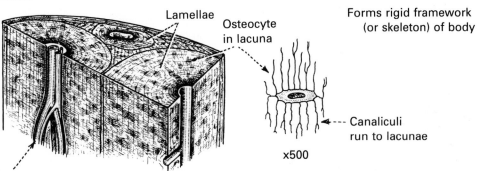

Lamellae

Osteocyte in lacuna

Forms rigid framework (or skeleton) of body

Canaliculi run to lacunae

x500

Haversian canal containing blood vessels.

x100

MUSCULAR TISSUES

All have **elongated** cells with special development of **contractility** and, as a result, provide motion, maintain posture and generate heat.

1. SMOOTH, NON-STRIATED, VISCERAL or INVOLUNTARY muscle

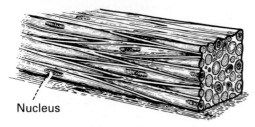

Least specialised. Not under voluntary control. Found in walls of blood vessels, airways to lungs, stomach and intestines. If connected by gap junctions, muscle contracts as a single unit. If gap junctions absent, fibres contract individually e.g. iris of eye.

Nucleus

2. CARDIAC or HEART muscle

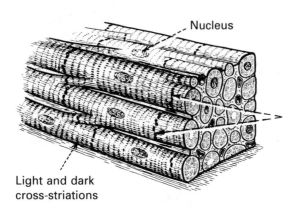

Nucleus

More highly specialised. Rapid rhythmical contraction (and relaxation) spreads through whole muscle mass. Not under voluntary control. Found only in heart wall.

Cells adhere, end to end, at intercalated discs to form long 'fibres' which branch and connect with adjacent 'fibres'.

There are GAP junctions and desmosomes (page 24) between the fibres.

Light and dark cross-striations

3. SKELETAL, STRIATED or VOLUNTARY muscle

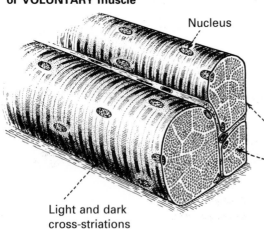

Nucleus

Most highly specialized. Very rapid, powerful contractions of individual fibres. Under voluntary control. Found in e.g. muscles of trunk, limbs, head.

Thick covering membrane (sarcolemma)

Many myofibrils embedded in sarcoplasm

Light and dark cross-striations (See page 000)

Cells are very long, multi-nucleated units. No branching.

NERVOUS TISSUES

Nervous tissue is divided into:-

(a) **Neurons or Nerve cells**
specialized in
IRRITABILITY
CONDUCTION
INTEGRATION

> MOTOR — pass messages from brain and spinal cord to effector organs (muscles and glands).
> ASSOCIATION — relay messages between neurons.
> SENSORY — receive and pass messages from environment to brain and spinal cord.

(b) **Accessory** or Supporting cells
Not RECEPTIVE
Not CONDUCTING

> NEUROGLIA in Central Nervous System (Brain and Spinal Cord).
> SHEATH (Schwann) cells on peripheral nerve fibres, i.e. outside CNS.
> SATELLITE cells in ganglia of peripheral nervous systems.

TYPICAL NERVE CELL (Motor)

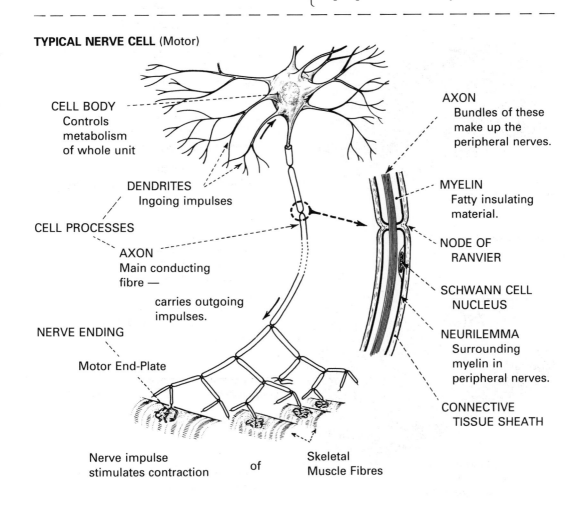

CELL BODY
Controls metabolism of whole unit

DENDRITES
Ingoing impulses

CELL PROCESSES

AXON
Main conducting fibre —

carries outgoing impulses.

NERVE ENDING

Motor End-Plate

AXON
Bundles of these make up the peripheral nerves.

MYELIN
Fatty insulating material.

NODE OF RANVIER

SCHWANN CELL NUCLEUS

NEURILEMMA
Surrounding myelin in peripheral nerves.

CONNECTIVE TISSUE SHEATH

Nerve impulse stimulates contraction of Skeletal Muscle Fibres

NERVOUS TISSUES

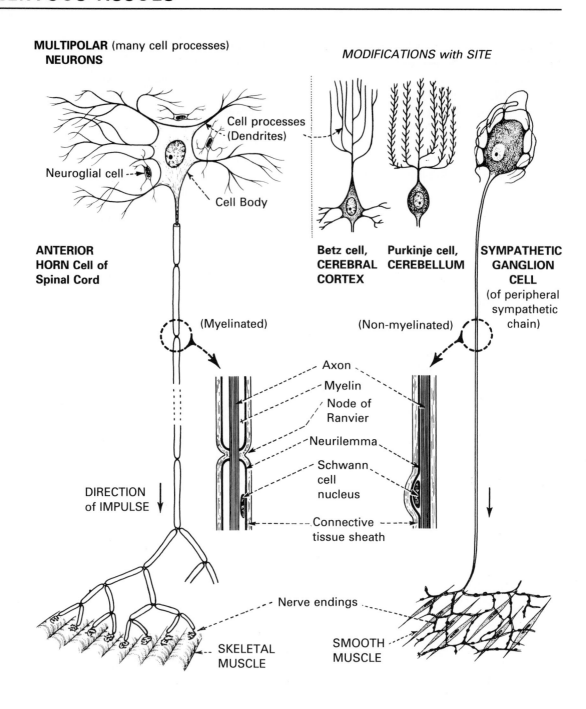

MULTIPOLAR (many cell processes) **NEURONS**

MODIFICATIONS with SITE

Cell processes (Dendrites)

Neuroglial cell

Cell Body

ANTERIOR HORN Cell of Spinal Cord

Betz cell, **CEREBRAL CORTEX**

Purkinje cell, **CEREBELLUM**

SYMPATHETIC GANGLION CELL (of peripheral sympathetic chain)

(Myelinated)

(Non-myelinated)

Axon

Myelin

Node of Ranvier

Neurilemma

Schwann cell nucleus

DIRECTION of IMPULSE

Connective tissue sheath

Nerve endings

SKELETAL MUSCLE

SMOOTH MUSCLE

Most multipolar neurons are **motor** (efferent) or **association** in function.

NERVOUS TISSUES

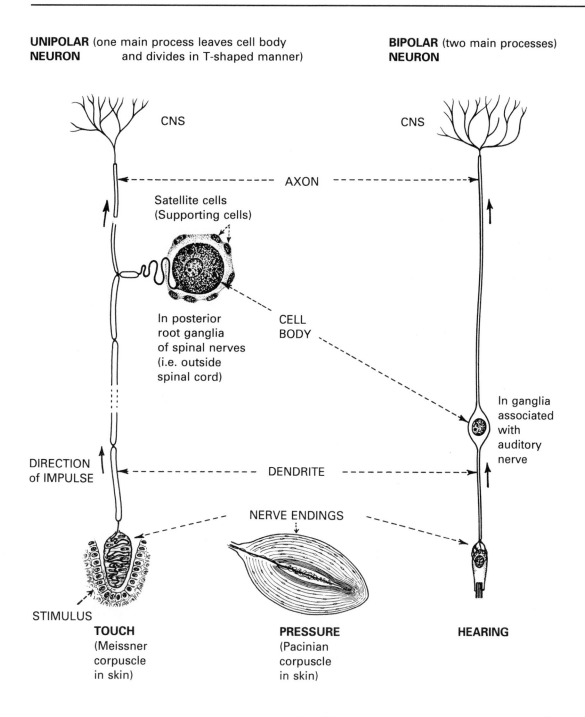

UNIPOLAR (one main process leaves cell body
NEURON   and divides in T-shaped manner)

BIPOLAR (two main processes)
NEURON

CNS

CNS

AXON

Satellite cells
(Supporting cells)

In posterior
root ganglia
of spinal nerves
(i.e. outside
spinal cord)

CELL
BODY

In ganglia
associated
with
auditory
nerve

DIRECTION
of IMPULSE

DENDRITE

NERVE ENDINGS

STIMULUS

TOUCH
(Meissner
corpuscle
in skin)

PRESSURE
(Pacinian
corpuscle
in skin)

HEARING

All unipolar and bipolar neurons are **sensory (afferent)** in function i.e. carry information
TO the Central Nervous System (CNS).

23

JUNCTIONS BETWEEN CELLS

Epithelial cells, cardiac muscle, some smooth muscle and some nerve cells are joined by 3 specialized types of membrane junction: 1. Tight Junctions, 2. Gap junctions, 3. Desmosomes.

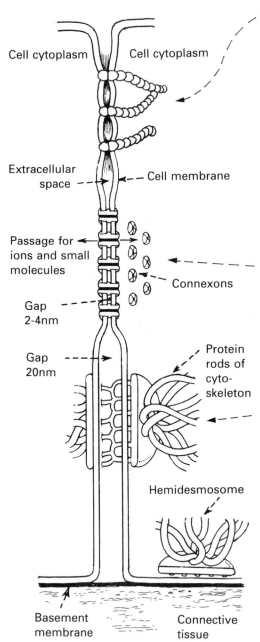

Cell cytoplasm

Cell cytoplasm

Extracellular space

Cell membrane

Passage for ions and small molecules

Connexons

Gap 2-4nm

Gap 20nm

Protein rods of cyto-skeleton

Hemidesmosome

Basement membrane

Connective tissue

TIGHT JUNCTIONS These are found just below the free surface of adjacent cells. Formed by a network of protein strands in the plasma membrane of adjacent cells which interlock and fuse at points around the entire circumference of the cells like teeth in a zip fastener. Between the sites of fusion intercellular separation remains. Common in epithelial cells of kidney, intestine and bladder. Tight junctions restrict the movement of molecules between the cells but they have a variable leakiness to ions and water. The movement of molecules is thus directed through the cell membranes which are able to control the types and amounts of substances absorbed.

GAP JUNCTIONS consist of cylindrical tubes of protein called CONNEXONS which span the membranes of adjacent cells and the 2-4 nanometre gap between them. They allow the direct passage of ions and small molecules, and hence of electrical signals, from cell to cell in cardiac muscle, some smooth muscle, some nerve cells and bone forming cells.

DESMOSOMES consist of dense intracellular proteins which form disc-shaped thickenings of the inner layers of the two cell membranes. A 20 nanometre gap between the cells at the discs has many fine filaments that connect the two cells together. The inner surface of the discs is attached to filaments of the cytoskeleton (internal cell skeleton made of protein rods). Desmosomes form firm attachments between cells somewhat like spot welds. HEMIDESMOSOMES — look like half a desmosome — anchor the basal (bottom) cell plasma membrane to the extracellular basement membrane.

(1 million nanometres = 1 millimetre)

CELL DIVISION (MEIOSIS)

New individuals develop after fusion of 2 specialized cells — the **gametes**. During their formation the **ovum** (female) and the **spermatozoon** (male) undergo two special cell divisions to reduce the chromosome content of each to the haploid number of 23. In fusion, the mingling of male and female chromosomes restores the normal diploid number — 46.

MATURATION of the MALE GAMETES (only one pair of chromosomes in a nucleus and no cytoplasm are illustrated)

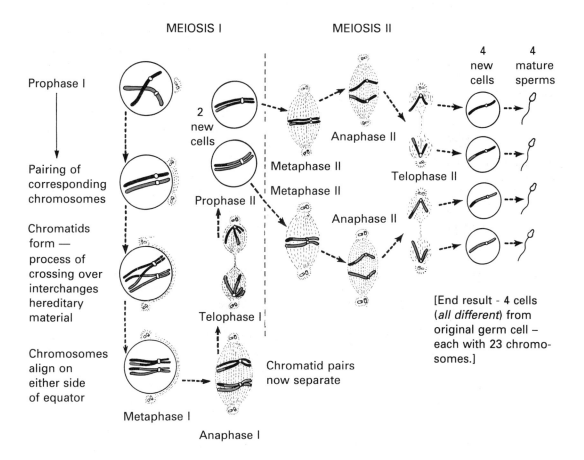

MEIOSIS I

MEIOSIS II

Prophase I

Pairing of corresponding chromosomes

Chromatids form — process of crossing over interchanges hereditary material

Chromosomes align on either side of equator

Metaphase I

Anaphase I

2 new cells

Prophase II

Telophase I

Metaphase II

Metaphase II

Chromatid pairs now separate

Anaphase II

Anaphase II

Telophase II

4 new cells

4 mature sperms

[End result - 4 cells (*all different*) from original germ cell – each with 23 chromosomes.]

In the **female**, three of the 'cells' are small polar bodies which are discarded and disintegrate.

One single mature **ovum** receives most of the cytoplasm.

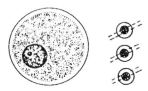

DEVELOPMENT OF THE INDIVIDUAL

All tissues of the human body are derived from the single cell — the **fertilized ovum**.

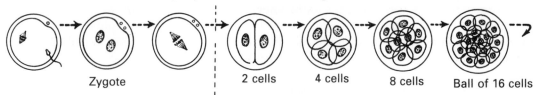

Zygote   2 cells   4 cells   8 cells   Ball of 16 cells

FERTILIZATION

Fusion of ovum and spermatozoon (gametes)

CLEAVAGE

Repeated mitotic divisions: each cell receives equal number of *maternal* and *paternal* chromosomes.

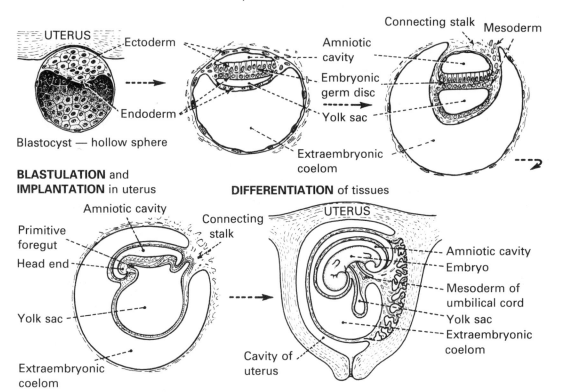

BLASTULATION and
IMPLANTATION in uterus

DIFFERENTIATION of tissues

EMBRYONIC GERM DISC

Ectoderm
gives rise to
- Epithelia of *external* surfaces, oral cavity and salivary glands.
- Nervous tissues.

Mesoderm
gives rise to
- Muscular tissues.
- Connective tissues.
- Kidneys, ureters and gonads.
- Lining of body cavities and blood vessels.

Endoderm
gives rise to
- Epithelia of most *internal* surfaces.
- Some glands (e.g. liver, pancreas, thyroid, parathyroid, urinary bladder, liver and gall bladder).

THE BODY SYSTEMS

The tissues are arranged to form **organs**.
Organs are grouped into **systems**.

THE ESSENTIAL LIFE PROCESSES — — — — — are delegated to — — — — — **SEPARATE SYSTEMS**

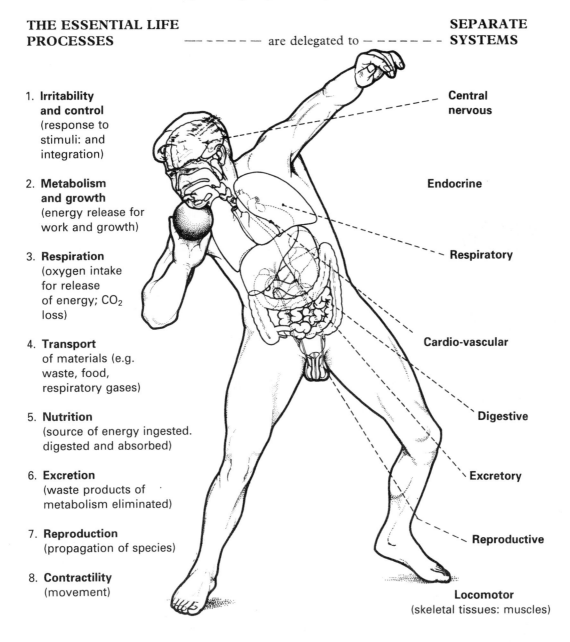

1. **Irritability and control** (response to stimuli: and integration)

2. **Metabolism and growth** (energy release for work and growth)

3. **Respiration** (oxygen intake for release of energy; CO_2 loss)

4. **Transport** of materials (e.g. waste, food, respiratory gases)

5. **Nutrition** (source of energy ingested. digested and absorbed)

6. **Excretion** (waste products of metabolism eliminated)

7. **Reproduction** (propagation of species)

8. **Contractility** (movement)

Central nervous

Endocrine

Respiratory

Cardio-vascular

Digestive

Excretory

Reproductive

Locomotor
(skeletal tissues: muscles)

The systems do not work independently. The body works as a whole. Health and well-being depend on the coordinated effort of every part.

CHAPTER 2

NUTRITION AND METABOLISM: THE SOURCES, RELEASE AND USES OF ENERGY

CARBOHYDRATES

Carbohydrates consist of atoms of C, H and O. They are a major energy source for the body.

MONOSACCHARIDES (sugars) are the simplest. Most common in the diet are the **hexoses**, which have six carbon atoms, e.g. **glucose, fructose** and **galactose**. Four or five carbon atoms lie in a flat plane, linked with an oxygen atom. Remaining atoms form side groups projecting above or below the ring.

GLUCOSE

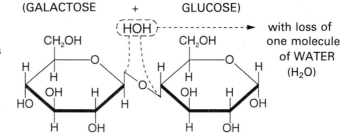

usually written →

Glucose is the major fuel required by cells to provide energy.

NB: The carbon atoms are numbered **1-6**

   Very large organic molecules can be made by linking together smaller molecular subunits forming chains known as **polymers**.
   Larger carbohydrate molecules can be formed by linking monosaccharides together.

DISACCHARIDES   Two monosaccharide molecules linked together, e.g.
   galactose + glucose = lactose (milk sugar),
   glucose + fructose = sucrose (table sugar).

LACTOSE   (GALACTOSE   +   GLUCOSE)

[NB: Same constituent elements as glucose but difference in orientation of H and O groups on carbon 4.]

HOH - - - - - - - - - - - → with loss of one molecule of WATER (H_2O)

POLYSACCHARIDES Long chains of **glucose** units can form **glycogen, starch** and **cellulose**.

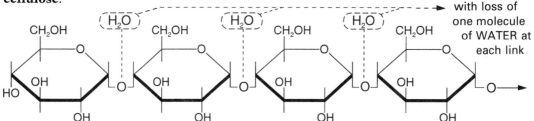

with loss of one molecule of WATER at each link

Cellulose is a straight chain without branches; important in the structure of plants.
Glycogen is a chain of glucose units with frequent branches along the molecule; it is the form in which **animals** store glucose.
Starch is less branched; it is the form in which plants store glucose.

LIPIDS

LIPIDS can be subdivided into three classes: (1) **Triglycerides** (Triacylglycerols or Neutral Fats), (2) **Phospholipids** and (3) **Steroids**. They all contain mainly H and C and are insoluble in water.

TRIGLYCERIDES — the most common form of fat in the body. They consist of one molecule of **glycerol** linked with 3 molecules of **fatty acid**. The three fatty acids may all be the same or they may be different. A fatty acid consists of a chain of carbon atoms with a carboxyl group at one end. In triglycerides the carboxyl group is linked to a hydroxyl group of glycerol.

GLYCEROL FATTY ACIDS

CH_2O [H+HO] $OCCH_2CH_2CH_2CH_2CH_2CH_2CH_2CH_2CH_2CH_2CH_2CH_2CH_2CH_2CH_2CH_3$
|
CHO [H+HO] $OCCH_2CH_2CH_2CH_2CH_2CH_2CH_2CH_2CH_2CH_2CH_2CH_2CH_2CH_2CH_2CH_3$
|
CH_2O [H+HO] $OCCH_2CH_2CH_2CH_2CH_2CH_2CH_2CH_2CH_2CH_2CH_2CH_2CH_2CH_2CH_2CH_3$

with the loss of three molecules of H_2O

When all the carbons in a fatty acid chain are linked by single bonds, the fatty acid is said to be **saturated** with hydrogen bonds. If the fatty acid chain contains double bonds it is **unsaturated**. If it contains more than one double bond, it is **polyunsaturated**. Animal fats contain saturated fatty acids and vegetable fats contain polyunsaturated fatty acids.

PHOSPHOLIPIDS – In these lipids glycerol is linked to two fatty acids and the third hydroxyl group of the glycerol molecule is linked to a phosphate group which in turn is linked to a nitrogen containing molecule. They line up tails-to-tails in cell membranes and micelles.

CH_2O [H+HO] $OCCH_2CH_2$ – – – – fatty acid – – – – CH_3
C_2HO [H+HO] $OCCH_2CH_2$ – – – – fatty acid – – – – CH_3

The tails - can interact only with other lipids.

$$CH_2O - \overset{O}{\underset{O}{\overset{\|}{\underset{|}{P}}}} - O\text{-}CH_2\text{-}CH_2\text{-}\overset{\oplus}{N}\text{-}(CH_3)_3 \quad \leftarrow \text{ The head.}$$

Both the phosphate and nitrogen groups are electrically charged. Can form hydrogen bonds with water.

STEROIDS – Four interconnected rings of carbon atoms form the basic structure of all steroids. The steroid family includes cholesterol, bile acids, some hormones (e.g. oestrogen and testosterone) and some vitamins.

The cyclopentanoperhydrophenanthrene nucleus.

EICOSANOIDS – These lipids are derived from arachidonic acid, a 20 carbon fatty acid. They include prostaglandins, prostacyclin, thromboxanes and leucotrienes. Important in a wide variety of body functions e.g. hyperaemia, airway resistance, immune responses and inflammation. They are modified fatty acids.

31

PROTEINS

PROTEINS are the chief organic material of all protoplasm — plant or animal. They are part of many body structures; may function as enzymes, antibodies etc. They are composed of atoms of C, H, O, N and sometimes S. Protein molecules are assembled by linking subunits called **amino acids**, i.e. they are **polymers** of amino acids.

All the 20 or so amino acids found in nature have an amino group, a carboxyl group and each has a different **amino acid side chain**.

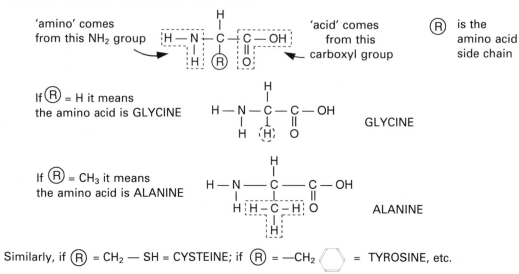

'amino' comes from this NH_2 group

'acid' comes from this carboxyl group

(R) is the amino acid side chain

If (R) = H it means the amino acid is GLYCINE

GLYCINE

If (R) = CH_3 it means the amino acid is ALANINE

ALANINE

Similarly, if (R) = $CH_2 — SH$ = CYSTEINE; if (R) = $—CH_2$ ⬡ = TYROSINE, etc.

In a protein molecule the amino acids are linked by combination of the amino group from one amino acid with the carboxyl group of the next amino acid with the loss of a molecule of water. This junction is a **peptide bond** or **link**.

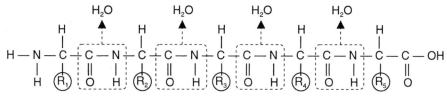

Thus a **polypeptide chain** is formed. If there are fewer than 50 amino acids in the chain the molecule is a **peptide**; if there are more than 50 the polypeptide is a **protein**.

Since each (R) in the above diagram can be any one of the 20 amino acids found in nature thousands of different kinds of protein can be formed. Thus differences between proteins depend on which amino acids are present and on their number and arrangement.

Although proteins are made up of a chain of units they have also a three-dimensional shape which is determined by hydrogen bonds (see page 4) between charged groups on the chain. The three-dimensional shape of proteins is functionally important.

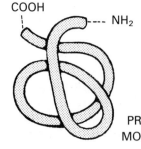

COOH

NH$_2$

PROTEIN MOLECULE

NUCLEIC ACIDS 1 – DNA

NUCLEIC ACIDS (so-called because they were first discovered in the nuclei of cells) store genetic information and pass it from cell to cell and from one generation to the next. There are 2 types of nucleic acid: **Deoxyribonucleic Acid (DNA)** and **Ribonucleic Acid (RNA)**. Both consist of linked chains of subunits called **nucleotides**, each of which has a phosphate group, a sugar and a ring consisting of carbon and nitrogen atoms called a **Base** (because it can accept hydrogen ions).

DNA

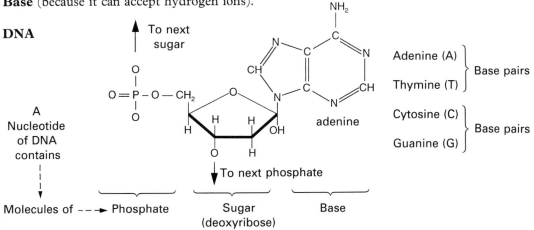

A Nucleotide of DNA contains

Molecules of – – → Phosphate   Sugar (deoxyribose)   Base

To next sugar

To next phosphate

adenine

Adenine (A) ⎱
Thymine (T) ⎰ Base pairs

Cytosine (C) ⎱
Guanine (G) ⎰ Base pairs

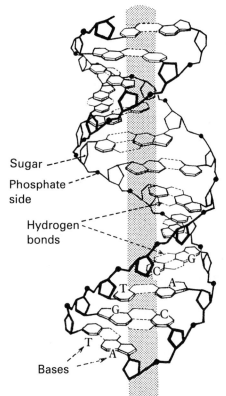

Sugar ---

Phosphate side

Hydrogen bonds

Bases ---

Millions of phosphate and sugar groups of adjacent nucleotides are joined to form a chain. Each DNA molecule has two such chains arranged in parallel. The alternating phosphate and deoxyribose groups form what is like two sides of a flexible 'ladder'. Each 'rung' of the ladder consists of a pair of bases, one from each chain, joined by weak hydrogen bonds. Adenine (A) always pairs with thymine (T) and *vice versa*; cystine (C) always pairs with guanine (G) and *vice versa*. This is called complementary base pairing. The rungs are joined to the sides of the ladder by rotatable joints. The ladder is coiled like a corkscrew, to the right, round an imaginary axis running through the hydrogen bonds and thus forms a double helix (a spiral curve).

DNA is copied by first breaking the rungs at the hydrogen bonds, then using the protruding bases from each side as a template for the construction of a new second strand of nucleotides with bases complementary to the exposed bases. The sequence of the bases serves as a code which determines the assembly of amino acids in the correct order for the synthesis of specific polypeptides.

A GENE is a segment of DNA which acts as a template for the synthesis of a particular polypeptide.

33

NUCLEIC ACIDS 2 – RNA AND MIXED ORGANIC MOLECULES

RNA — a single chain of nucleotides similar to DNA but in which the sugar is ribose instead of deoxyribose, and the base thymine in DNA is replaced in RNA by the base uracil (U).

NB: Ribose has OH where deoxyribose has H.

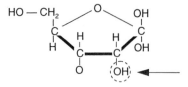

Ribose

RNA is smaller than DNA and can pass through the nuclear membrane into the cytosol.

DNA chains   RNA chain

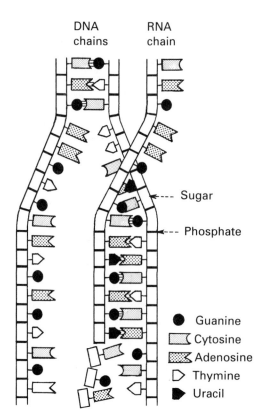

- ---- Sugar
- ---- Phosphate

● Guanine
▭ Cytosine
▨ Adenosine
▷ Thymine
◀ Uracil

To assemble an RNA molecule the two linked chains of DNA must first be separated. Then one of the two chains serves as a template for the assembly of nucleotides into a molecule of RNA. Thus is formed an RNA chain of bases, complementary to but specified by the bases of the DNA chain. Next, the RNA chain is released as an independent molecule and at the same time the two DNA chains which were separated are rejoined. The released RNA now undergoes processing into either messenger RNA (mRNA) or ribosomal RNA (rRNA) (see page 10) and then moves from the nucleus into the cytoplasm. mRNA goes to a ribosome to be used as a template. In addition, amino acids are carried to the ribosome by tRNA for assembly into a polypeptide or protein in a sequence determined by the sequence of bases on the mRNA.

MIXED ORGANIC MOLECULES

Glycoproteins (protein plus carbohydrate). Most integral proteins in cell membranes (see page 10) are glycoproteins, as are several homones.

Lipoproteins (lipid molecules coated with a layer of protein). Involved in the transport of lipids by the blood.

Glycolipids (lipid plus monosaccharides). Found in plasma membrane facing the extracellular fluid. Involved in recognition of cells by defence cells and viruses, etc. Important for adhesion among cells and tissues. Mediate cell recognition and communication.

SOURCE OF ENERGY: PHOTOSYNTHESIS

The essential life processes or the phenomena which characterize life depend on the use of **energy**. The **SUN** is the **source** of energy for **all** living things.

Only green **plants** can **trap** and **store** the sun's energy and build simple **carbohydrates** from carbon dioxide and water. This process is called **photosynthesis**. These simple carbohydrates are converted by additional metabolic processes of the plant into lipids, proteins, nucleic acids, etc. Thus PLANTS are the primary source of the energy-rich body building compounds required by **protoplasm**.

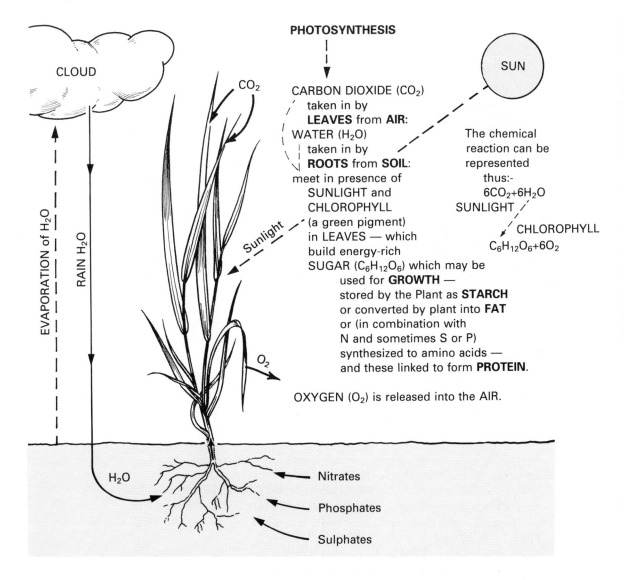

PHOTOSYNTHESIS

CLOUD

CO_2

SUN

CARBON DIOXIDE (CO_2)
taken in by
LEAVES from **AIR**:
WATER (H_2O)
taken in by
ROOTS from **SOIL**:
meet in presence of
SUNLIGHT and
CHLOROPHYLL
(a green pigment)
in LEAVES — which
build energy-rich
SUGAR ($C_6H_{12}O_6$) which may be
used for **GROWTH** —
stored by the Plant as **STARCH**
or converted by plant into **FAT**
or (in combination with
N and sometimes S or P)
synthesized to amino acids —
and these linked to form **PROTEIN**.

The chemical
reaction can be
represented
thus:-
$6CO_2+6H_2O$
SUNLIGHT
CHLOROPHYLL
$C_6H_{12}O_6+6O_2$

EVAPORATION of H_2O

RAIN H_2O

Sunlight

O_2

OXYGEN (O_2) is released into the AIR.

H_2O

Nitrates

Phosphates

Sulphates

When plants or their products are eaten this stored energy becomes available to animals and man.

CARBON 'CYCLE' IN NATURE

Animal bodies are unable to build proteins, carbohydrates or fats directly from **atoms**.
They must be built up for them by **plants**.
Carbon is the basic building unit of all these compounds.

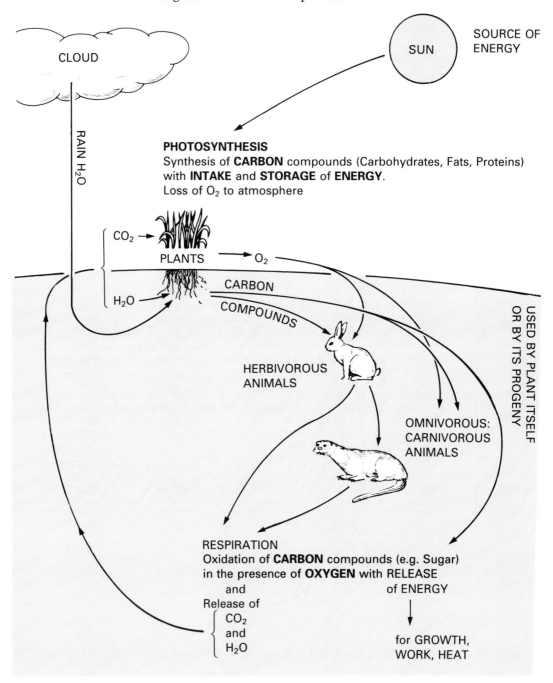

CLOUD

SUN

SOURCE OF ENERGY

RAIN H_2O

PHOTOSYNTHESIS
Synthesis of **CARBON** compounds (Carbohydrates, Fats, Proteins)
with **INTAKE** and **STORAGE** of **ENERGY**.
Loss of O_2 to atmosphere

CO_2 →

PLANTS

→ O_2 —

CARBON

COMPOUNDS

H_2O →

HERBIVOROUS
ANIMALS

OMNIVOROUS:
CARNIVOROUS
ANIMALS

USED BY PLANT ITSELF OR BY ITS PROGENY

RESPIRATION
Oxidation of **CARBON** compounds (e.g. Sugar)
in the presence of **OXYGEN** with RELEASE
    and   of ENERGY
Release of
    CO_2
    and
    H_2O

for GROWTH,
WORK, HEAT

NITROGEN 'CYCLE' IN NATURE

Although **animals** are surrounded by **nitrogen** in the air they cannot use that nitrogen to build nitrogen-containing compounds. They can only use the nitrogen trapped by plants to make these compounds.

NITROGEN in the **Atmosphere**

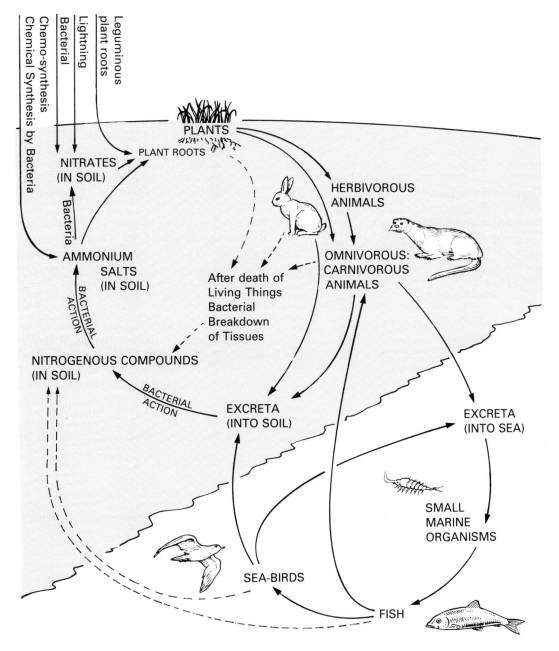

NUTRITION

Man eats **FOOD**, the substance which **plants** (and, through them, **animals**) have made.
These are broken down in man's body into simpler chemical units which **provide**

BUILDING and PROTECTIVE MATERIALS

Man requires more or less the same elements as plants. (Some, such as the minerals iodine, sodium, iron, calcium, he assimilates in **inorganic form**.)

Most must be built up for him by plants:-

Organically combined
Carbon, Nitrogen, and Sulphur, etc.
Essential amino acids

Essential fatty acids
Certain **vitamins**

These are
used to
BUILD, MAINTAIN or REPAIR
PROTOPLASM
— — — — — — — — — — —
Body-building requirements
of the individual determine

QUALITY
of DIET

ENERGY

Stored originally
by plants
RELEASED in man's cells
by
OXIDATION

When food is 'burned' it gives up
its stored energy

Proteins yield 17 kJ (4kcal) ⎫ units of
Carbohydrates yield 17 kJ (4 kcal) ⎬ Energy
Fats yield 38 kJ (9 kcal) ⎭ per gram

Most of this appears as HEAT
and is used for
KEEPING BODY WARM;
some is used for WORK of CELLS
— — — — — — — — — — —
Energy requirements
of the individual determine

QUANTITY
of DIET

For a
BALANCED DIET
TOTAL INTAKE
of
Essential Constituents and Energy Units
must balance . . .
. . . amounts *stored* plus amounts *lost* from body plus amounts *used*
as Work or Heat.

1 kilocalorie (kcal) = 4.2 kilojoules (kJ)
1000 kilojoules = 1 megajoule (MJ)

ENERGY-GIVING FOODS

All the main foodstuffs yield **energy** — the energy originally trapped by plants.
Carbohydrates and **fats** are the chief energy-giving foods. **Proteins** can give energy but are mainly used for building and repairing protoplasm.

CARBOHYDRATES are the
    PRIMARY SOURCE of ENERGY —
More easily and quickly digested
and utilized than fats.

PLANT SOURCES:
    SUGAR is found in
    leaves, fruit and **roots** of **plants** *and in*

foods made from
them by man
e.g. jam, treacle,
sweets, syrup
i.e. especially those products
made by plants for development
of next generation.
    Sugar can be stored in plants as
    — — — — — CARBOHYDRATE or converted to FAT and stored as such

FATS are a
    SECONDARY SOURCE of ENERGY –
Ideal energy storage material. Weight
for weight, give twice as many energy
units as carbohydrates

STARCH is found in
grain, seeds and **roots** of plants
e.g.   e.g.
wheat   potatoes

OILS in
seeds   **nuts**
e.g. olives,   e.g. peanuts,
cotton seeds   coconuts
sun flowers

and in
foods made from them by man
flour e.g. bread, cakes, cereals e.g.
cornflakes, crisps, chips.   *cooking fats*   *peanut butter*

ANIMAL SOURCES
SUGAR (glucose) is found in **tissues** and **blood** of **animals** and in
    foods made from them by man
                 e.g. hamburger

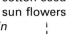
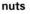

    e.g. chop

and in products made by animals for themselves or the next generation
Milk sugar (lactose) — — — — — —   **milk fat**

Honey (fructose)

MILK   — — — — — — butter, cheese

Sugar can be stored in animals as
    | — — CARBOHYDRATE or converted to FAT and stored (together with fat
ANIMAL STARCH (glycogen)   built from dietary fatty acids and
is found in **muscles**   Glycerol) in **fat depots** of body.
           e.g. steak   e.g. suet, lard, mutton-fat, vegetable oil

                 liver

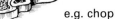

and in **foods** made from them by man
    e.g. sausages   e.g. margarine

39

BODY-BUILDING TISSUES

PROTEIN is the chief body-building food. Because it is the chief constitutent of protoplasm, tissues of plants and animals are the richest sources.

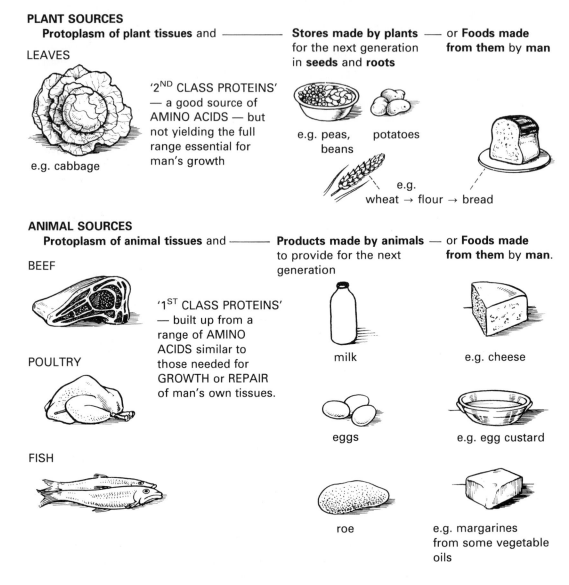

PLANT SOURCES

Protoplasm of plant tissues and ———— Stores made by plants — or Foods made
for the next generation   **from them** by **man**
in **seeds** and **roots**

LEAVES

'2ND CLASS PROTEINS'
— a good source of
AMINO ACIDS — but
not yielding the full
range essential for
man's growth

e.g. cabbage

e.g. peas,   potatoes
beans

e.g.
wheat → flour → bread

ANIMAL SOURCES

Protoplasm of animal tissues and ———— Products made by animals — or Foods made
to provide for the next   **from them** by **man**.
generation

BEEF

'1ST CLASS PROTEINS'
— built up from a
range of AMINO
ACIDS similar to
those needed for
GROWTH or REPAIR
of man's own tissues.

POULTRY

milk   e.g. cheese

eggs   e.g. egg custard

FISH

roe   e.g. margarines
from some vegetable
oils

These foods between them also contain other important body-building elements:-
e.g. **calcium** and **phosphorus** for making **bones** and **teeth** hard; **iron** for building
haemoglobin — the **oxygen carrying** substance in **red blood** corpuscles; iodine for
building the thyroid hormone.

VITAMINS – 1

Body-building and energy-giving foods cannot maintain growth and normal metabolism in the absence of organic substances called vitamins. Most of these substances cannot be manufactured in the body. They were thought to be 'amines essential to life'; hence named vitamines. This name was changed to 'vitamin' when it was found that they were not all amines. Most vitamins function as coenzymes. (Enzyme = a protein + non-protein portion which is either a metal ion or an organic molecule called a coenzyme). Vitamin deficient diets can cause specific metabolic defects.

	FUNCTION	SOURCE	DEFICIENCY
FAT SOLUBLE VITAMINS A (RETINOL)	Maintains health of epithelial cells, especially skin, front of eye and lining of the digestive and respiratory tracts. Essential for regeneration of photopigments in retina. ? Cancer prevention. Is an antioxidant.	*PLANT*: Formed in G.I. tract from provitamin CAROTENE in green and yellow vegetables (esp. spinach and kale). Yellow maize, peas, beans, carrots. *ANIMAL*: Stored in liver of animals and fish, milk, egg yolk, butter, cream.	Atrophy and keratinization of epithelia; dry skin; night blindness. **XEROPHTHALMIA** Corneal epithelium thickened, dry and infected.
D 1, 25 $(OH)_2 D_3$ (CALCITRIOL)	(Also D_3) Important in Ca^{2+} and P metabolism. Essential for deposition of Ca^{2+} and P in bones and teeth Promotes absorption of Ca^{2+} and P from G.I. tract. Calcitriol or $1,25(OH)_2 D_3$ is the active from of vitamin D.	*PLANT*: Vegetables, fruits and cereals contain negligible amounts. *ANIMAL*: Sunlight converts 7-dehydro-cholesterol to cholecalciferol (Vitamin D_3) in the skin. In the liver, cholecalciferol is converted to 25-hydroxycholecalciferol and, in the kidneys, this is hydroxylated to 1,25-dihydroxycholecalciferol (calcitriol). Found in liver of fish and animals, egg yolk and milk.	Slow and faulty development of bones and teeth. **RICKETS** in children. **OSTEOMALACIA** in ADULTS. Bones become soft and deformed.
E TOCOPHEROLS	Inhibits breakdown of fatty acids that help form cell membranes. Involved in red blood corpuscle, DNA and RNA formation. Is an antioxidant. Helps normal structure and function of nervous system and wound healing.	*PLANT*: Green leaves (e.g. lettuce), peas. Richest source – germ of various cereals e.g. wheat germ, seed oils. *ANIMAL*: Stored in liver, adipose tissue and muscle. Small amounts in meat and dairy products.	Causes muscle dystrophy in monkeys and sterility in rats. May cause abnormalities of mitochondria, lysosomes and plasma membrane.

VITAMINS – 2

	FUNCTION	SOURCE	DEFICIENCY
Fat Soluble vitamins (continued) **K**	Essential for the production of Prothrombin and Factors VII, IX and X in liver – important for normal blood clotting.	*PLANTS*: Spinach, kale, cabbage, cereals, tomatoes, carrots, potatoes. *ANIMAL*: Synthesized by bacteria in man's intestine then absorbed in presence of bile salts.	Antibiotic drugs cause deficient absorption from intestine and lead to delayed blood clotting time.
WATER SOLUBLE VITAMINS **B$_1$** (THIAMINE)	Coenzyme for enzymes that break bonds between carbon atoms. Involved in metabolism of pyruvic acid to CO_2 and H_2O and in synthesis of acetylcholine.	*PLANTS*: Whole grain products. Pulses e.g. green peas. Seeds and outer coats of grain e.g. rice, wheat. Nuts e.g. peanuts. Yeast and yeast extracts. *ANIMAL*: Eggs, liver, pork.	Decreased ATP formation in muscle and nerve, hence: 1. **BERI-BERI:** Partial paralysis of G.I. tract: paralysis and atrophy of skeletal muscles.⟶ 2. **POLYNEURITIS:** Touch sense and intestinal motility decreased.
B$_2$ (RIBOFLAVIN)	Component of coenzymes concerned with carbohydrate and protein metabolism in cells of eye, intestinal mucosa and blood.	Most is excreted in urine. G.I. tract bacteria produce a little. *PLANTS*: Whole grain products, asparagus, peas, yeast and peanuts. *ANIMAL*: Liver, fish, meat.	**RIBOFLAVINOSIS** Roughening of the skin. Cornea becomes cloudy. Cracks and fissures around lips and tongue.
NIACIN (NICOTINIC ACID)	Component of coenzymes concerned with citric acid cycle. Inhibits production of cholesterol. Assists triglyceride breakdown.	Derived from tryptophan. *PLANT*: Yeast, whole grain, peas, beans, nuts. *ANIMAL*: Liver, fish, meats.	**NIACIN PELLAGRA** Roughening and reddening of the skin. Tongue red and sore in severe cases – gastrointestinal upsets and mental derangement.
B$_6$ (PYRIDOXINE)	Coenzyme for amino acid metabolism. Helps produce circulating antibodies. Coenzyme in triglyceride metabolism.	G.I. tract bacteria synthesize. *PLANT*: Yeast, tomatoes, spinach, whole grain products. *ANIMAL*: Salmon, liver, yoghurt.	Dermatitis of eyes, mouth, nose; nausea.

VITAMINS – 3

	FUNCTION	SOURCE	DEFICIENCY
Water soluble vitamins (continued) **PANTOTHENIC ACID**	Constituent of coenzyme A which transfers pyruvic acid into citric acid cycle; converts lipids and amino acids to glucose; helps synthesis of steroid hormones.	Produced by G.I. tract bacteria. *PLANTS*: Green vegetables, cereal, yeast. *ANIMAL*: Liver and kidney.	Produces fatigue, muscle spasm, neuromuscular degeneration. Adrenal cortical hormone deficiency.
BIOTIN	Coenzyme to form oxaloacetic acid from pyruvic acid and synthesis of fatty acids and purines.	Produced by G.I. tract bacteria. *PLANTS*: Yeast. *ANIMAL*: Liver, kidneys and egg yolk.	Dermatitis: muscular fatigue; mental depression; nausea.
FOLIC ACID	Coenzyme for synthesis of purine and pyrimidine bases for DNA and RNA. Production of red and white blood cells.	Produced by G.I. tract bacteria. *PLANTS*: Green leafy vegetables. *ANIMAL*: Liver.	Macrocytic anaemia; spina bifida in fetus.
B$_{12}$ (CYANOCOBALAMINE)	Coenzyme for RBC and methionine formation, entrance of amino acids to citric acid cycle – synthesis of acetylcholine.	Contains cobalt. Absorption from G.I. tract depends on HCl and intrinsic factor secreted by gastric mucosa. *ANIMAL*: Liver, kidney, milk, cheese, eggs, meat.	**PERNICIOUS ANAEMIA** Memory loss, ataxia, mood changes, abnormal sensations. Impaired osteoblast activity.
C (ASCORBIC ACID)	Coenzyme involved in forming a constituent of collagen. Essential for formation and maintenance of intercellular cement and connective tissue. Especially necessary for healthy blood vessels, wound healing, bone growth. Functions as an antioxidant. ? Cancer prevention.	Rapidly destroyed by heat. *PLANTS*: Green vegetables, e.g. parsley, peas, green peppers. Citrus fruits e.g. lemons, oranges, limes grapefruits. Tomatoes, rosehips, blackcurrants, red peppers, turnips and potatoes. *ANIMAL*: Stored in body – high concentration in adrenal glands. Found in meat, liver. Secreted in milk.	**SCURVY** Intercellular cement breaks down. Capillary walls leak → haemorrhages into tissues, e.g. gums swell and bleed easily. Wounds heal slowly.

DIGESTION

The organic substances of man's food are chemically *similar* to those which his body will form from them. They differ only in detail.

Conversion of FOOD **SUBSTANCE** ——— to ——— **BODY SUBSTANCE**

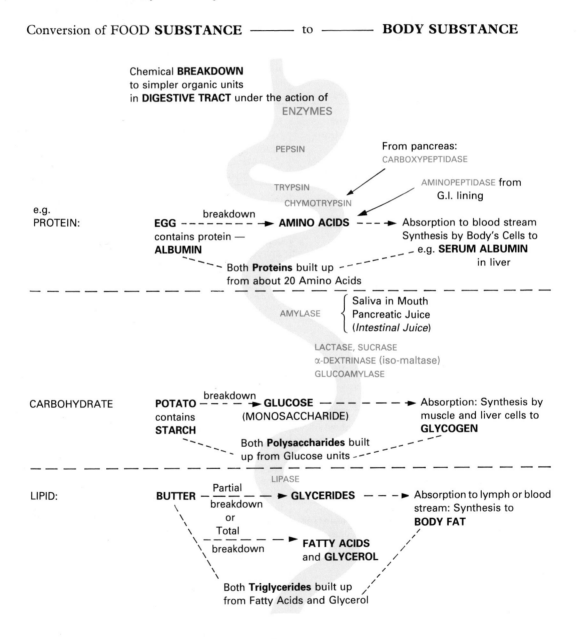

Chemical **BREAKDOWN**
to simpler organic units
in **DIGESTIVE TRACT** under the action of
ENZYMES

PEPSIN

From pancreas:
CARBOXYPEPTIDASE

TRYPSIN

AMINOPEPTIDASE from
G.I. lining

CHYMOTRYPSIN

e.g.
PROTEIN:

breakdown
EGG - - - - - - - - ▶ **AMINO ACIDS** - - - ▶ Absorption to blood stream
contains protein — Synthesis by Body's Cells to
ALBUMIN e.g. **SERUM ALBUMIN**
in liver

Both **Proteins** built up
from about 20 Amino Acids

AMYLASE { Saliva in Mouth
Pancreatic Juice
(*Intestinal Juice*)

LACTASE, SUCRASE
α-DEXTRINASE (iso-maltase)
GLUCOAMYLASE

CARBOHYDRATE

breakdown
POTATO - - - - ▶ **GLUCOSE** — — — — ▶ Absorption: Synthesis by
contains (MONOSACCHARIDE) muscle and liver cells to
STARCH **GLYCOGEN**

Both **Polysaccharides** built
up from Glucose units

LIPASE

LIPID:

Partial
BUTTER - - - - ▶ **GLYCERIDES** - - - ▶ Absorption to lymph or blood
breakdown stream: Synthesis to
or **BODY FAT**
Total
- - - - ▶ **FATTY ACIDS**
breakdown and **GLYCEROL**

Both **Triglycerides** built up
from Fatty Acids and Glycerol

DIGESTION is brought about by **SPECIFIC ENZYMES** themselves made of **Protein** — each acts as a **CATALYST** for speeding up one particular chemical breakdown without effect on any others.

PROTEIN METABOLISM

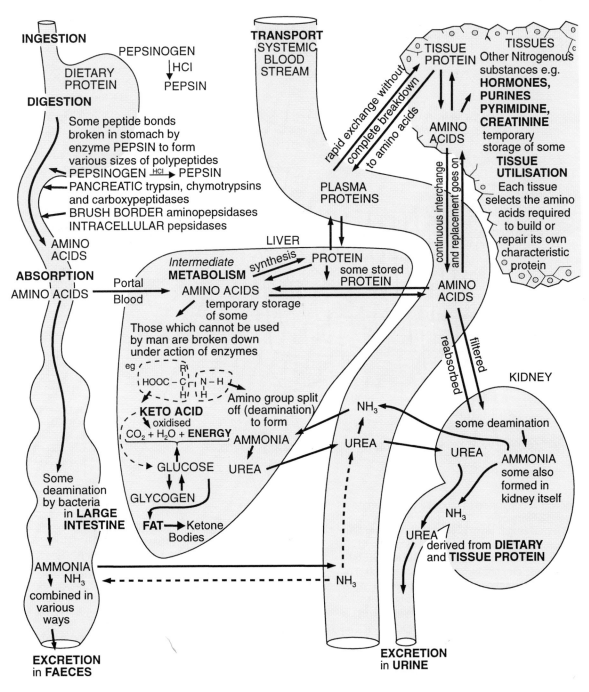

Growth hormone (somatotrophin) from the anterior pituitary enhances the entrance of amino acids into cells and stimulates building them into protein. These actions favour growth.

CARBOHYDRATE METABOLISM

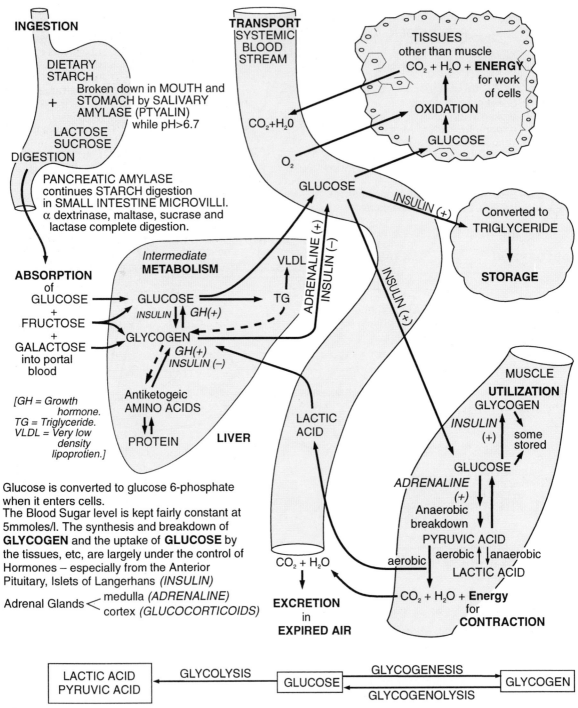

INGESTION

DIETARY STARCH
Broken down in MOUTH and STOMACH by SALIVARY AMYLASE (PTYALIN) while pH>6.7
+
LACTOSE SUCROSE
DIGESTION

PANCREATIC AMYLASE continues STARCH digestion in SMALL INTESTINE MICROVILLI. α dextrinase, maltase, sucrase and lactase complete digestion.

ABSORPTION
of
GLUCOSE
+
FRUCTOSE
+
GALACTOSE
into portal blood

[GH = Growth hormone.
TG = Triglyceride.
VLDL = Very low density lipoprotien.]

Intermediate **METABOLISM**

GLUCOSE
INSULIN ↕ *GH(+)*
GLYCOGEN
GH(+)
INSULIN (−)
Antiketogeic AMINO ACIDS
↕
PROTEIN   **LIVER**

VLDL
TG

TRANSPORT
SYSTEMIC BLOOD STREAM

CO_2+H_2O

O_2

GLUCOSE

ADRENALINE (+)
INSULIN (−)

INSULIN (+)

TISSUES
other than muscle
$CO_2 + H_2O$ + **ENERGY**
for work of cells

OXIDATION

GLUCOSE

INSULIN (+)

Converted to TRIGLYCERIDE

STORAGE

LACTIC ACID

MUSCLE
UTILIZATION
GLYCOGEN
INSULIN
(+)   some stored

GLUCOSE

ADRENALINE
(+)
Anaerobic breakdown
PYRUVIC ACID
aerobic   aerobic ↕ anaerobic
LACTIC ACID
$CO_2 + H_2O$ + **Energy**
for **CONTRACTION**

$CO_2 + H_2O$

EXCRETION
in
EXPIRED AIR

Glucose is converted to glucose 6-phosphate when it enters cells.
The Blood Sugar level is kept fairly constant at 5mmoles/l. The synthesis and breakdown of **GLYCOGEN** and the uptake of **GLUCOSE** by the tissues, etc, are largely under the control of Hormones – especially from the Anterior Pituitary, Islets of Langerhans *(INSULIN)*

Adrenal Glands < medulla *(ADRENALINE)*
cortex *(GLUCOCORTICOIDS)*

LACTIC ACID PYRUVIC ACID ← GLYCOLYSIS ← GLUCOSE → GLYCOGENESIS → GLYCOGEN
GLYCOGENOLYSIS

FAT METABOLISM

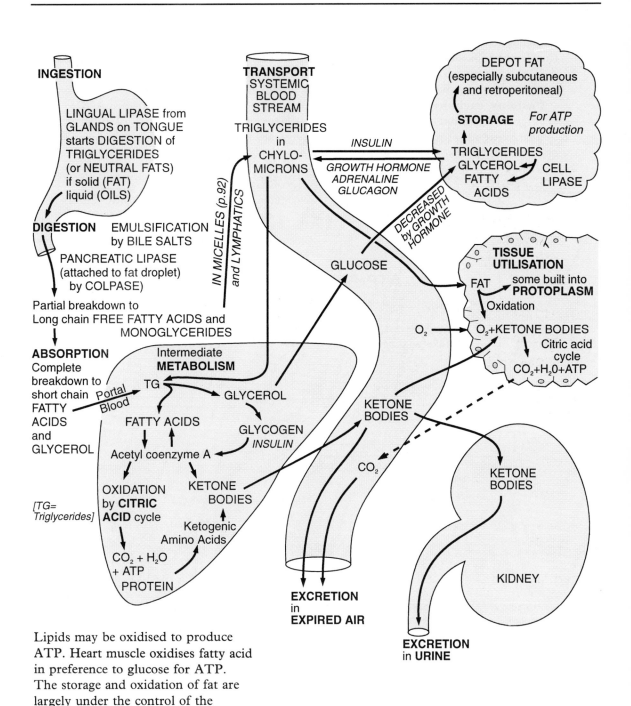

INGESTION

LINGUAL LIPASE from GLANDS on TONGUE starts DIGESTION of TRIGLYCERIDES (or NEUTRAL FATS) if solid (FAT) liquid (OILS)

DIGESTION EMULSIFICATION by BILE SALTS

PANCREATIC LIPASE (attached to fat droplet) by COLPASE)

Partial breakdown to Long chain FREE FATTY ACIDS and MONOGLYCERIDES

ABSORPTION Complete breakdown to short chain FATTY ACIDS and GLYCEROL

Portal Blood

[TG= Triglycerides]

Intermediate **METABOLISM**

TG

FATTY ACIDS

GLYCEROL

GLYCOGEN
INSULIN

Acetyl coenzyme A

OXIDATION by **CITRIC ACID** cycle

KETONE BODIES

Ketogenic Amino Acids

$CO_2 + H_2O$ + ATP

PROTEIN

TRANSPORT SYSTEMIC BLOOD STREAM

TRIGLYCERIDES in CHYLO-MICRONS

IN MICELLES (p.92) and LYMPHATICS

INSULIN

GROWTH HORMONE ADRENALINE GLUCAGON

DECREASED by GROWTH HORMONE

GLUCOSE

O_2

KETONE BODIES

CO_2

EXCRETION in **EXPIRED AIR**

EXCRETION in **URINE**

DEPOT FAT (especially subcutaneous and retroperitoneal)

STORAGE *For ATP production*

TRIGLYCERIDES GLYCEROL FATTY ACIDS

CELL LIPASE

TISSUE UTILISATION

FAT some built into **PROTOPLASM**

Oxidation

O_2+KETONE BODIES

Citric acid cycle

$CO_2 + H_2O$+ATP

KETONE BODIES

KIDNEY

Lipids may be oxidised to produce ATP. Heart muscle oxidises fatty acid in preference to glucose for ATP. The storage and oxidation of fat are largely under the control of the endocrine system. Growth hormone exerts its effect by the production of somatomedins by the liver.

ENERGY FROM FOOD

Organic molecules have chemical energy locked in their structure. This energy can be transferred to adenosine triphosphate (ATP) when food molecules are broken down. From ATP the energy can be transferred to operate energy-requiring cell functions, e.g. muscle contraction, the active transport of molecules across membranes, etc.

Proteins, carbohydrates and **fats** can all provide energy for cells through ATP synthesis. In addition the products (**intermediates**) of *each* of these types of molecule can, to a large extent, provide the raw materials necessary to synthesize members of other classes. NB: the *two-way* arrows:

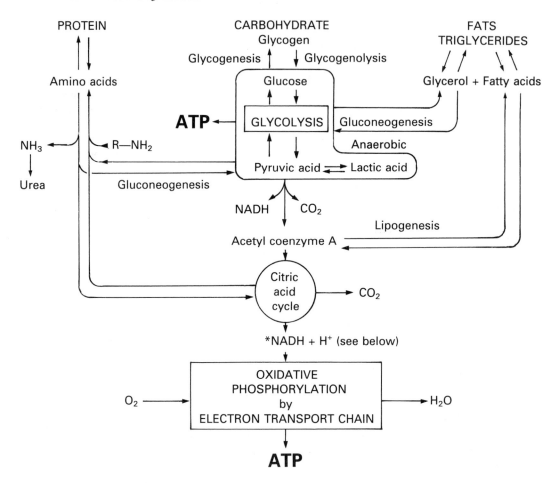

* The oxidised form of the coenzyme nicotinamide adenine dinucleotide (NAD^+) receives, in the citric acid cycle, two H^+ and two electrons, thus reducing it to $NADH + H^+$. The H^+ is released into the surrounding solution. NADH supplies electrons to the electron transport chain.

The main mechanism for producing ATP is **OXIDATIVE PHOSPHORYLATION**. This occurs when **oxygen** is available. ATP can also be produced by **GLYCOLYSIS**, a process in which carbohydrate is broken down to pyruvic acid.

FORMATION OF ATP

ENZYME SYSTEMS exist within cells which can convert (in a series of steps) Fats, Proteins and Carbohydrates into intermediate compounds suitable for entering the **'ENERGY-PRODUCING' CITRIC ACID CYCLE** (Krebs cycle).

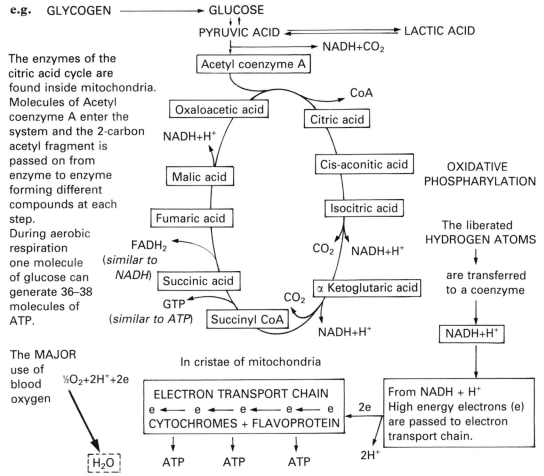

e.g. GLYCOGEN ⟶ GLUCOSE

PYRUVIC ACID ⇌ LACTIC ACID

⟶ NADH+CO_2

Acetyl coenzyme A

The enzymes of the citric acid cycle are found inside mitochondria. Molecules of Acetyl coenzyme A enter the system and the 2-carbon acetyl fragment is passed on from enzyme to enzyme forming different compounds at each step.

During aerobic respiration one molecule of glucose can generate 36–38 molecules of ATP.

CoA

Oxaloacetic acid

Citric acid

NADH+H^+

Cis-aconitic acid

Malic acid

Isocitric acid

Fumaric acid

CO_2 / NADH+H^+

FADH$_2$
(similar to NADH)

Succinic acid

α Ketoglutaric acid

CO_2

GTP
(similar to ATP)

Succinyl CoA

NADH+H^+

OXIDATIVE PHOSPHARYLATION

The liberated HYDROGEN ATOMS

are transferred to a coenzyme

NADH+H^+

The MAJOR use of blood oxygen

½O_2+2H^++2e

In cristae of mitochondria

ELECTRON TRANSPORT CHAIN
e ⟵ e ⟵ e ⟵ e ⟵ e
CYTOCHROMES + FLAVOPROTEIN

2e

From NADH + H^+
High energy electrons (e) are passed to electron transport chain.

H_2O

ATP   ATP   ATP

2H^+

The **ENERGY** produced in the electron transport chain is used to link inorganic phosphate to ADP (adenosine diphosphate) to form the energy-rich compound ATP. The energy 'trapped' in ATP is used as required.

For example:

(a) for MEMBRANE TRANSPORT. Sodium, potassium etc. require the expenditure of energy to transport them across cell membranes.

(b) for SYNTHESIS of CHEMICAL COMPOUNDS. Many thousands of ATP molecules must release their energy to form one protein molecule.

(c) for MECHANICAL WORK. Contraction of a muscle fibre requires expenditure of tremendous quantities of ATP.

The energy stored in food is thus released by cells to make their own energy-rich phosphorus compound — **ADENOSINE TRIPHOSPHATE** (ATP).

49

HEAT BALANCE

Heat is produced by all metabolic processes, food intake and muscular activity. The body temperature is kept relatively constant (with a slight fluctuation throughout the 24 hours) in spite of wide variations in environmental temperature and heat production.

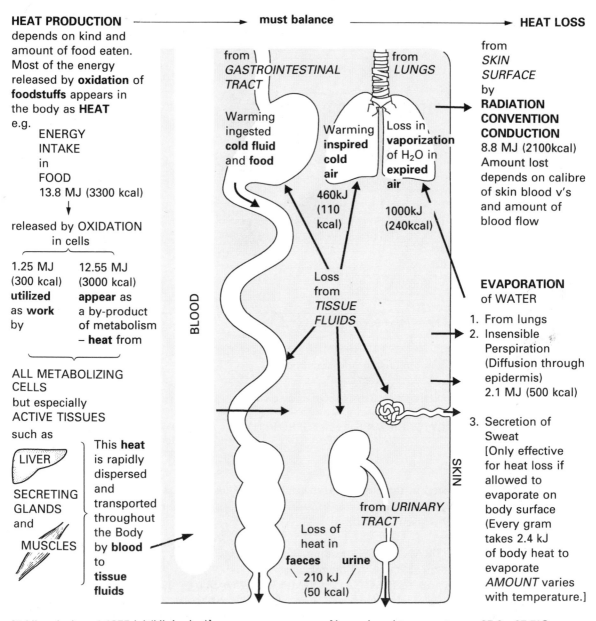

HEAT PRODUCTION ──────► **must balance** ──────► **HEAT LOSS**

depends on kind and amount of food eaten. Most of the energy released by **oxidation** of **foodstuffs** appears in the body as **HEAT** e.g.

ENERGY
INTAKE
in
FOOD
13.8 MJ (3300 kcal)
↓
released by OXIDATION
in cells

| 1.25 MJ (300 kcal) **utilized** as **work** by | 12.55 MJ (3000 kcal) **appear** as a by-product of metabolism – **heat** from |

ALL METABOLIZING CELLS
but especially
ACTIVE TISSUES
such as

LIVER

SECRETING GLANDS
and

MUSCLES

This **heat** is rapidly dispersed and transported throughout the Body by **blood** to **tissue fluids**

BLOOD

from \ \
GASTROINTESTINAL TRACT

Warming ingested **cold fluid** and **food**

from
LUNGS

Warming **inspired cold air**

Loss in **vaporization** of H_2O in **expired air**

460kJ (110 kcal)

1000kJ (240kcal)

Loss from *TISSUE FLUIDS*

SKIN

from *URINARY TRACT*

Loss of heat in **faeces** **urine**
\ 210 kJ /
(50 kcal)

from *SKIN SURFACE* by **RADIATION CONVENTION CONDUCTION** 8.8 MJ (2100kcal) Amount lost depends on calibre of skin blood v's and amount of blood flow

EVAPORATION of WATER

1. From lungs
2. Insensible Perspiration (Diffusion through epidermis) 2.1 MJ (500 kcal)

3. Secretion of Sweat [Only effective for heat loss if allowed to evaporate on body surface (Every gram takes 2.4 kJ of body heat to evaporate *AMOUNT* varies with temperature.]

[1 kilocalorie = 4.1855 kJ (kilojoules)]

Normal oral temperature = 35.8 - 37.7°C

MAINTENANCE OF BODY TEMPERATURE

Any tendency for the **body temperature** to *rise*
as by

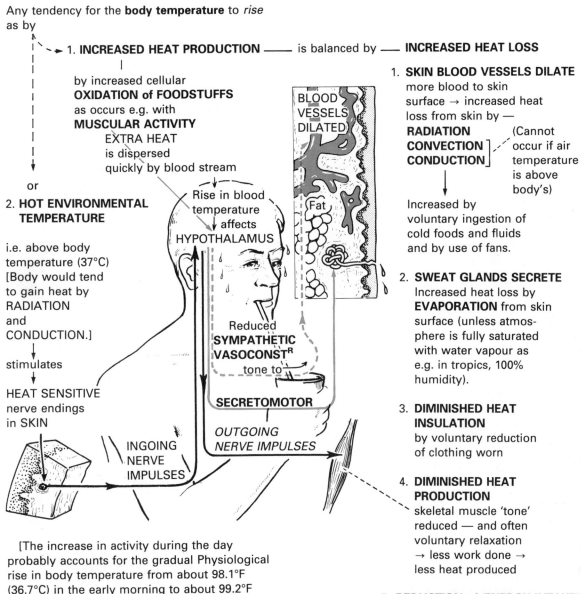

1. **INCREASED HEAT PRODUCTION** —— is balanced by —— **INCREASED HEAT LOSS**

by increased cellular
OXIDATION of FOODSTUFFS
as occurs e.g. with
MUSCULAR ACTIVITY
EXTRA HEAT
is dispersed
quickly by blood stream

or

2. **HOT ENVIRONMENTAL TEMPERATURE**

i.e. above body
temperature (37°C)
[Body would tend
to gain heat by
RADIATION
and
CONDUCTION.]

stimulates

HEAT SENSITIVE
nerve endings
in SKIN

BLOOD
VESSELS
DILATED)

Fat

Rise in blood
temperature
affects
HYPOTHALAMUS

Reduced
**SYMPATHETIC
VASOCONST^R**
tone to

SECRETOMOTOR

*OUTGOING
NERVE IMPULSES*

INGOING
NERVE
IMPULSES

1. **SKIN BLOOD VESSELS DILATE**
more blood to skin
surface → increased heat
loss from skin by —
**RADIATION
CONVECTION
CONDUCTION**⎤ (Cannot
　　　　　　　⎦ occur if air
　　　　　　temperature
　　　　　　is above
　　　　　　body's)

Increased by
voluntary ingestion of
cold foods and fluids
and by use of fans.

2. **SWEAT GLANDS SECRETE**
Increased heat loss by
EVAPORATION from skin
surface (unless atmos-
phere is fully saturated
with water vapour as
e.g. in tropics, 100%
humidity).

3. **DIMINISHED HEAT
INSULATION**
by voluntary reduction
of clothing worn

4. **DIMINISHED HEAT
PRODUCTION**
skeletal muscle 'tone'
reduced — and often
voluntary relaxation
→ less work done →
less heat produced

5. **REDUCTION** of 'ENERGY INTAKE'
by voluntary restriction of
protein in diet

[The increase in activity during the day
probably accounts for the gradual Physiological
rise in body temperature from about 98.1°F
(36.7°C) in the early morning to about 99.2°F
(37.3°C) in the late afternoon.]
Normal oral temperature is 97 to 99°F (36.1–37.2°C).
Rectal temperature is about 0.5°C higher.

Unless exercise is very strenuous or environment
is very hot and humid these measures ———→ **RESTORE BODY TEMPERATURE**
to **normal**

MAINTENANCE OF BODY TEMPERATURE

Any tendency for the **body temperature** to *fall*
as by

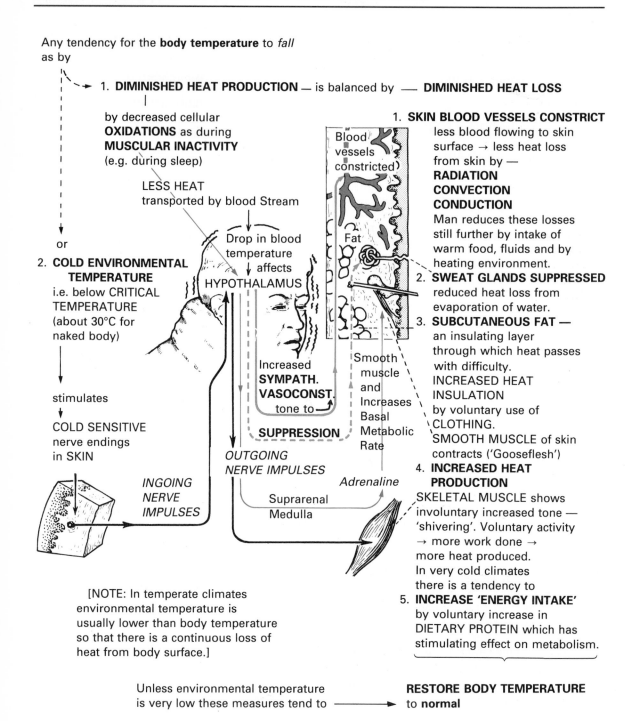

1. **DIMINISHED HEAT PRODUCTION** — is balanced by — **DIMINISHED HEAT LOSS**

by decreased cellular
OXIDATIONS as during
MUSCULAR INACTIVITY
(e.g. during sleep)

LESS HEAT
transported by blood Stream

or

2. **COLD ENVIRONMENTAL
   TEMPERATURE**
   i.e. below CRITICAL
   TEMPERATURE
   (about 30°C for
   naked body)

stimulates

COLD SENSITIVE
nerve endings
in SKIN

Blood
vessels
constricted

Drop in blood
temperature
↓ affects
HYPOTHALAMUS

Fat

Increased
**SYMPATH.
VASOCONST.**
tone to

SUPPRESSION

*OUTGOING
NERVE IMPULSES*

*INGOING
NERVE
IMPULSES*

Smooth
muscle
and
Increases
Basal
Metabolic
Rate

Adrenaline

Suprarenal
Medulla

1. **SKIN BLOOD VESSELS CONSTRICT**
   less blood flowing to skin
   surface → less heat loss
   from skin by —
   **RADIATION
   CONVECTION
   CONDUCTION**
   Man reduces these losses
   still further by intake of
   warm food, fluids and by
   heating environment.

2. **SWEAT GLANDS SUPPRESSED**
   reduced heat loss from
   evaporation of water.

3. **SUBCUTANEOUS FAT** —
   an insulating layer
   through which heat passes
   with difficulty.
   INCREASED HEAT
   INSULATION
   by voluntary use of
   CLOTHING.
   SMOOTH MUSCLE of skin
   contracts ('Gooseflesh')

4. **INCREASED HEAT
   PRODUCTION**
   SKELETAL MUSCLE shows
   involuntary increased tone —
   'shivering'. Voluntary activity
   → more work done →
   more heat produced.
   In very cold climates
   there is a tendency to

5. **INCREASE 'ENERGY INTAKE'**
   by voluntary increase in
   DIETARY PROTEIN which has
   stimulating effect on metabolism.

[NOTE: In temperate climates
environmental temperature is
usually lower than body temperature
so that there is a continuous loss of
heat from body surface.]

Unless environmental temperature
is very low these measures tend to ⟶ **RESTORE BODY TEMPERATURE**
to **normal**

GROWTH

Each individual grows, by repeated cell divisions, from a single cell to a total of 75 trillion or more cells. Growth is most rapid before birth and during 1st year of life.

The proportion of ENERGY INTAKE in food used to build and maintain tissue	INFANCY		CHILDHOOD		
	At Birth	3 months	1 year	2 years	9-11 years
	40%	40%	20%	20%	4-10%
Average WEIGHT	3 kg	5 kg	10.4 kg	12.4 kg	27.1 kg
Average HEIGHT	50 cm	58 cm	73 cm	84 cm	129 cm

A baby is born with epithelia, connective tissues, muscles, nerves and organs all present and formed — but all tissues do not grow at the same rate.

Differential growth and **functional development** of **tissues** lead to **change** in **body proportions**

e.g. Rapid growth of skeletal tissue during childhood.
Nervous tissue develops rapidly in first 2 years.
Most rapid growth is first at the head then legs begin to lengthen.
Chiefly **PROTEIN** being laid down or retained

Lymphoid Tissue Growth Spurt

10 YEARS

2 YEARS

1 YEAR

3 MONTHS

At BIRTH

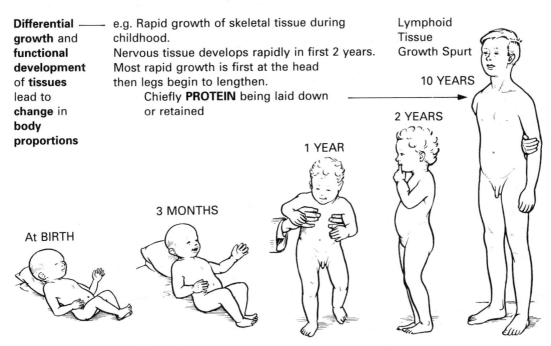

FIRST (Neutral) GROWTH PHASE (Infancy to Puberty). No marked difference between sexes — Regulated by Growth Hormone of Anterior Pituitary — stimulates Growth of all Tissues and Organs. Thyroid hormone essential for brain development especially in first year.

FACTORS INFLUENCING NORMAL GROWTH:

Genetic: To large extent rate of growth/sequence of events is determined. Inherited factors control pattern and limitations of growth.

Environment: Nutrition: For optimal growth the body requires an adequate and balanced diet.

Endocrine glands: Especially growth hormone, thyroid hormone, insulin, adrenal androgens, testicular testosterone, oestrogens.

53

GROWTH

GROWTH SPURT 11–12 years	ADOLESCENCE ⟶		ADULTHOOD ⟶	
	GIRL	BOY	WOMAN	MAN
	13 years	15 years	17 years	19 years
	10–15%	10–15%	4%	4%
	42.8 kg	51.1 kg	54.8 kg	65 kg
	152 cm	163 cm	162 cm	173 cm

Growth and development of reproductive organs

More **FAT** being deposited now

Apart from **protein** replacement in **repair**, weight increase is now by deposition of **FAT**.

SEXUAL GROWTH PHASE (Puberty to Maturity)

REPRODUCTIVE PHASE

Marked difference between sexes is initiated by gonadotrophin releasing hormone, luteinising hormone and follicle stimulating hormone of the anterior pituitary acting on sex glands and stimulating their production of oestrogen and testosterone. These hormones are largely responsible for development of secondary sex characteristics and development of reproductive organs.

– – – – – – These hormones maintain secondary sex characteristics and reproductive ability during reproductive phase of adult life.

ENERGY REQUIREMENTS – MALE

DAILY FOOD INTAKE
must supply **total
energy requirements
for**
1. ACTIVITY
   SPECIAL — individual
requirements vary with
type of work or play and
the **intensity** of **work**
and frequency and
length of **rest pauses**.
   EVERYDAY
         ACTIVITIES —
such as **sitting, standing,**
walking, etc.

**2. SPECIFIC DYNAMIC
ACTION of FOOD (S.D.A.)**
The mere taking of food
stimulates metabolism
of cells so that heat
production increases
(30% by protein,
6% by carbohydrate
and 4% by fat).
Must allow 10% above ‐ ‐ ‐ ➔
basal requirements on
average mixed diet.

3. BASAL METABOLISM
Energy expenditure of cells
measured when subject has
fasted overnight; is resting
comfortably but not sleeping
e.g. tasks involved
in **respiration,
circulation, digestion,
excretion,
secretion,
synthesis** of
special substances,
**keeping body
temperature** at 37°C,
growth and **repair**.

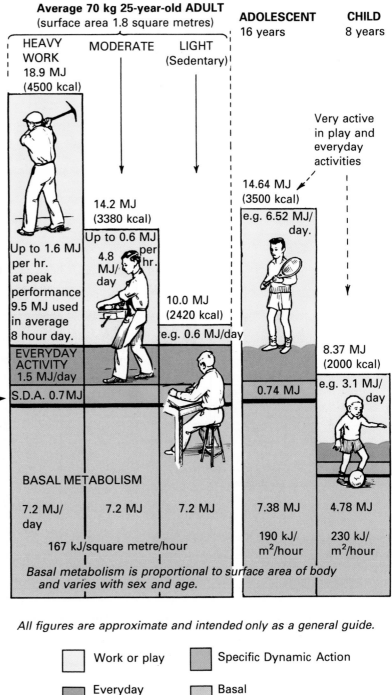

Average 70 kg 25-year-old ADULT
(surface area 1.8 square metres)

ADOLESCENT
16 years

CHILD
8 years

HEAVY
WORK
18.9 MJ
(4500 kcal)

MODERATE

LIGHT
(Sedentary)

Very active
in play and
everyday
activities

14.64 MJ
(3500 kcal)

e.g. 6.52 MJ/
day.

14.2 MJ
(3380 kcal)

Up to 1.6 MJ
per hr.
at peak
performance
9.5 MJ used
in average
8 hour day.

Up to 0.6 MJ
per
4.8 hr.
MJ/
day

10.0 MJ
(2420 kcal)

e.g. 0.6 MJ/day

8.37 MJ
(2000 kcal)

EVERYDAY
ACTIVITY
1.5 MJ/day

S.D.A. 0.7 MJ

0.74 MJ

e.g. 3.1 MJ/
day

BASAL METABOLISM

7.2 MJ/
day

7.2 MJ

7.2 MJ

7.38 MJ

190 kJ/
m²/hour

4.78 MJ

230 kJ/
m²/hour

167 kJ/square metre/hour

*Basal metabolism is proportional to surface area of body
and varies with sex and age.*

All figures are approximate and intended only as a general guide.

☐ Work or play   ☐ Specific Dynamic Action

☐ Everyday
   activities

☐ Basal
   Metabolism

55

ENERGY REQUIREMENTS – FEMALE

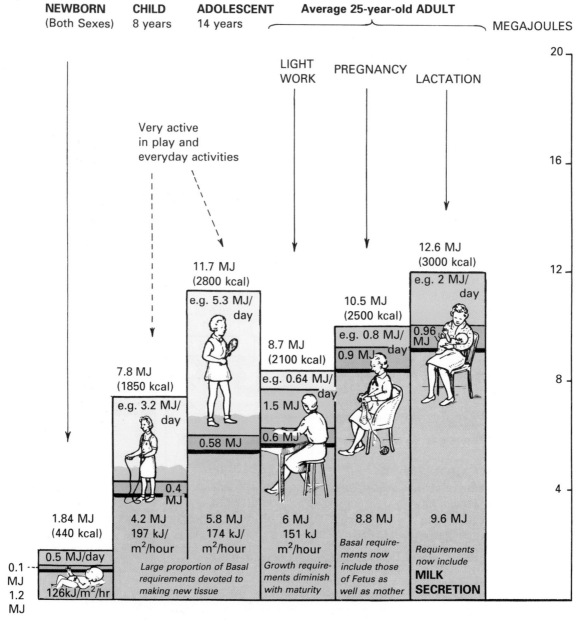

NEWBORN (Both Sexes)

CHILD 8 years

ADOLESCENT 14 years

Average 25-year-old ADULT

MEGAJOULES

LIGHT WORK

PREGNANCY

LACTATION

Very active in play and everyday activities

12.6 MJ (3000 kcal)

e.g. 2 MJ/ day

11.7 MJ (2800 kcal)

e.g. 5.3 MJ/ day

10.5 MJ (2500 kcal)

e.g. 0.8 MJ/ day

0.96 MJ

8.7 MJ (2100 kcal)

e.g. 0.64 MJ/ day

0.9 MJ

7.8 MJ (1850 kcal)

e.g. 3.2 MJ/ day

1.5 MJ

0.58 MJ

0.6 MJ

0.4 MJ

1.84 MJ (440 kcal)

0.5 MJ/day

126kJ/m²/hr

4.2 MJ 197 kJ/ m²/hour

Large proportion of Basal requirements devoted to making new tissue

5.8 MJ 174 kJ/ m²/hour

6 MJ 151 kJ m²/hour

Growth requirements diminish with maturity

8.8 MJ

Basal requirements now include those of Fetus as well as mother

9.6 MJ

Requirements now include **MILK SECRETION**

0.1 MJ
1.2 MJ

Proportion needed for growth diminishes in both sexes with age.

1 MJ = 239 kcal; 1000 kcal = 4.185 MJ

Because a person's Basal Metabolic Rate is not constant, to find total daily energy expenditure, some researchers now measure Resting Metabolic Rate (in bed) = 293 × (body weight in kg)$^{0.75}$ + energy output at work + non-occupational work output.

BALANCED DIET

The individual's daily energy requirements are best obtained by eating well-balanced meals which contain carbohydrates, fat and protein plus vitamins, minerals and water. Diet should contain about 70g protein, no more than 75g fat for men (53g for women) and 300-500g carbohydrate per day.

MEAT, FISH and DAIRY FOODS

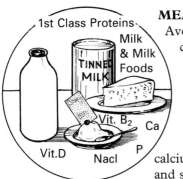

Avoid excess fat; causes obesity and coronary heart disease. Choose lean, red meat. Remove fatty skin from chicken. White fish is low in fat. Oily fish contains essential fatty acids. Milk and dairy foods are important sources of calcium. Low fat varieties cut fat intake and still provide vitamins and minerals.

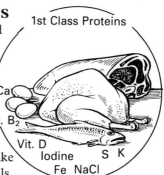

FRUIT and VEGETABLES

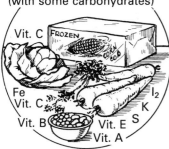
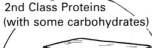

Eat as much as you like — at least 400 grams per day (5 portions). The more you eat the better. Contain vitamins A, C, E — the antioxidants — which may protect against cancer. Also high in fibre and minerals.

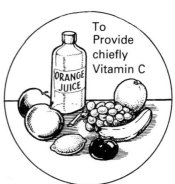

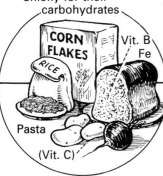

Intake high
Bread, cereals potatoes, rice, pasta should provide 50-70% of our calories. Gives fibre, vitamins, minerals and essential fatty acids.

Keep intake low
Saturated fats (animal fats and butter). Polyunsaturated fats (vegetable oil products) also salt and sugar.

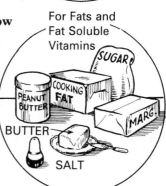

Daily additional water requirement is about 1 litre. This varies with sweat loss, etc. (See Index under 'Water Balance'.)

CHAPTER 3

CELL MEMBRANE FUNCTIONS

TRANSPORT THROUGH MEMBRANES I – DIFFUSION

The PLASMA MEMBRANE of a cell is semipermeable and consists of a double layer of phospholipids with protein molecules embedded in it (see p. 10). Transport through membranes takes several forms.

SIMPLE DIFFUSION

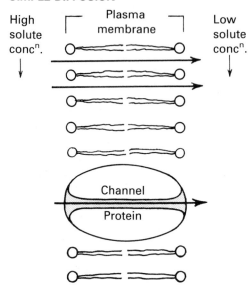

Small uncharged molecules can diffuse between the phospholipid molecules of the membrane by random thermal motion. This requires a **concentration** gradient. Ions can move down both a concentration and an electrical gradient, i.e. an **electrochemical** gradient. Because of their charge, ions *cannot* move between the phospholipid molecules. However some membrane proteins span the whole membrane and can form in their structure water-filled **channels** or **pores** which allow the passage of ions across the membrane, e.g. Na^+, K^+, Cl^-, Ca^{2+}. Movement through some channels is altered by the membrane potential (see p. 64), i.e. **voltage-gated** channels. Other channels have receptors and are opened or closed by the binding of a hormone or neurotransmitter (**ligand-gated** channels) which alters the shape of the channel proteins. Many channels remain open permanently.

FACILITATED DIFFUSION

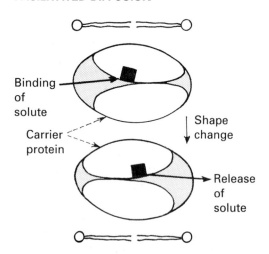

Other membrane proteins are called **carrier** proteins. The solute to be transported binds to the carrier which then changes its shape and by doing so moves the solute to the other side of the membrane. Glucose is an important substance transported by this mechanism. Little is known about the change in shape which takes place in the protein molecules. The diagram is not meant to indicate otherwise.

TRANSPORT THROUGH MEMBRANES II – ACTIVE TRANSPORT

PRIMARY ACTIVE TRANSPORT

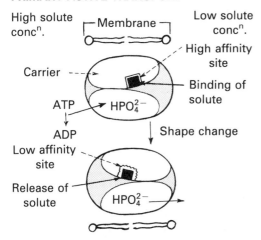

SECONDARY ACTIVE TRANSPORT

COTRANSPORT

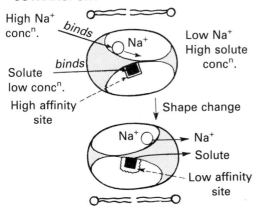

COUNTER TRANSPORT

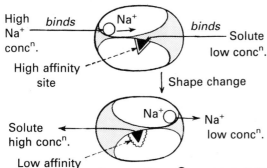

Carrier proteins are involved also in transporting molecules 'uphill' against an electrochemical gradient from a region of low concentration to a region of high concentration. Such a mechanism requires the energy of ATP and is called ACTIVE TRANSPORT. The process is called **PRIMARY ACTIVE TRANSPORT** if ATP is used in the mechanism. ATP produces a **high affinity** binding site on the carrier protein on the **low solute** concentration side of the membrane. The transported solute thus binds *tightly* to the carrier – the carrier then changes its shape – the binding site becomes a **low affinity site** on the opposite side of the membrane where the concentration of solute is *high* – the solute molecule can therefore dissociate into the high concentration. These active transport mechanisms are often referred to as PUMPS, e.g. NA^+, K^+-pump; Ca^{2+}-pump; H^+-pump. **SECONDARY ACTIVE TRANSPORT** uses the energy of a concentration gradient (often Na^+) to energize the carrier protein. This is similar to the use of a waterfall to energize a water wheel to perform work. The binding of Na^+ produces a **high affinity** solute binding site on the outside of the membrane where this time solute concentration is **low**. Na^+ and solute are transported to the inside of the membrane by a change in shape of the carrier. Na^+ dissociates – the solute binding site then becomes a **low affinity** site and solute dissociates. This is called COTRANSPORT. A solute can be transported in the *opposite* direction to Na^+. This is called COUNTER TRANSPORT. **ENDOCYTOSIS** is the transport of large molecules or particles in a membrane bound vesicle through the membrane from the *outside* to the *inside* of a cell. **EXOCYTOSIS** is similar but in the opposite direction.

IONS AND CHARGES

IONS have electrical charges which may be **positive** or **negative**. See page 4.

E.g. Na^+ is a **positive** ion called a CATION,

Cl^- is a **negative** ion called an ANION.

Like the poles of a magnet, *unlike* charges are *drawn towards* each other. *Like* charges *repel* each other.

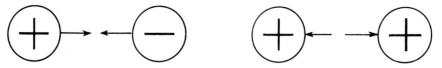

If the numbers of **positive** and **negative** charges inside a cell were equal the inside of the cell would be electrically neutral.

However, essentially all cells of the body have an *excess* of **negative** charges *inside* the cell and an *excess* of **positive** charges *outside*. Thus a POTENTIAL DIFFERENCE exists between the inside and the outside of the cell. Inside is **negative** to the outside.

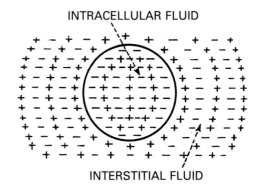

INTRACELLULAR FLUID

INTERSTITIAL FLUID

The excess **negative** charge *inside* the cell and the excess **positive** charges *outside* the cell are attracted to each other. Hence the excess ions collect in a thin layer on the inside and outside surfaces of the plasma membrane. The bulk of the interstitial and intracellular fluid is electrically neutral. The total number of positive and negative charges that account for the potential difference is a minute fraction of the K^+ and Na^+ present and therefore cannot be detected chemically. The potential difference across the membrane is measured in millivolts (mV).

When the cell is not stimulated, the difference in potential is called the resting membrane potential. However, nerve and muscle cells are 'excitable', i.e. their membrane potential can change rapidly in response to stimulation. Nerves employ such potential changes to transmit signals along their membranes.

EQUILIBRIUM POTENTIAL

To understand how the **resting membrane potential** of an excitable cell is established it is necessary to consider first what potential difference would be produced if the membrane were (a) permeable only to K^+ and (b) permeable only to Na^+.

(a) *Inside* an excitable cell there is a *high* concentration of K^+, and *outside* a *low* concentration. If the membrane was permeable only to K^+ some K^+ would diffuse out of the cell down this concentration gradient carrying **positive** charge thus leaving an excess of **negative** charges inside the cell.

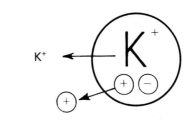

As K^+ moves out of the cell and the inside becomes more **negative** this **negativity**, by its attraction force, begins to oppose further outward movement of **positively** charged K^+. Positive charge **outside** also repels the outward movement of K^+. Thus the K^+ ions inside the cell are subjected to two forces: a concentration force tending to move them outwards and an electrical force tending to keep them inside the cell.

AT EQUILIBRIUM

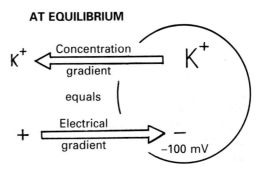

When the electric force *opposing* the outward movement of K^+ *equals* the force due to the K^+ concentration difference the potential difference across the membrane is said to be at the **equilibrium potential** for **potassium**. In a nerve or muscle cell this will occur when the *inside* is about 100 mV **negative** to the *outside*. Both greater permeability of the membrane to K^+ and a larger **concentration difference** cause more K^+ to leave the cell. The inside of the cell would then become **more negative** i.e. the potential *difference* would be *larger*.

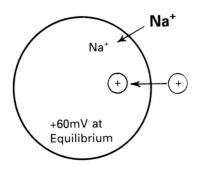

(b) There is a *high* concentration of Na^+ *outside* a cell and a *low* concentration *inside*. If the membrane was **permeable** only to Na^+, diffusion of Na^+ into the cell carrying **positive** charge would make the inside **positive** with respect to the outside. At the **equilibrium potential** for Na^+ (about $+60$ mV) the force due to the concentration difference moving Na^+ inward equals the electrical force repelling Na^+ from the inside of the cell.

63

RESTING POTENTIAL

A nerve or muscle cell at rest (not stimulated) has a **resting membrane potential**, the size of which depends mainly on the permeability of the cell membrane to K^+ and Na^+ and to the concentration of these two ions inside and outside the cell.

In the membrane there are separate **channel proteins** (page 60) for each type of ion. These may be *open* or *closed*. The more channels that are open the greater will be the permeability of the membrane.

The resting membrane is about 75 times more permeable to K^+ than to Na^+, so K^+ diffuses *out* of the cell making the inside **negative** with respect to the outside. At the same time a small amount of Na^+ diffuses *into* the cell cancelling the effect of an equivalent small number of K^+ ions. Because of this effect of Na^+ the resting membrane potential is *not* equal to the **equilibrium potential** for K^+ (-100 mV) but is much closer to that value than it is to the equilibrium potential for Na^+ ($+60$ mV). The resting membrane potential of a nerve cell is about -70mV and of a skeletal muscle cell about -90mV.

The concentrations of K^+ and Na^+ inside the cell are kept **constant** by the Na^+, K^+-ATPase pump which actively transports K^+ into the cell and Na^+ out of the cell to balance exactly the **diffusion** of Na^+ into and K^+ out of the cell.

OUTSIDE CELL

| + | 150 Na$^+$ | 4.5 K$^+$ | 125 Cl$^-$ | Na$^+$ | Concentrations mmol/l |

NERVE CELL MEMBRANE

Na$^+$K$^+$ PUMP

Channel protein

| − | Na$^+$ 15 | K$^+$ 150 | Cl$^-$ 9 | K$^+$ | Concentrations mmol/l |

INSIDE CELL

Most but not all cells are relatively permeable to Cl^-. They have Cl^- channels but do not have Cl^- pumps in their membrane. In such cells Cl^- does not help to establish the resting membrane potential. However the electrical force of the membrane potential moves Cl^- to the **positive** outside of the membrane until a concentration gradient of Cl^- builds up which has a diffusion force which equals the electrical force of the membrane potential and stops further net Cl^- movement. If the **permeability** of the membrane to Cl^- *increases*, since the Cl^- concentration outside the cell is higher than inside, more Cl^- will move into the cell making the cell **more negative**.

ELECTROTONIC POTENTIALS

The membrane potential of an excitable cell can be changed by stimulating the membrane. If the inside of the cell becomes **less negative** (i.e. the potential difference is decreased) the membrane is said to be **depolarized**. If the inside of the cell becomes **more negative** the membrane is said to be **hyperpolarized** (i.e. the potential difference is increased).

Small localized changes in the potential of a membrane can occur with **subthreshold** stimuli. This change spreads only a few millimetres from the point of stimulation and quickly dies out. This is called **electrotonic potential** or the local response.

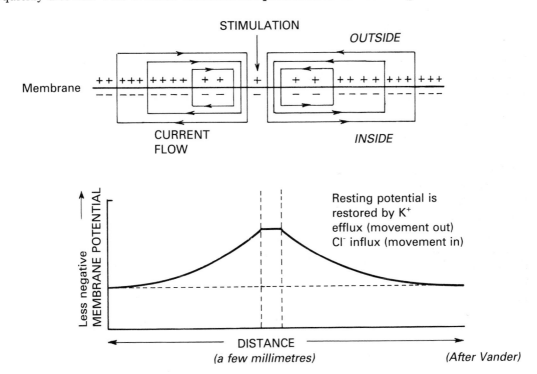

(After Vander)

When such a potential change occurs, current flows through the extracellular and intracellular fluids between the stimulated and unstimulated parts of the membrane. The direction of current flow is conventionally regarded as the direction in which **positive** ions move.

At the point of stimulation, Na^+ ions move into the cell and current will flow in the extracellular fluid, *outside* the membrane, *towards* the stimulation site (which is now less positive), and in the intracellular fluid, *inside* the membrane, *away from* the stimulation site (which is less negative, i.e. more positive).

Action potentials occur only when the membrane potential reaches a level at which depolarizing forces are *greater than* the repolarizing forces. The membrane potential at which this occurs is called the **threshold potential** or the **firing level**. A stimulus which is just sufficiently large to produce this change is a *threshold stimulus*.

THE ACTION POTENTIAL

An **action potential** is a rapid **reversal** of the resting membrane potential (inside becomes **positive** with respect to the outside). This is followed by a rapid return to the resting membrane potential.

The action potential is the result of changes in the permeability of the membrane, mainly to Na^+ and K^+ ions. In the resting membrane, most of the Na^+ channels are closed. Stimulation of the membrane causes opening of the Na^+ channels, followed slightly later by opening of the K^+ channels. Both these channel types are voltage-gated. As the membrane becomes less and less negative, more and more channels open.

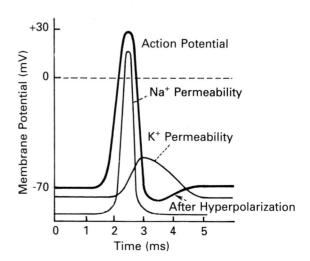

On stimulation of the membrane, its permeability to Na^+ increases several hundred fold. Na^+ rushes into the cell and, as it moves in, the inside rapidly becomes less and less negative; it reaches **zero** then becomes **positive** as Na^+ continues to enter the cell. The potential does *not* reach the **equilibrium potential** for Na^+ ($+60mV$) because *some* K^+ channels are *open* (allowing some K^+ to leave the cell and tending to make the inside **negative**).

Closure of the Na^+ channels now occurs, followed by rapid outflow of **positively** charged K^+ **ions**. The membrane potential is thus returned to its resting level. Indeed it may pass the resting level and produce an after **hyperpolarization** due to slow closure of some voltage-gated K^+ channels. The action potential in nerve axons lasts about 1 ms (millisecond).

Only a minute fraction of the Na^+ and K^+ in the cell is involved in the changes which occur during the action potential, hence many action potentials can occur without producing a significant change in intracellular ion concentrations. These are continuously being restored by Na^+, K^+ –ATPase pumps.

Ca^{2+} is involved in transporting **positive** charge through slow-conducting channels during the action potential in cardiac and smooth muscle.

Local anaesthetics can block nerve conduction by preventing the opening of fast Na^+ channels.

PROPAGATION OF THE NERVE IMPULSE

The **threshold** potential for most excitable cells is about 15 mV **less negative** than the **resting** membrane potential. In a nerve, if the membrane potential decreases from -70 mV to -55 mV the cell fires an action potential which **propagates** along the axon.

An action potential is propagated (i.e. 'handed on') with the same shape and size along the whole length of the axon or muscle cell.

One particular action potential does not itself travel along the membrane. Each action potential **activates** voltage-gated channels in the adjacent part of the membrane and a *new* action potential occurs there. This triggers the next region of the membrane and the process is repeated again and again right along the nerve.

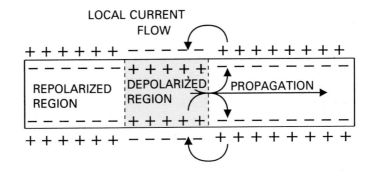

The **velocity** of propagation depends on the **diameter** of the nerve fibre and whether or not the fibre is **myelinated**. The *larger* the fibre the *faster* is the propagation.

In **MYELINATED NERVE FIBRES:**

Myelin makes it difficult for currents to flow between intracellular and extracellular fluid. Consequently action potentials only occur where the myelin is interrupted, i.e. at the **nodes of Ranvier**. Thus the nerve impulse is propagated by leaping from **node** to **node**. This method of propagation is called **saltatory conduction**.

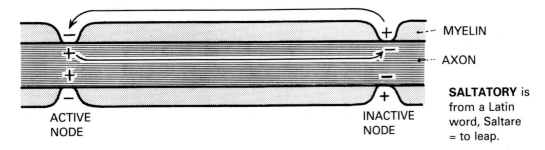

— MYELIN

— AXON

SALTATORY is from a Latin word, Saltare = to leap.

ACTIVE NODE

INACTIVE NODE

Saltatory conduction causes a more rapid propagation of the action potential than occurs in **non-myelinated** axons of the same diameter.

COMMUNICATION BETWEEN CELLS

Cells communicate with one another by sending *messages* in the form of *chemicals* to bring about a change in the activity of the target cell.

A variety of cell types including cardiac muscle and smooth muscle have small channels linking their membranes at **gap junctions** (p. 24). Small molecules and ions can pass through these gap junctions allowing the spread of electrical activity between the cells.

Gap junctions

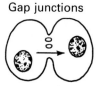

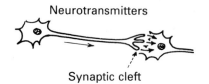

Neurotransmitters

Synaptic cleft

Messages can be passed long distances via impulses in nerve axons. The nerve impulses liberate a **neurotransmitter** at the nerve endings which diffuses across a small **synaptic cleft** and activates either another nerve or some other post-synaptic cell.

Other nerves secrete neurohormones from their endings into the blood stream. The blood conveys the hormone to cells elsewhere in the body. Such a mechanism is used, e.g. by neurons from the hypothalamus to deliver messages to the pituitary gland.

Neurohormone

Blood vessel

Hormone

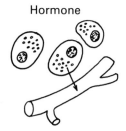

Endocrine glands secrete **hormones** directly into the blood stream which then delivers the message to a large number of cells which are widely distributed. Chemical messengers may be released by cells and diffuse to neighbouring cells through the **interstitial fluid**. Such messengers are called **paracrines**.

Paracrines

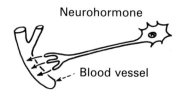

Autocrines

Similarly other chemical messengers act on the cell that secreted them. These are **autocrines**.

Chemical messages activate the correct target cells because the target cells have specific protein molecules called **receptors** (NB *not sensory* receptors, page 264) to which the chemical messenger binds. Many receptors are located in the plasma membrane but some are on the nucleus and some are elsewhere in the cell.

The number of receptors in the membrane is not constant. Excess messenger often causes the number of receptors for that messenger to decrease. This is **down regulation**. A deficiency of chemical messenger can increase the number of receptors. This is **up regulation**.

SECOND MESSENGERS – 1

When a chemical messenger e.g. a neurotransmitter or a hormone binds to a membrane receptor, this is just an initial step which leads, eventually, to a change in the activity of the cell. Such a change in activity may be e.g. an alteration in membrane permeability, electrical potential or molecular transport, or it may be a change in the cell's metabolism, its secretory state or, if the cell is a muscle cell, its contraction. All of these effects are brought about by an alteration in cell proteins e.g. a change in channel proteins can alter the ion permeability of the cell's membrane and hence its electrical potential; a change in the concentration of an enzyme can alter the cell's metabolism and changes in contractile proteins can alter muscle contraction (p.315). The chemical messenger which binds to the receptor is called a **first messenger** (or ligand). The **binding** process **activates** the receptor which may then alter the permeability of a channel protein (p.60) or it may interact with a **G protein** in the plasma membrane which in turn may interact with what is called an **effector protein** (or catalytic unit) in the plasma membrane.

The effector protein may itself be an ion channel, the permeability of which is altered. More commonly the effector protein changes the concentration of a mediator inside the cell which in turn alters the cell's activity. The intracellular mediator is called a **second messenger**. One important second messenger is adenosine 3′, 5′–cyclic monophosphate (**cAMP**) which is formed from ATP by the action of the enzyme adenylate cyclase. cAMP is inactivated by the enzyme phosphodiesterase.

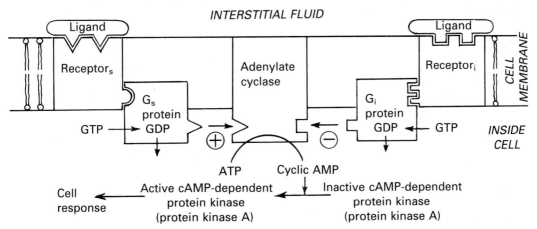

Intercellular cAMP is increased when a ligand binds to a stimulatory receptor which then activates a G_s protein (subscript 's' = stimulatory) which in turn activates the effector protein adenylate cyclase. This enzyme catalyses the conversion of ATP in the cytosol to cAMP which then activates a cAMP-dependent protein kinase (protein kinase A). Protein kinase A phosphorylates proteins which mediate the cell's response. A **reduction** of cAMP occurs when adenylate cyclase is **inhibited** by the binding of a ligand to an **inhibitory receptor** which in turn **inhibits** adenylate cyclase.

When a ligand binds to a receptor which is coupled to a G protein, activation of the G protein occurs by guanosine triphosphate (GTP) displacing guanosine diphosphate (GDP) which is bound to the G protein when it is inactive. The GTP is then converted back to GDP by GTPase and the effect of the G protein is terminated.

G proteins are so-called because they strongly bind guanosine nucleotides (p.33).

SECOND MESSENGERS – 2

Adenylate cyclase is the most widely distributed effector protein and is responsible for converting ATP to the second messenger cAMP (p.69). A similar effector protein, **guanylate** cyclase, generates guanosine 3′, 5′ cyclic monophosphate **(cGMP)**, another second messenger, which activates cGMP-dependent protein kinase (protein kinase G). This second messenger system is not linked to so many receptors as the adenylate cyclase-cAMP system. Another important second messenger system is the Ca^{2+} **system** which includes as second messengers not only Ca^{2+} but also inositol triphosphate (IP_3) and diacylglycerol (**DAG**).

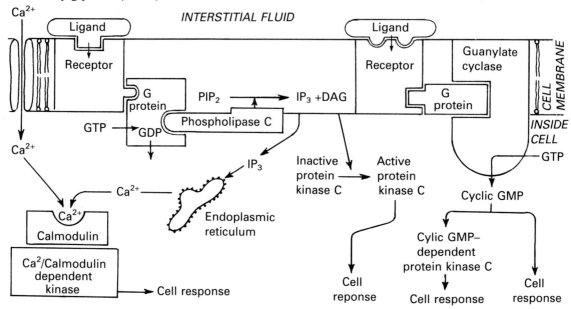

The concentration of Ca^{2+} inside a cell can be increased firstly by diffusion of Ca^{2+} into the cell through ligand or voltage-gated channels (p.60). Secondly, a ligand may bind to a receptor which can activate, via a G protein, the membrane effector enzyme phospholipase C, which catalyses the formation of diacylglycerol (DAG) and inositol triphosphate (IP_3) from phosphatidylinositol 4,5-diphosphate (PIP_2). IP_3 acts as a second messenger and releases Ca^{2+} from the endoplasmic reticulum. Ca^{2+} inside the cell then binds to a Ca^{2+}-binding protein calmodulin (in e.g. smooth muscle) or troponin (in e.g. skeletal muscle) and this **complex** alters cellular activity. DAG activates protein kinase C which leads to altered cellular activity.

Protein kinases are a class of enzymes that **phosphorylate** other proteins by transferring to them a phosphate group from ATP and, by so doing, alter their activity. This in turn alters the activity of the cell. At each step in the process the number of molecules produced is multiplied by about one hundred times.

Noradrenaline increases intracellular cAMP via β_1 and β_2 adrenergic receptors and inhibits cAMP via α_1 adrenergic receptors. Noradrenaline increases IP_3 and DAG via α_1 adrenergic receptors. Angiotensin II and vasopressin also increase IP_3 and DAG. Intracellular cGMP is increased by atrial natriuretic peptide (ANP) (p.183) and nitric oxide (endothelium-derived relaxing factor EDRF).

DIGESTIVE SYSTEM

DIGESTIVE SYSTEM

The **ALIMENTARY CANAL** and **ASSOCIATED GLANDS** } Special System for dealing with **FOOD** and **FLUIDS**

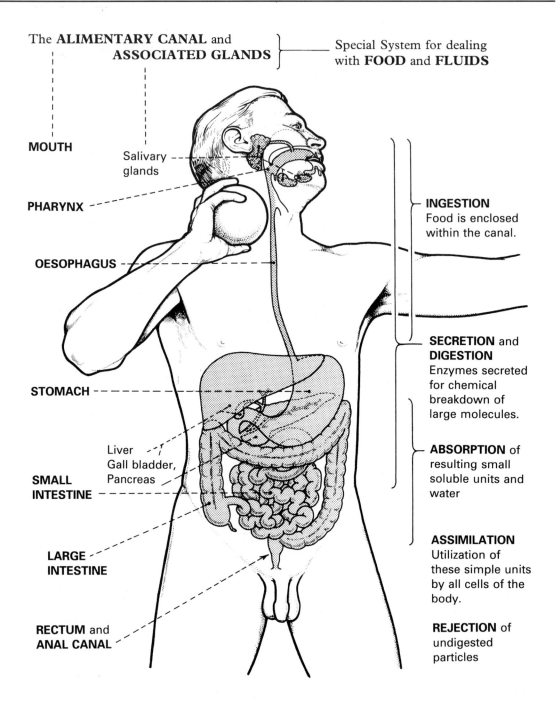

MOUTH

Salivary glands

PHARYNX

OESOPHAGUS

STOMACH

Liver
Gall bladder,
Pancreas

SMALL INTESTINE

LARGE INTESTINE

RECTUM and ANAL CANAL

INGESTION
Food is enclosed within the canal.

SECRETION and **DIGESTION**
Enzymes secreted for chemical breakdown of large molecules.

ABSORPTION of resulting small soluble units and water

ASSIMILATION
Utilization of these simple units by all cells of the body.

REJECTION of undigested particles

PROGRESS OF FOOD ALONG ALIMENTARY CANAL

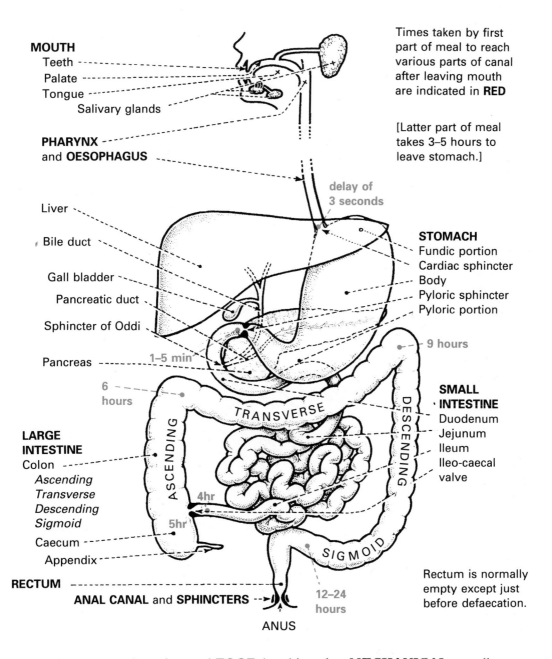

MOUTH
  Teeth
  Palate
  Tongue
    Salivary glands

PHARYNX
and **OESOPHAGUS**

Liver

Bile duct

Gall bladder

Pancreatic duct

Sphincter of Oddi

Pancreas

6 hours

1–5 min

LARGE INTESTINE
Colon
  Ascending
  Transverse
  Descending
  Sigmoid
Caecum
  Appendix

RECTUM

ANAL CANAL and SPHINCTERS

ANUS

Times taken by first part of meal to reach various parts of canal after leaving mouth are indicated in **RED**

[Latter part of meal takes 3–5 hours to leave stomach.]

delay of 3 seconds

STOMACH
  Fundic portion
  Cardiac sphincter
  Body
  Pyloric sphincter
  Pyloric portion

9 hours

SMALL INTESTINE
  Duodenum
  Jejunum
  Ileum
  Ileo-caecal valve

TRANSVERSE

ASCENDING

DESCENDING

4hr

5hr

SIGMOID

12–24 hours

Rectum is normally empty except just before defaecation.

During its progress along the canal **FOOD** is subjected to **MECHANICAL** as well as **CHEMICAL** changes to render it suitable for absorption and assimilation.

DIGESTION IN THE MOUTH

MECHANICAL PROCESSES

MASTICATION

Chewing movements of **teeth,** **tongue,** **cheeks,** **lips,** **lower jaw,** break down food, mix it with **saliva** and roll it into a moist soft mass (**bolus**) suitable for **swallowing**

[Mastication is a reflex behaviour but subject to voluntary control]

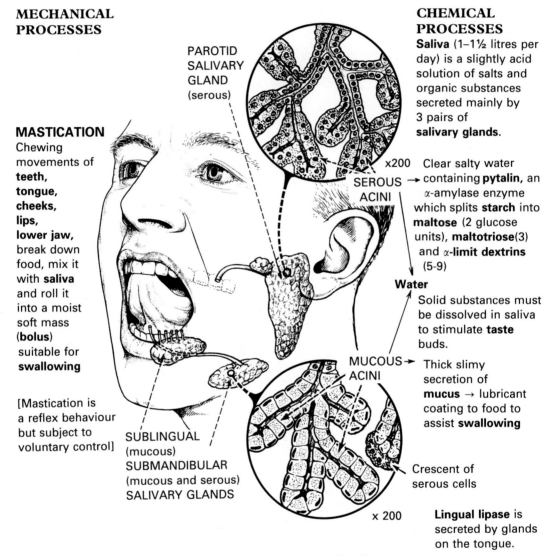

PAROTID SALIVARY GLAND (serous)

x200

SEROUS ACINI

MUCOUS ACINI

SUBLINGUAL (mucous)
SUBMANDIBULAR (mucous and serous)
SALIVARY GLANDS

x 200

Crescent of serous cells

CHEMICAL PROCESSES

Saliva (1–1½ litres per day) is a slightly acid solution of salts and organic substances secreted mainly by 3 pairs of **salivary glands.**

Clear salty water containing **pytalin,** an α-amylase enzyme which splits **starch** into **maltose** (2 glucose units), **maltotriose**(3) and α-**limit dextrins** (5-9)

Water

Solid substances must be dissolved in saliva to stimulate **taste** buds.

Thick slimy secretion of **mucus** → lubricant coating to food to assist **swallowing**

Lingual lipase is secreted by glands on the tongue.

Other important (non-digestive) functions of **saliva**:–

CLEANSING – Mouth and teeth kept free of debris, etc.

PROTECTION – Leucocytes, the enzyme lysozyme and antibodies act against some bacteria.

MOISTENING and **LUBRICATING** – Soft parts of mouth kept pliable for **speech**. Cells of oral mucosa protected from drying.

EXCRETORY – Many organic substances (e.g. urea, sugar) and inorganic substances (e.g. mercury, lead) can be excreted in saliva.

CONTROL OF SALIVARY SECRETION

Increased secretion at meal times is **reflex** (involuntary).
Salivary reflexes are of two types:–

(a) **UNCONDITIONED** (inborn)

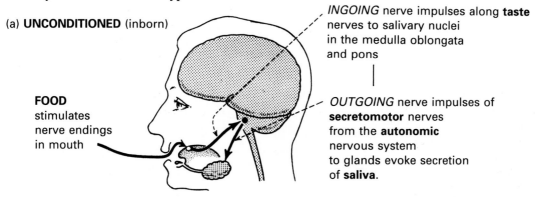

INGOING nerve impulses along **taste** nerves to salivary nuclei in the medulla oblongata and pons

FOOD stimulates nerve endings in mouth

OUTGOING nerve impulses of **secretomotor** nerves from the **autonomic** nervous system to glands evoke secretion of **saliva**.

(b) **CONDITIONED** (depend on experience)

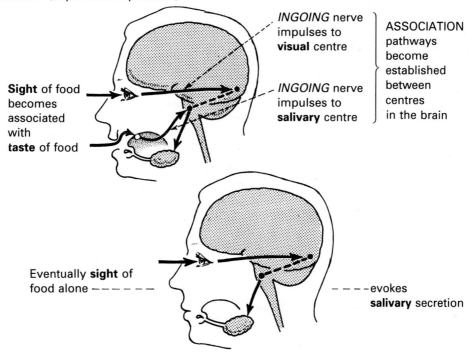

INGOING nerve impulses to **visual** centre

INGOING nerve impulses to **salivary** centre

ASSOCIATION pathways become established between centres in the brain

Sight of food becomes associated with **taste** of food

Eventually **sight** of food alone – – – – –   – – – –evokes **salivary** secretion

Similar conditioned reflexes are established by smell, by thought of food, and even by the sounds of its preparation.

Parasympathetic nerve releases (a) **acetylcholine** which greatly increases salivary secretion and (b) **vasoactive intestinal polypeptide (VIP)** which dilates the salivary gland blood vessels.

Sympathetic nerves cause secretion of small amounts of saliva rich in protein and glycoprotein.

OESOPHAGUS

The oesophagus is a muscular tube about 25 cm long which conveys ingested food and fluid from the lower end of the pharynx to the stomach.

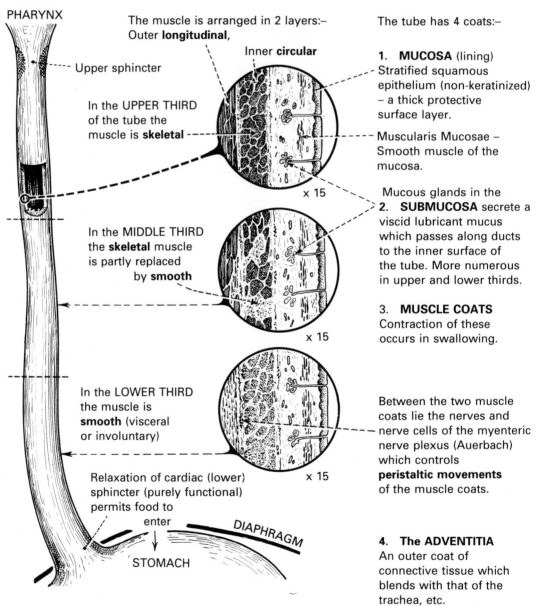

PHARYNX

The muscle is arranged in 2 layers:–
Outer **longitudinal**,
Inner **circular**

Upper sphincter

In the UPPER THIRD of the tube the muscle is **skeletal**

x 15

In the MIDDLE THIRD the **skeletal** muscle is partly replaced by **smooth**

x 15

In the LOWER THIRD the muscle is **smooth** (visceral or involuntary)

x 15

Relaxation of cardiac (lower) sphincter (purely functional) permits food to enter

DIAPHRAGM

STOMACH

The tube has 4 coats:–

1. **MUCOSA** (lining) Stratified squamous epithelium (non-keratinized) – a thick protective surface layer.

Muscularis Mucosae – Smooth muscle of the mucosa.

Mucous glands in the
2. **SUBMUCOSA** secrete a viscid lubricant mucus which passes along ducts to the inner surface of the tube. More numerous in upper and lower thirds.

3. **MUSCLE COATS** Contraction of these occurs in swallowing.

Between the two muscle coats lie the nerves and nerve cells of the myenteric nerve plexus (Auerbach) which controls **peristaltic movements** of the muscle coats.

4. **The ADVENTITIA** An outer coat of connective tissue which blends with that of the trachea, etc.

Except during passage of food the oesophagus is flattened and closed. If the pressure in stomach rises e.g. during pregnancy or after a large meal, gastric contents can enter the lower oesophagus and cause a burning sensation – **heartburn**.

SWALLOWING

Swallowing is a complex act initiated **voluntarily** and completed **involuntarily** (or **reflexly**).

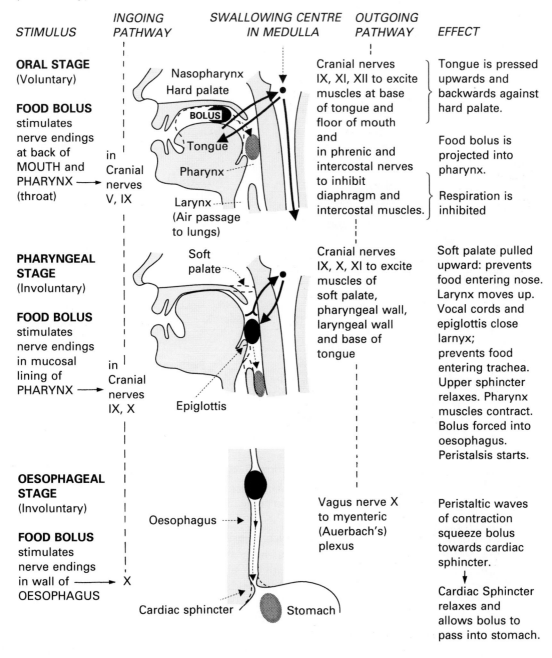

STIMULUS	*INGOING PATHWAY*	*SWALLOWING CENTRE IN MEDULLA*	*OUTGOING PATHWAY*	*EFFECT*
ORAL STAGE (Voluntary) **FOOD BOLUS** stimulates nerve endings at back of MOUTH and PHARYNX (throat) →	in Cranial nerves V, IX	Nasopharynx, Hard palate, BOLUS, Tongue, Pharynx, Larynx (Air passage to lungs)	Cranial nerves IX, XI, XII to excite muscles at base of tongue and floor of mouth and in phrenic and intercostal nerves to inhibit diaphragm and intercostal muscles.	Tongue is pressed upwards and backwards against hard palate. Food bolus is projected into pharynx. Respiration is inhibited
PHARYNGEAL STAGE (Involuntary) **FOOD BOLUS** stimulates nerve endings in mucosal lining of PHARYNX →	in Cranial nerves IX, X	Soft palate, Epiglottis	Cranial nerves IX, X, XI to excite muscles of soft palate, pharyngeal wall, laryngeal wall and base of tongue	Soft palate pulled upward: prevents food entering nose. Larynx moves up. Vocal cords and epiglottis close larnyx; prevents food entering trachea. Upper sphincter relaxes. Pharynx muscles contract. Bolus forced into oesophagus. Peristalsis starts.
OESOPHAGEAL STAGE (Involuntary) **FOOD BOLUS** stimulates nerve endings in wall of OESOPHAGUS → X		Oesophagus, Cardiac sphincter, Stomach	Vagus nerve X to myenteric (Auerbach's) plexus	Peristaltic waves of contraction squeeze bolus towards cardiac sphincter. ↓ Cardiac Sphincter relaxes and allows bolus to pass into stomach.

STOMACH

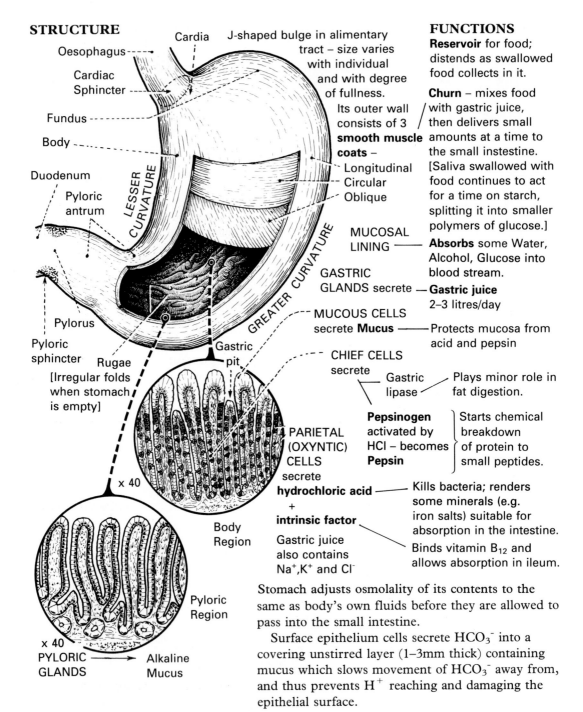

STRUCTURE

Cardia

Oesophagus ----

Cardiac Sphincter ----

Fundus ----

Body ----

Duodenum

Pyloric antrum

LESSER CURVATURE

Pylorus

Pyloric sphincter

Rugae [Irregular folds when stomach is empty]

Gastric pit

× 40

Body Region

× 40
PYLORIC GLANDS —— Alkaline Mucus

Pyloric Region

J-shaped bulge in alimentary tract – size varies with individual and with degree of fullness.

Its outer wall consists of 3 **smooth muscle coats** –
-- Longitudinal
-- Circular
-- Oblique

GREATER CURVATURE

MUCOSAL LINING ——

GASTRIC GLANDS secrete ——

MUCOUS CELLS secrete **Mucus** ——

CHIEF CELLS secrete —
— Gastric lipase

PARIETAL (OXYNTIC) CELLS secrete
hydrochloric acid
+
intrinsic factor

Gastric juice also contains Na^+, K^+ and Cl^-

FUNCTIONS

Reservoir for food; distends as swallowed food collects in it.

Churn – mixes food with gastric juice, then delivers small amounts at a time to the small instestine. [Saliva swallowed with food continues to act for a time on starch, splitting it into smaller polymers of glucose.]

Absorbs some Water, Alcohol, Glucose into blood stream.

Gastric juice 2–3 litres/day

Protects mucosa from acid and pepsin

Plays minor role in fat digestion.

Pepsinogen activated by HCl – becomes **Pepsin** } Starts chemical breakdown of protein to small peptides.

Kills bacteria; renders some minerals (e.g. iron salts) suitable for absorption in the intestine.

Binds vitamin B_{12} and allows absorption in ileum.

Stomach adjusts osmolality of its contents to the same as body's own fluids before they are allowed to pass into the small intestine.

Surface epithelium cells secrete HCO_3^- into a covering unstirred layer (1–3mm thick) containing mucus which slows movement of HCO_3^- away from, and thus prevents H^+ reaching and damaging the epithelial surface.

'G' cells in antrum secrete **gastrin** which stimulates growth of gastric glands and secretion of large amounts of gastric juice.

GASTRIC SECRETION AND MOTILITY

Secretion of gastric juice and gastric motility are under 2 types of control:

(a) **NERVOUS** – Messages are conveyed rapidly from hypothalamic feeding centre in brain to medulla and by **autonomic nervous system** for *immediate* effect, e.g. stimulation of vagus nerves produces secretion of a **highly acid juice** containing enzymes from **gastric glands** and increased motility.

(b) **HUMORAL** – Message is **chemical** and carried via **blood stream** to the gastric glands for *slower* and longer-lasting effect.

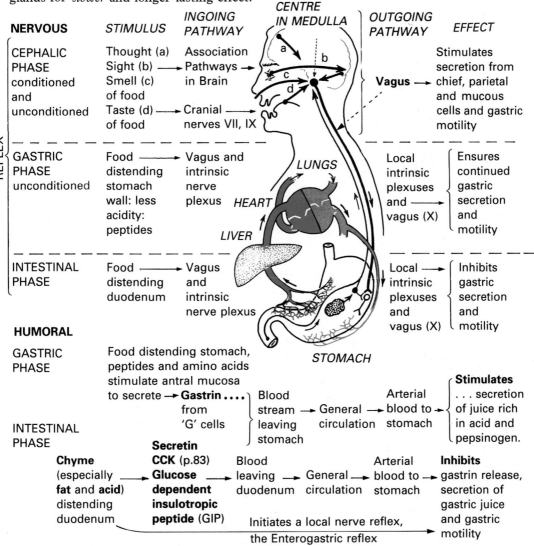

NERVOUS	*STIMULUS*	*INGOING PATHWAY*	*CENTRE IN MEDULLA*	*OUTGOING PATHWAY*	*EFFECT*

REFLEX

| | **CEPHALIC PHASE** conditioned and unconditioned | Thought (a) Sight (b) Smell (c) of food | Association Pathways in Brain | | **Vagus** → | Stimulates secretion from chief, parietal and mucous cells and gastric motility |
| | | Taste (d) of food | Cranial nerves VII, IX | | | |

| | **GASTRIC PHASE** unconditioned | Food distending stomach wall: less acidity: peptides | Vagus and intrinsic nerve plexus | Local intrinsic plexuses and vagus (X) | Ensures continued gastric secretion and motility |

| | **INTESTINAL PHASE** | Food distending duodenum | Vagus and intrinsic nerve plexus | Local intrinsic plexuses and vagus (X) | Inhibits gastric secretion and motility |

HUMORAL

| **GASTRIC PHASE** | Food distending stomach, peptides and amino acids stimulate antral mucosa to secrete → **Gastrin** .... from 'G' cells | Blood stream leaving stomach | General circulation | Arterial blood to → stomach | **Stimulates** . . . secretion of juice rich in acid and pepsinogen. |

| **INTESTINAL PHASE** | **Chyme** (especially **fat** and **acid**) distending duodenum | **Secretin CCK** (p.83) **Glucose dependent insulotropic peptide** (GIP) | Blood leaving duodenum | General circulation | Arterial blood to → stomach | **Inhibits** gastrin release, secretion of gastric juice and gastric motility |

Initiates a local nerve reflex, the Enterogastric reflex

Histamine acts on H_2 receptors on parietal cells to enhance acid secreting effect of acetylcholine and gastrin. Blocked by H_2 blocking agents. Gastrin secretion is inhibited when the pH of gastric contents falls to 2. Fear, anger, anxiety and sympathetic nerve stimulation **inhibit** gastric secretions.

MOVEMENTS OF THE STOMACH

Very little movement is seen in empty stomach until onset of **hunger**. During fasting, stomach's capacity is 50ml.

FILLING

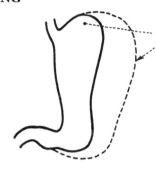

FUNDUS and GREATER CURVATURE bulge and lengthen as stomach fills with food. This is '**receptive relaxation**' – the smooth muscle cells relax so that the pressure in the stomach does not rise until the organ's capacity is 1.5 litres. This is a **nervous reflex** triggered by movement of the pharynx and oesophagus and involves vagal fibres which release an inhibitory neurotransmitter.

PERISTALSIS occurs while food is in the stomach.

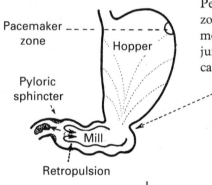

Pacemaker zone

Hopper

Pyloric sphincter

Mill

Retropulsion

Peristaltic contractions orginate from the pacemaker zone on the greater curvature of the stomach. Food moves towards the antrum and is mixed with gastric juice. The mixture becomes semifluid and is then called **chyme**.

From INCISURA ANGULARIS vigorous waves of contraction carry chyme through the PYLORUS in small squirts. The sphincter then contracts forcing chyme back by **retropulsion** and mixes the food with digestive juices.

GASTRIC SLOW WAVES

Waves of depolarization and repolarization originate in pacemaker cells.

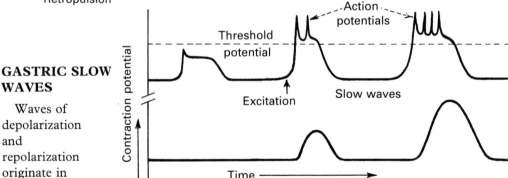

Contraction potential

Threshold potential

Action potentials

Excitation

Slow waves

Time

One wave every 20secs is conducted through gap junctions of smooth muscle to pylorus – **basic electrical rhythm**. If neural or hormonal input is absent, waves are too small to reach threshold. Stimulation by nerves or hormones can take potential above threshold and action potentials are generated at peak of slow wave cycle. Number of AP's determine strength of contraction. Force of contraction is increased by **gastric** distension, gastrin and vagus nerve stimulation, and is inhibited by duodenal distension, fat, acid, hypertonicity and decreased vagal or increased sympathetic activity.

VOMITING

Vomiting is a **complex reflex** coordinated by a centre in the region of the brain called the medulla oblongata. It starts with profuse salivation and the sensation of nausea.

Nerve pathways involved:

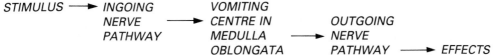

STIMULUS ⟶ INGOING NERVE PATHWAY ⟶ VOMITING CENTRE IN MEDULLA OBLONGATA ⟶ OUTGOING NERVE PATHWAY ⟶ EFFECTS

PSYCHIC INFLUENCES
e.g. fear, unpleasant sights and smells.
INCREASED PRESSURE inside skull.
DISCORDANT INGOING IMPULSES from eyes and LABYRINTH of EARS e.g. stimulation of nerve endings of utricle in motion sickness.

Excessive **DISTENSION** or **IRRITATION** of the stomach or small intestine.
Disease in pharynx, oesophagus, stomach, intestine (especially appendix), gall bladder and uterus.
Intense pain in any organ of the body.

BLOOD-BORNE EFFECTS
Certain EMETIC DRUGS or other chemicals stimulating a CHEMORECEPTOR TRIGGER ZONE in the brain.
METABOLIC DISTURBANCES e.g. in pregnancy and fatigue

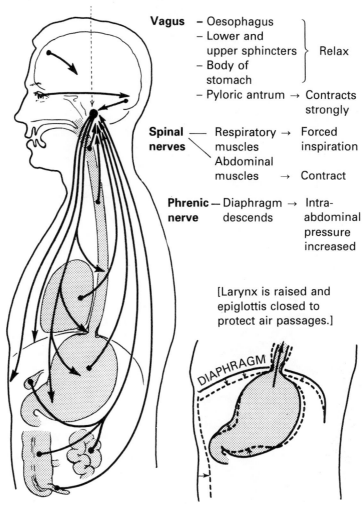

Vagus
– Oesophagus
– Lower and upper sphincters ⎫
– Body of stomach ⎭ Relax
– Pyloric antrum → Contracts strongly

Spinal nerves — Respiratory muscles → Forced inspiration
Abdominal muscles → Contract

Phrenic nerve — Diaphragm descends → Intra-abdominal pressure increased

[Larynx is raised and epiglottis closed to protect air passages.]

DIAPHRAGM

As a result of these changes the stomach is compressed and contents emptied into oesophagus → pharynx → mouth.

In **retching,** the initial stages of vomiting occur and gastric contents are forced into the oesophagus but they do not enter the pharynx.

81

PANCREAS

The pancreas is a large gland lying across the posterior abdominal wall. It has 2 secretions – a digestive secretion (exocrine) poured into the duodenum, and a hormonal secretion (endocrine) passed into the blood stream.

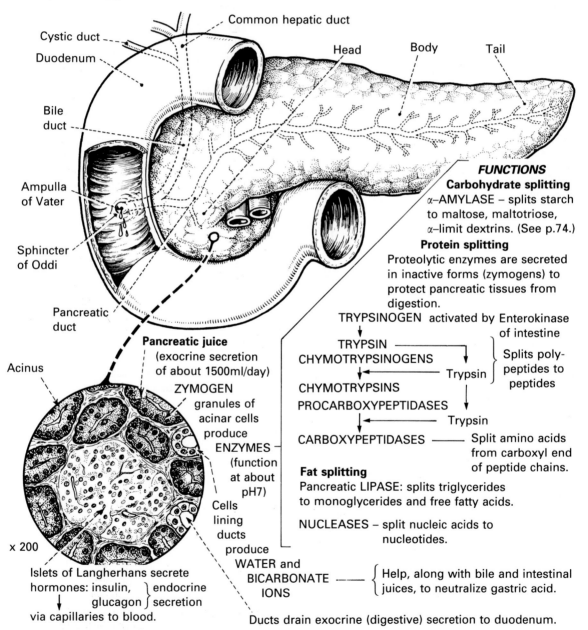

Common hepatic duct

Cystic duct

Duodenum

Head   Body   Tail

Bile duct

Ampulla of Vater

Sphincter of Oddi

Pancreatic duct

Acinus

x 200

Pancreatic juice (exocrine secretion of about 1500ml/day)

ZYMOGEN granules of acinar cells produce ENZYMES (function at about pH7)

Cells lining ducts produce WATER and BICARBONATE IONS

Islets of Langherhans secrete hormones: insulin, glucagon } endocrine secretion via capillaries to blood.

FUNCTIONS

Carbohydrate splitting
α–AMYLASE – splits starch to maltose, maltotriose, α–limit dextrins. (See p.74.)

Protein splitting
Proteolytic enzymes are secreted in inactive forms (zymogens) to protect pancreatic tissues from digestion.

TRYPSINOGEN activated by Enterokinase of intestine
↓
TRYPSIN
CHYMOTRYPSINOGENS
↓   ← Trypsin
CHYMOTRYPSINS
PROCARBOXYPEPTIDASES
↓ ← Trypsin
CARBOXYPEPTIDASES ——— Split amino acids from carboxyl end of peptide chains.

} Splits poly-peptides to peptides

Fat splitting
Pancreatic LIPASE: splits triglycerides to monoglycerides and free fatty acids.

NUCLEASES – split nucleic acids to nucleotides.

{ Help, along with bile and intestinal juices, to neutralize gastric acid.

Ducts drain exocrine (digestive) secretion to duodenum.

A **trypsin inhibitor** is also secreted by the pancreas and prevents premature activation of proteolytic enzymes in pancreatic ducts. Lipase deficiency leads to deficient fat digestion (steatorrhoea).

PANCREATIC JUICE

Secretion of pancreatic juice is under 2 types of control:– **nervous** and **humoral**. The humoral mechanism is the more important.

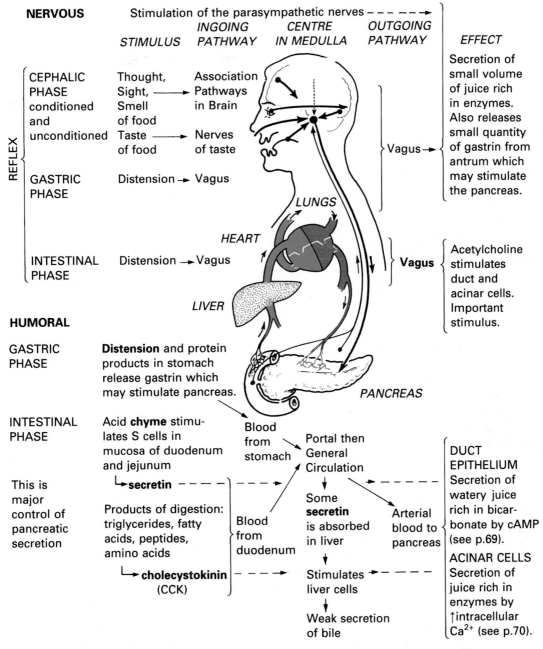

NERVOUS Stimulation of the parasympathetic nerves – – – – →

| | *STIMULUS* | *INGOING PATHWAY* | *CENTRE IN MEDULLA* | *OUTGOING PATHWAY* | *EFFECT* |

REFLEX

CEPHALIC PHASE conditioned and unconditioned — Thought, Sight, Smell of food → Association Pathways in Brain; Taste of food → Nerves of taste

GASTRIC PHASE — Distension → Vagus

INTESTINAL PHASE — Distension → Vagus

Vagus → Secretion of small volume of juice rich in enzymes. Also releases small quantity of gastrin from antrum which may stimulate the pancreas.

Vagus { Acetylcholine stimulates duct and acinar cells. Important stimulus.

LUNGS
HEART
LIVER
PANCREAS

HUMORAL

GASTRIC PHASE — **Distension** and protein products in stomach release gastrin which may stimulate pancreas.

INTESTINAL PHASE — Acid **chyme** stimulates S cells in mucosa of duodenum and jejunum

This is major control of pancreatic secretion

↳ **secretin** – – – –

Products of digestion: triglycerides, fatty acids, peptides, amino acids

↳ **cholecystokinin** (CCK) – – – →

Blood from stomach → Portal then General Circulation → Some **secretin** is absorbed in liver → Arterial blood to pancreas

Blood from duodenum

Stimulates liver cells → Weak secretion of bile

DUCT EPITHELIUM Secretion of watery juice rich in bicarbonate by cAMP (see p.69).

ACINAR CELLS Secretion of juice rich in enzymes by ↑intracellular Ca^{2+} (see p.70).

Inhibitors of pancreatic secretion include: **Pancreatone** from colon mucosa; **Glucagon** and **Somatostatin** from cells of pancreatic islets and intestinal mucosa.

LIVER FUNCTIONS

The **LIVER** has the following important metabolic and digestive functions.

Carbohydrate metabolism

Maintains normal blood glucose level. Converts glucose to glycogen and glycogen to glucose. Converts amino acids, lactic acid, fructose and galactose to glucose. Converts glucose to triglycerides.

Removal of drugs, hormones etc.

Detoxifies drugs, hormones, waste products of metabolism and other foreign chemicals.

Storage

Glycogen, fats, vitamins A, B_{12}, D, E, K, copper and iron (combined with a protein, apoferritin, in a combination called ferritin).

Lipid metabolism

Stores triglycerides. Converts fatty acids to acetylcoenzyme A, then to ketone bodies. Synthesizes lipoproteins which transport fatty acids, triglycerides and cholesterol. Synthesizes cholesterol which is used to make bile salts and also is released into the blood stream.

Phagocytosis

Kuppfer cells phagocytize old red and white blood cells and bacteria.

LIVER

Endocrine functions

Secretes insulin-like growth factor I (IGF-I, somatomedin C) in response to growth hormone. Forms T_3 from T_4 (p.195). Secretes angiotensinogen.

Activation of vitamin D

First, the liver adds an OH group to vitamin D. Then the kidney adds another to form active vitamin D (dihydroxy vitamin D_3).

Protein metabolism

Removes NH_2 from (deaminates) amino acids which can then be used to form ATP or converted to fats or carbohydrates. Converts toxic NH_3 to the less toxic urea – excreted in urine. Synthesizes plasma proteins. Can transfer an amino group to convert one amino acid into another.

Aids blood clotting

Produces prothrombin and fibrinogen. Bile salts promote absorption of vitamin K from gut.

Digestive functions

Secretes bile, rich in HCO_3 which helps neutralize acid in duodenum. Synthesizes bile salts from cholesterol. These aid absorption of fats, cholesterol, phospholipids and lipoproteins from the intestine. Synthesizes bile pigments from haem of haemoglobin. Excretes plasma cholesterol and lecithin (a phospholipid).

LIVER AND GALL BLADDER

The liver is a large highly complex organ with many functions. One of these is the production of **bile** (500–1000 ml/day).

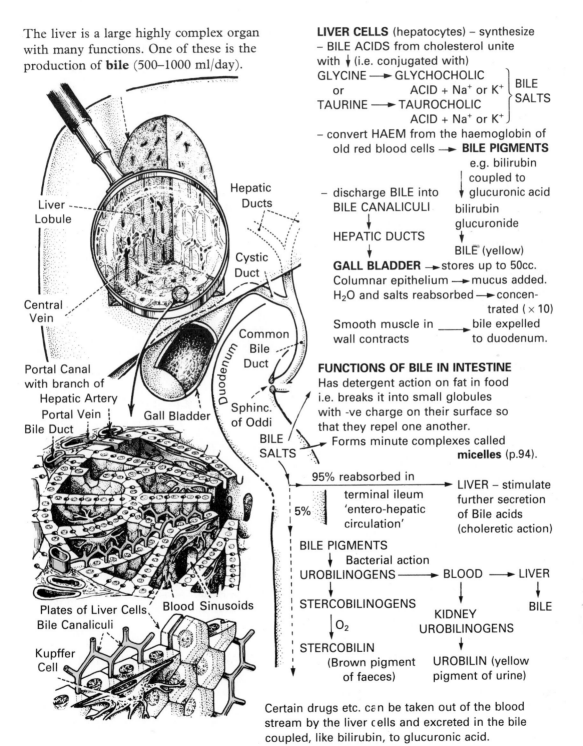

Hepatic Ducts

Liver Lobule

Central Vein

Cystic Duct

Portal Canal with branch of Hepatic Artery
Portal Vein
Bile Duct

Gall Bladder

Duodenum

Common Bile Duct

Sphinc. of Oddi

BILE SALTS

Plates of Liver Cells
Bile Canaliculi

Blood Sinusoids

Kupffer Cell

LIVER CELLS (hepatocytes) – synthesize
– BILE ACIDS from cholesterol unite
with ↓ (i.e. conjugated with)

GLYCINE ⟶ GLYCHOCHOLIC
  or   ACID + Na$^+$ or K$^+$ } BILE
TAURINE ⟶ TAUROCHOLIC   } SALTS
           ACID + Na$^+$ or K$^+$ }

– convert HAEM from the haemoglobin of
  old red blood cells ⟶ **BILE PIGMENTS**
                           e.g. bilirubin
                         ↓ coupled to
– discharge BILE into   ↓ glucuronic acid
  BILE CANALICULI   bilirubin
       ↓   glucuronide
  HEPATIC DUCTS   ↓
       ↓   BILE (yellow)

GALL BLADDER ⟶ stores up to 50cc.
Columnar epithelium ⟶ mucus added.
H$_2$O and salts reabsorbed ⟶ concen-
                              trated (× 10)
Smooth muscle in ⟶ bile expelled
wall contracts   to duodenum.

FUNCTIONS OF BILE IN INTESTINE
Has detergent action on fat in food
i.e. breaks it into small globules
with -ve charge on their surface so
that they repel one another.
⟶ Forms minute complexes called
              micelles (p.94).

95% reabsorbed in
         terminal ileum   ⟶ LIVER – stimulate
5%   'entero-hepatic   further secretion
         circulation'   of Bile acids
                                  (choleretic action)

BILE PIGMENTS
↓   Bacterial action
UROBILINOGENS ⟶ BLOOD ⟶ LIVER
↓   ↓   ↓
STERCOBILINOGENS KIDNEY   BILE
↓ O$_2$ UROBILINOGENS
STERCOBILIN   ↓
(Brown pigment   UROBILIN (yellow
of faeces)   pigment of urine)

Certain drugs etc. can be taken out of the blood
stream by the liver cells and excreted in the bile
coupled, like bilirubin, to glucuronic acid.

85

EXPULSION OF BILE (FROM THE GALL BLADDER)

Bile is necessary for the digestion and absorption of fat. Its bicarbonate content helps neutralize acid chyme in the duodenum. Bile is stored and concentrated in the gall bladder. During a meal it is discharged into the duodenum. Nervous and humoral factors influence this expulsion:

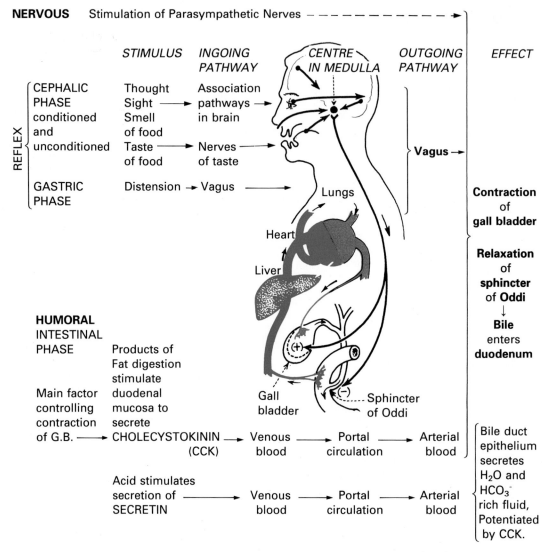

NERVOUS Stimulation of Parasympathetic Nerves – – – – – – – – – – – ➤

| STIMULUS | INGOING PATHWAY | CENTRE IN MEDULLA | OUTGOING PATHWAY | EFFECT |

REFLEX

CEPHALIC PHASE conditioned and unconditioned
Thought
Sight → Association pathways → in brain
Smell of food
Taste of food → Nerves of taste →

GASTRIC PHASE
Distension → Vagus →

Lungs

Heart

Liver

Vagus →

Contraction of gall bladder

Relaxation of sphincter of Oddi
↓
Bile enters duodenum

HUMORAL
INTESTINAL PHASE
Products of Fat digestion stimulate

Main factor controlling contraction of G.B. ──→
duodenal mucosa to secrete CHOLECYSTOKININ (CCK) → Venous blood → Portal circulation → Arterial blood

Gall bladder

Sphincter of Oddi

Acid stimulates secretion of ──→ SECRETIN → Venous blood → Portal circulation → Arterial blood

Bile duct epithelium secretes H_2O and HCO_3^- rich fluid, Potentiated by CCK.

During and just after meals bile salts are absorbed in the distal ileum and carried via the portal blood to the liver where they stimulate bile salt secretion but inhibit bile salt synthesis. Between meals since release of bile to the duodenum is low, there is a low concentration of bile salts in the portal blood, producing inhibition of bile salt secretion and stimulation of bile salt synthesis. Nerve fibres containing vasoactive intestinal peptide (VIP) and sympathetic nerves in the wall of the gall bladder inhibit its contraction.

SMALL INTESTINE

The small intestine is a long muscular tube – approximately 275 cm long in life and 700 cm after death. It receives **chyme** in small quantities from the stomach; **pancreatic juice** from the pancreas; **bile** from the gall bladder.

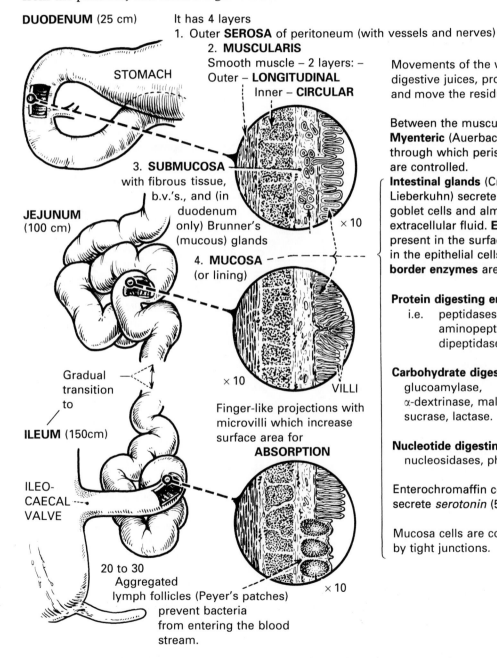

DUODENUM (25 cm)

STOMACH

JEJUNUM (100 cm)

Gradual transition to

ILEUM (150cm)

ILEO-CAECAL VALVE

20 to 30 Aggregated lymph follicles (Peyer's patches) prevent bacteria from entering the blood stream.

It has 4 layers
1. Outer **SEROSA** of peritoneum (with vessels and nerves)
2. **MUSCULARIS**
   Smooth muscle – 2 layers: –
   Outer – **LONGITUDINAL**
   Inner – **CIRCULAR**

3. **SUBMUCOSA**
   with fibrous tissue, b.v.'s, and (in duodenum only) Brunner's (mucous) glands

× 10

4. **MUCOSA** (or lining)

× 10

VILLI

Finger-like projections with microvilli which increase surface area for **ABSORPTION**

× 10

Movements of the wall mix food with digestive juices, promote absorption and move the residue along the tube.

Between the muscular layers lies the **Myenteric** (Auerbach's) **nerve plexus** through which peristaltic movements are controlled.

Intestinal glands (Crypts of Lieberkuhn) secrete **mucus** from goblet cells and almost pure extracellular fluid. **Enzymes** are present in the surface microvilli and in the epithelial cells. These **brush border enzymes** are:

Protein digesting enzymes –
   i.e.   peptidases –
          aminopeptidase, dipeptidase.

Carbohydrate digesting enzymes –
   glucoamylase, α-dextrinase, maltase, sucrase, lactase.

Nucleotide digesting enzymes –
   nucleosidases, phosphatases.

Enterochromaffin cells secrete *serotonin* (5HT)

Mucosa cells are connected by tight junctions.

THE BASIC PATTERN OF THE GUT WALL

The wall of the digestive tube shows a basic structural pattern. 4 layers are seen in transverse section.

STRUCTURE

1. MUCOSA
SURFACE EPITHELIUM with its glands –
type varies with site and function.
LOOSE FIBROUS TISSUE (lamina propria)
with capillaries and lymphatic vessels.

MUSCULARIS MUCOSAE
(thin layers of
smooth muscle)

LYMPHATIC TISSUE

2. SUBMUCOSA
DENSE FIBROUS TISSUE
in which lie blood vessels,
lymphatic vessels and SUBMUCOUS
(Meissner's) nerve plexus

[Glands in oesophagus
and 1st part of duodenum]
LYMPHATIC TISSUE

3. MUSCULARIS
SMOOTH MUSCLE
LAYERS
Inner – Circular arrangement
Outer – Longitudinal
arrangement
Between them blood and
lymphatic vessels and
MYENTERIC (Auerbach's)
nerve plexus
· [Some striated muscle in oesophagus]

4. SEROSA
FIBROUS TISSUE
with fat, blood and lymphatic vessels

MESOTHELIUM
Where tube is suspended by a **mesentery**
the serosa is formed by visceral layer of Peritoneum.

[Where there is no mesentery – replaced by
fibrous tissue which merges with surrounding fibrous tissue]

FUNCTION

Layer in close contact with gut
contents: specialized for –
SECRETION
ABSORPTION – nutrients and
hormones to blood stream.

MOBILITY (can continually
change degree of folding and the
surface area of contact with
gut contents.

DEFENCE against bacteria.

STRONG LAYER of SUPPLY
to specialized mucosa
(Blood vessels supply
needs and remove
absorbed materials).

COORDINATION of motor
and secretory activities
of mucosa.

MOVEMENT

Controls diameter of tube.
Mixes contents.
Propagates contents
along tube.

Nervous elements
coordinate secretory and
muscular activities,
Carries nerves, blood and
lymphatic vessels to and
from mesentery.

↓

Forms smooth, moist
membrane which reduces
friction between contacting
surfaces in the peritoneal
cavity.

INTESTINAL SECRETIONS

The mucosa of the intestine secretes over 2 litres/day of mucus, electrolytes and water into the lumen. Mucus protects the mucosa from mechanical damage. The nature and control of secretions differ in each part of the intestine.

DUODENUM First part is at risk from gastric acid and liable to peptic ulceration. Small coiled BRUNNER'S GLANDS in the submucosa secrete a thick alkaline mucus to protect this region.

Stimuli for secretion of intestinal juice:
(a) Tactile or irritating stimuli of the overlying mucosa act via intrinsic nerve plexuses.
(b) Vagal stimulation.
(c) Intestinal hormones, especially secretin and CCK have a minor role. Brunner's glands are inhibited by sympathetic stimulation.

SMALL INTESTINE

Mucus from GOBLET CELLS is secreted, in response to tactile stimuli, throughout the intestine. Mucus from CRYPTS of LIEBERKUHN is secreted in response to local nerve reflexes. Also from crypts a fluid like pure extracellular fluid is secreted. Provides a medium for absorption of food products. Mechanism involves active Cl^- and HCO_3^- transport into the lumen. Na^+, K^+ and water follow passively via the tight junctions, the paracellular pathway (compare page 172). Cholera and *E.coli* toxins somehow stimulate Cl^- transport and thus a severe watery diarrhoea is produced.

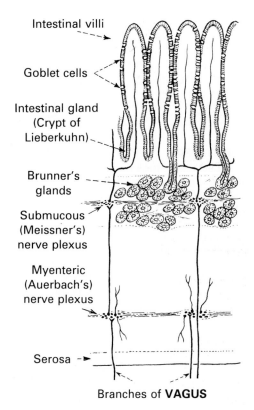

Intestinal villi

Goblet cells

Intestinal gland (Crypt of Lieberkuhn)

Brunner's glands

Submucous (Meissner's) nerve plexus

Myenteric (Auerbach's) nerve plexus

Serosa

Branches of **VAGUS**

COLON

There are no villi here. Secretion is rich in **mucus**, bicarbonate and potassium. Mechanical irritation, bacterial toxins and cholinergic nerves stimulate secretion. Sympathetic nerves inhibit it.

MOVEMENTS OF SMALL INTESTINE

The duodenum receives food in small quantities from the stomach. The mixture of food and digestive juices – chyme – is passed along the length of the small intestine.

TWO TYPES of MOVEMENT

SEGMENTATION

Rhythmical alternating contractions and relaxations – the most frequent type of movement.

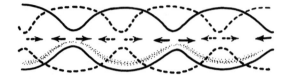

These 'shuttling' movements serve to mix **chyme** and to bring it into contact with the absorptive mucosa, i.e. **digestion** and **absorption** are promoted.

This type of movement is **myogenic**, i.e it is the property of the smooth muscle cells. It does not depend on a nervous mechanism.

PERISTALSIS

Food acts as a stretch stimulus detected by neurons containing calcitonin gene-related polypeptide (CGRP).

Waves of this contraction move the food along the canal.

The contraction behind the bolus sweeps it into the portion of the tube ahead.

Circular muscle behind bolus **contracts** due to acetylcholine and substance P.

Muscle in front of bolus may **relax** due to vasoactive intestinal polypeptide (VIP)

This type of movement is **neurogenic**, i.e. it is carried out through a 'local' reflex mediated through **intrinsic** nerve plexuses within the wall of the tube.

The extrinsic nerve supply influences it { Parasympathetic stimulation → ↑ contractions
Sympathetic stimulation → ↓ motility

EMPTYING

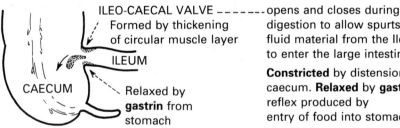

ILEO-CAECAL VALVE ------- opens and closes during digestion to allow spurts of fluid material from the Ileum to enter the large intestine.

Formed by thickening of circular muscle layer

ILEUM

CAECUM

Relaxed by **gastrin** from stomach

Constricted by distension of caecum. **Relaxed** by **gastro-ileal** reflex produced by entry of food into stomach.

Meals of different composition travel along the intestine at different rates. **Digestion** and **absorption** of food are usually complete by the time the residue reaches the ileo-caecal valve.

Contractions of the small intestine are coordinated by slow waves of depolarization which travel in the smooth muscle from the duodenum to the ileum at a frequency of 9–12/minute (see p. 80).

ABSORPTION IN SMALL INTESTINE

Absorption of most digested foodstuffs occurs in the small intestine through the microvilli which form the brush border on the free edges of the cells of the epithelium of the villi.

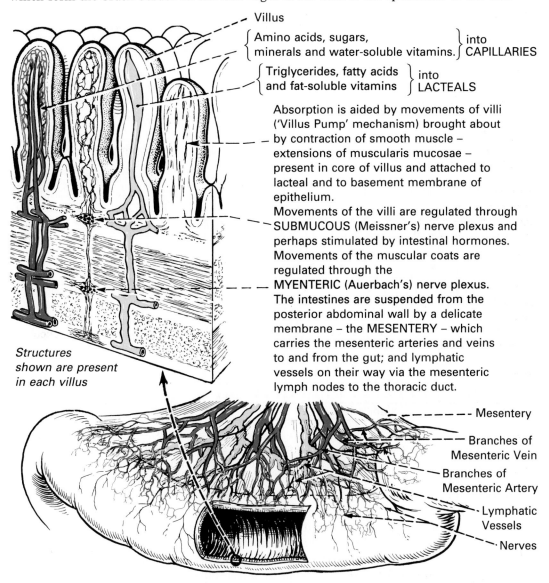

Villus

Amino acids, sugars, minerals and water-soluble vitamins. } into CAPILLARIES

Triglycerides, fatty acids and fat-soluble vitamins } into LACTEALS

Absorption is aided by movements of villi ('Villus Pump' mechanism) brought about by contraction of smooth muscle – extensions of muscularis mucosae – present in core of villus and attached to lacteal and to basement membrane of epithelium.
Movements of the villi are regulated through SUBMUCOUS (Meissner's) nerve plexus and perhaps stimulated by intestinal hormones.
Movements of the muscular coats are regulated through the MYENTERIC (Auerbach's) nerve plexus.
The intestines are suspended from the posterior abdominal wall by a delicate membrane – the MESENTERY – which carries the mesenteric arteries and veins to and from the gut; and lymphatic vessels on their way via the mesenteric lymph nodes to the thoracic duct.

Structures shown are present in each villus

Mesentery

Branches of Mesenteric Vein

Branches of Mesenteric Artery

Lymphatic Vessels

Nerves

Absorption of sugars and amino acids is by cotransport with Na^+; water is absorbed by osmosis secondary to Na^+ absorption; fatty acids and monoglycerides are absorbed by diffusion along with fat-soluble vitamins; Na^+, Ca^{2+} and Mg^{2+} are absorbed by active transport and Cl^- and K^+ by passive transport.

FOOD ABSORPTION BY CELLS OF THE SMALL INTESTINE

Digestion of food continues as it is absorbed through the **brush border** and **cystosol** of the endothelial cells of the small intestine.

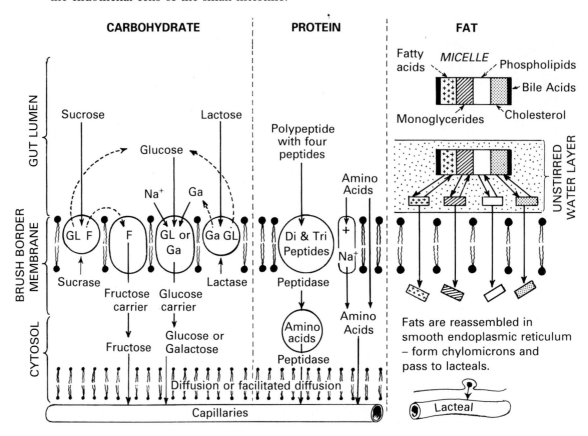

Small **carbohydrates** are broken down by enzymes (e.g. **sucrase, lactase**) in the brush border, then **fructose** (F) is transported by a fructose carrier into the cytosol. Glucose (GL) competes with galactose (Ga) for another carrier which cotransports the sugar with Na^+. From the cytosol the monosaccharides pass by diffusion or facilitated diffusion through the basolateral membrane into the capillaries.

Some free amino acids in the intestinal lumen diffuse passively through the plasma membrane. Others are cotransported with Na^+ into the cytosol. Some polypeptides are split by the brush border peptidases (p.87) into amino acids. Some di- and tripeptides are actively transported into the cytosol and split by intracellular peptidases to amino acids. From the cytosol amino acids pass by simple or facilitated diffusion through the cell membrane to the blood stream.

Micelles transport fatty acids, phospholipids, cholesterol, monoglycerides and sometimes fat-soluble vitamins across the **unstirred water layer** which lies next to the membrane. From there, these substances diffuse across the membrane into the cytosol where triglycerides are reassembled, coated with protein, cholesterol and phospholipids, forming **chylomicrons** which pass by exocytosis through the basal membrane into the lacteals.

TRANSPORT OF ABSORBED FOODSTUFFS

After absorption the **nutrients** are transported in:–

(a) **BLOOD** through
Mesenteric Veins
to
Portal Vein
to
LIVER ——→ Many substances
  via   undergo further
  ↓   changes;
Sinusoids   some are stored;
  ↓   some are passed on
Central vein via
  ↓   ↓
  Hepatic Veins → Inferior
            Vena Cava
            Heart and
            Systemic
            Circulation

(b) **LYMPH** in
Lymphatic Vessels
to
THORACIC DUCT
and via a large vein
(the innominate) in
the root of the neck
to the
Systemic Circulation
    ↓
which then distributes
Food to **all tissues** of
the **body**.

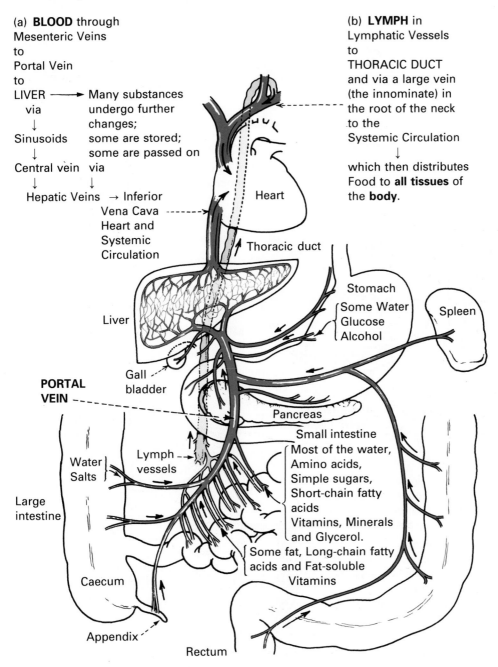

Heart

Thoracic duct

Liver

Stomach
{ Some Water
Glucose
Alcohol

Spleen

Gall
bladder

**PORTAL
VEIN** -----

Pancreas

Lymph
vessels

Water
Salts {

Large
intestine

Small intestine
{ Most of the water,
Amino acids,
Simple sugars,
Short-chain fatty
acids
Vitamins, Minerals
and Glycerol.
{ Some fat, Long-chain fatty
acids and Fat-soluble
Vitamins

Caecum

Appendix

Rectum

LARGE INTESTINE

Total length about 100 cm – living,
150 cm – at autopsy.

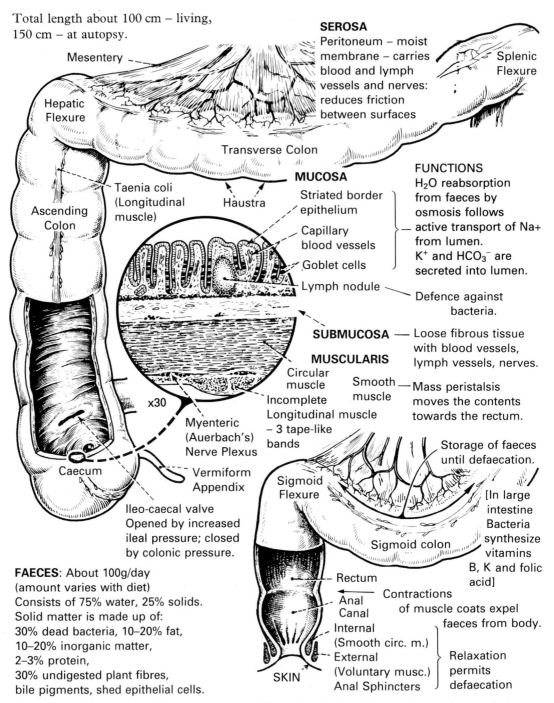

Mesentery

Hepatic Flexure

Ascending Colon

Taenia coli (Longitudinal muscle)

Haustra

Caecum

x30

SEROSA
Peritoneum – moist membrane – carries blood and lymph vessels and nerves: reduces friction between surfaces

Splenic Flexure

Transverse Colon

MUCOSA
Striated border epithelium
Capillary blood vessels
Goblet cells
Lymph nodule

FUNCTIONS
H_2O reabsorption from faeces by osmosis follows active transport of Na^+ from lumen.
K^+ and HCO_3^- are secreted into lumen.

Defence against bacteria.

SUBMUCOSA — Loose fibrous tissue with blood vessels, lymph vessels, nerves.

MUSCULARIS
Circular muscle
Incomplete Longitudinal muscle – 3 tape-like bands

Smooth muscle

Mass peristalsis moves the contents towards the rectum.

Storage of faeces until defaecation.

[In large intestine Bacteria synthesize vitamins B, K and folic acid]

Myenteric (Auerbach's) Nerve Plexus

Vermiform Appendix

Ileo-caecal valve
Opened by increased ileal pressure; closed by colonic pressure.

Sigmoid Flexure

Sigmoid colon

Rectum
Anal Canal
Internal (Smooth circ. m.)
External (Voluntary musc.)
Anal Sphincters

Contractions of muscle coats expel faeces from body.

Relaxation permits defaecation

SKIN

FAECES: About 100g/day (amount varies with diet)
Consists of 75% water, 25% solids.
Solid matter is made up of:
30% dead bacteria, 10–20% fat,
10–20% inorganic matter,
2–3% protein,
30% undigested plant fibres,
bile pigments, shed epithelial cells.

Taeniae coli broaden and fuse to form a uniform longitudinal layer of smooth muscle in rectum and lower sigmoid.

MOVEMENTS OF THE LARGE INTESTINE

The ileocaecal valve is usually closed. When food leaves the stomach the caecum relaxes and chyme passes through the ileocaecal valve (**gastro-ileal reflex**). Also, short range peristalsis in the ileum causes brief relaxations of the sphincter and allows squirts of chyme into the caecum. While in the colon, faecal matter is subjected to the following movements:

SEGMENTATION (p. 90) – – – – – – – →
Long-lasting myogenic contraction rings of circular muscle which divide colon into deep pockets (haustra). In ascending colon, waves running backward from hepatic flexure to caecum predominate.

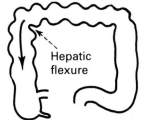

Hepatic flexure

Prolongs contact of contents with mucosa and promotes absorption of water and salt from faeces. In **transverse** and **descending** colons haustration and peristaltic contractions which move faeces short distances towards rectum predominate.

MASS PERISTALSIS – – – – – – – – – →
(or Mass Movement) Single powerful, long-lasting peristaltic contractions of circular smooth muscle that moves faeces over long distances.

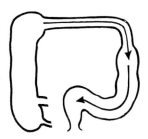

Occurs 1 to 3 times daily throughout the colon. **Sigmoid** and **rectum** have little rhythmic peristalsis and rare mass peristalsis. This reflex is often initiated by passage of food into stomach (the **gastro-colic reflex**).

EMPTYING
(DEFAECATION)

Complex **reflex** act.

Stimulus:
Passage of faeces into the rectum distends wall and initiates the reflex which is prolonged by the passage of faeces through anal canal.

(−)
(+)

SYMPATHETIC

FAECES

Pelvic nerves

PARASYMP

SPINAL CORD

(−) (+)

Pudendal nerves

(−)

The **urge** to defaecate reaches **consciousness** at rectal pressure of 18 mm Hg. **Internal** sphincter relaxes reflexly. Voluntary **contraction** of external sphincter stops reflex unless rectal pressure reaches 55 mm Hg when both sphincters relax. Voluntary **relaxation** of internal sphincter permits reflex evacuation. Outgoing nerve impulses → powerful contractions of descending and sigmoid colon and rectum, assisted by increased intra-abdominal pressure by contraction of diaphragm and abdominal muscles.
Pelvic floor relaxes.

Evacuation of faeces.

INNERVATION OF THE GUT WALL

In the wall of the gut there is an **intrinsic nervous system** called the enteric nervous system i.e. myenteric (Auerbach's) and submucous (Meissner's) plexuses (p.89) which control most gut movements and secretions. It is made up of the following types of neuron: (a) postganglionic parasympathetic, (b) secretory - controlling secretions from the mucosal cells, (c) sensory afferents from mechanoreceptors and chemoreceptors in mucosa and (d) interneurons. Many substances are secreted by these intrinsic neurons e.g. acetylcholine, serotonin, GABA and many polypeptides including e.g. **vasoactive intestinal peptide** (VIP) - inhibits smooth muscle; substance P - contracts smooth muscle; gastrin-releasing peptide (GRP); calcitonin gene-related peptide (CGRP); neurotensin etc.

   Extrinsic autonomic nerves control the level of activity of the **enteric nervous system**. The **sympathetic decreases** and the **parasympathetic increases** gut movement and secretions.

Sympathetic nerves when stimulated release at their ganglia a chemical substance **acetylcholine,** and at their post-ganglionic endings **noradrenaline**. Sympathetic post-ganglionic nerves to the gut terminate in the enteric nervous system and on smooth muscle in blood vessels. The noradrenaline released inhibits (-) transmission in the myenteric plexus thus decreasing gut movements. It constricts some sphincters (+) and some blood vessels (+). Fibres of the enteric nervous system dilate blood vessels during digestion by releasing ?VIP.

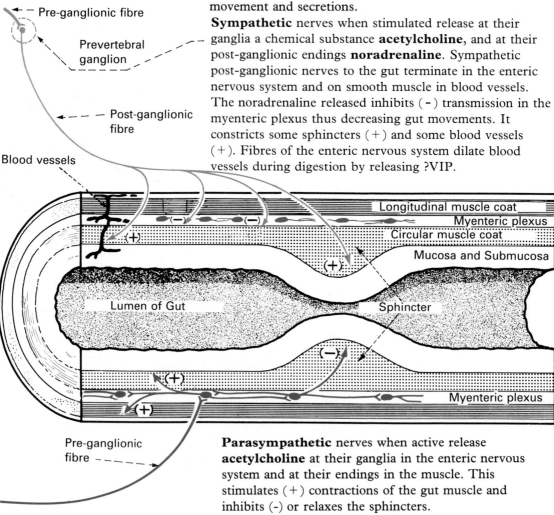

Pre-ganglionic fibre

Prevertebral ganglion

Post-ganglionic fibre

Blood vessels

Longitudinal muscle coat
Myenteric plexus
Circular muscle coat
Mucosa and Submucosa

Lumen of Gut

Sphincter

Myenteric plexus

Pre-ganglionic fibre

Parasympathetic nerves when active release **acetylcholine** at their ganglia in the enteric nervous system and at their endings in the muscle. This stimulates (+) contractions of the gut muscle and inhibits (-) or relaxes the sphincters.

NERVOUS CONTROL OF GUT MOVEMENTS

Movements in the wall of the gastro-intestinal tract are either

(a) **myogenic** – a property of the smooth muscle, e.g segmentation or
(b) **neurogenic** – dependent on the enteric nervous system e.g. peristalsis.

These movements can occur even after extrinsic nerves to the tract have been cut. Normally, however, impulses travelling in the **sympathetic** and **parasympathetic nerves**, from the **controlling centres** of the **autonomic nervous system** in the brain and spinal cord, influence and coordinate events in the whole tract.

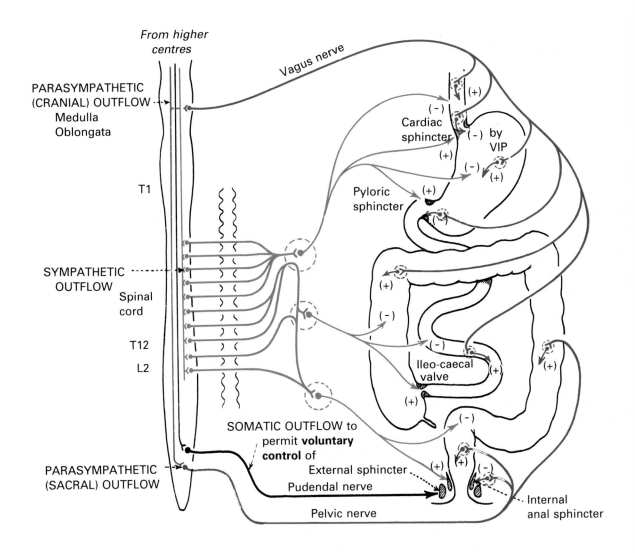

CHAPTER 5

TRANSPORT SYSTEM
THE HEART, BLOOD VESSELS AND BODY
FLUIDS: HAEMOPOIETIC SYSTEM

CARDIOVASCULAR SYSTEM

The **CIRCULATORY** System

Chief **TRANSPORT** System
of the body

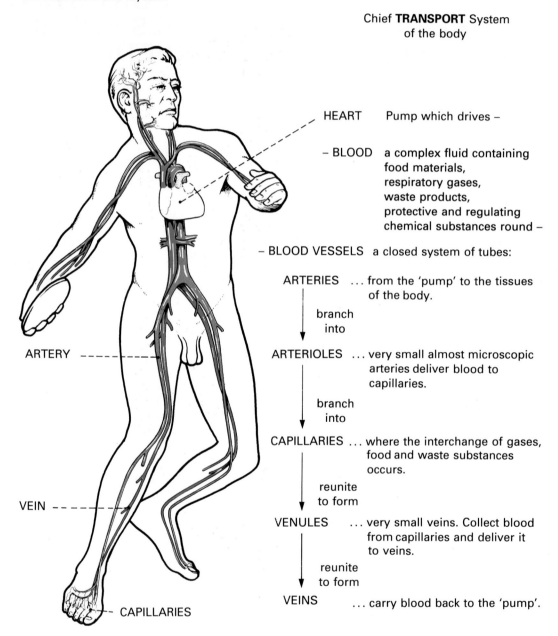

HEART   Pump which drives –

– BLOOD   a complex fluid containing
food materials,
respiratory gases,
waste products,
protective and regulating
chemical substances round –

– BLOOD VESSELS   a closed system of tubes:

ARTERIES   ... from the 'pump' to the tissues
of the body.

branch
into

ARTERIOLES   ... very small almost microscopic
arteries deliver blood to
capillaries.

branch
into

CAPILLARIES   ... where the interchange of gases,
food and waste substances
occurs.

reunite
to form

VENULES   ... very small veins. Collect blood
from capillaries and deliver it
to veins.

reunite
to form

VEINS   ... carry blood back to the 'pump'.

ARTERY

VEIN

CAPILLARIES

GENERAL COURSE OF THE CIRCULATION

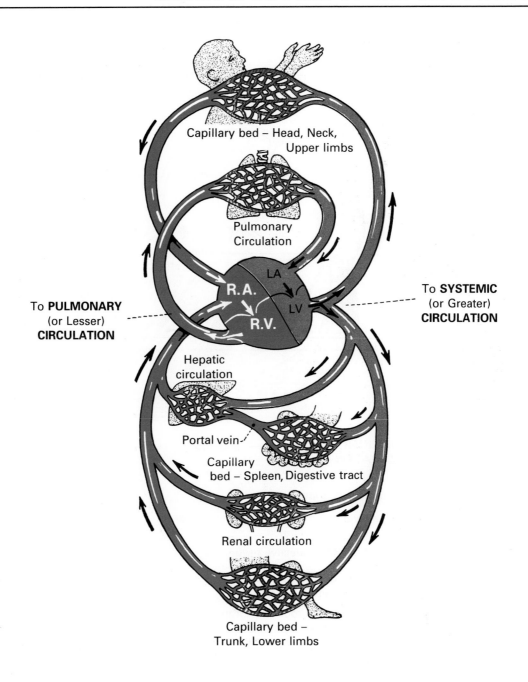

Capillary bed – Head, Neck, Upper limbs

Pulmonary Circulation

LA

R.A.

LV

To **PULMONARY** (or Lesser) **CIRCULATION**

R.V.

To **SYSTEMIC** (or Greater) **CIRCULATION**

Hepatic circulation

Portal vein

Capillary bed – Spleen, Digestive tract

Renal circulation

Capillary bed – Trunk, Lower limbs

HEART

The HEART has 4 chambers

2 UPPER CHAMBERS ———————————————— with thin walls of **cardiac muscle**
(of equal capacity)   separated by thin **interatrial septum**.

which
contract
to expel
Blood
into

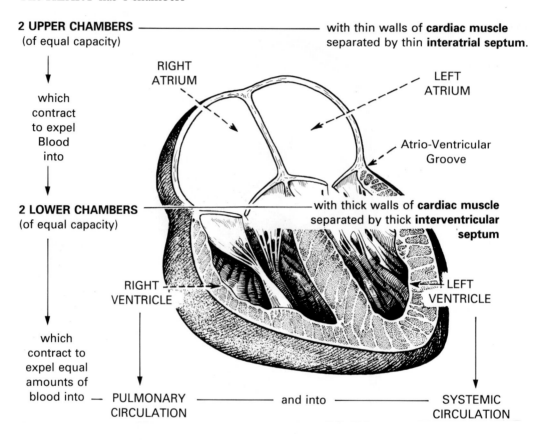

RIGHT
ATRIUM

LEFT
ATRIUM

Atrio-Ventricular
Groove

2 LOWER CHAMBERS ———————— with thick walls of **cardiac muscle**
(of equal capacity)   separated by thick **interventricular
septum**

RIGHT
VENTRICLE

LEFT
VENTRICLE

which
contract to
expel equal
amounts of
blood into — PULMONARY ———————— and into ———————— SYSTEMIC
CIRCULATION   CIRCULATION

The wall of each chamber has 3 layers

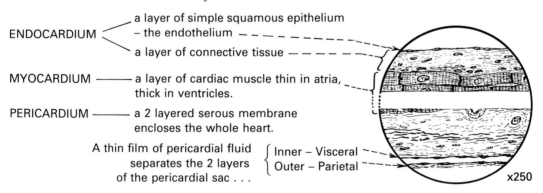

ENDOCARDIUM
a layer of simple squamous epithelium
– the endothelium – – – – –
a layer of connective tissue – – – – –

MYOCARDIUM ——— a layer of cardiac muscle thin in atria,
thick in ventricles.

PERICARDIUM ——— a 2 layered serous membrane
encloses the whole heart.

A thin film of pericardial fluid
separates the 2 layers
of the pericardial sac . . .

Inner – Visceral – – –
Outer – Parietal – – –

x250

The cardiac muscle of the atria is completely separated from the cardiac muscle of the
ventricles, at the atrio-ventricular groove, by a **fibrous skeleton** which consists of **4 rings**
of dense connective tissue joined together. Each ring is called an **annulus fibrosus** and
has a heart valve attached to it.

HEART

This is a diagrammatic section through the heart.

HEART VALVES have a core of fibrous tissue
covered on both sides with **Endothelium**

Extensions from
**ATRIO-VENTRICULAR (AV)
FIBROUS RING**

Designed to
allow blood to
flow in one
direction only –
from **atrium** to
ventricle – and
on into **arteries**

The AV valves are
attached by thin
CHORDAE
TENDINEAE
to
extensions of **cardiac
muscle** –
PAPILLARY MUSCLES

These contract when
ventricles contract
and pull on Chordae
Tendineae so that
valve flaps cannot be
everted into atria.

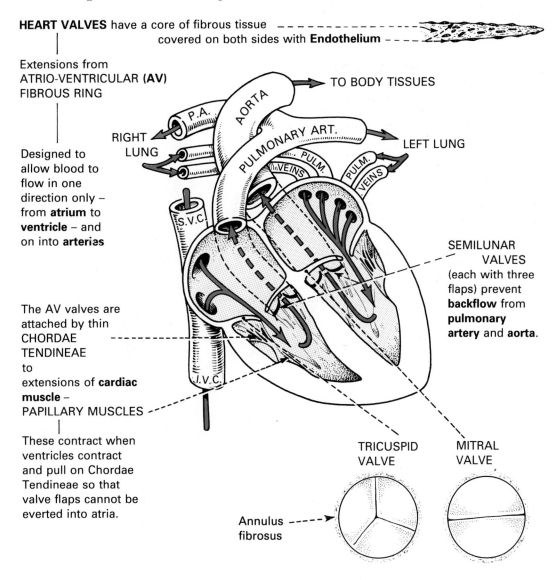

TO BODY TISSUES

P.A.

AORTA

PULMONARY ART.

RIGHT
LUNG

LEFT LUNG

PULM.
VEINS

PULM.
VEINS

S.V.C.

I.V.C.

SEMILUNAR
VALVES
(each with three
flaps) prevent
backflow from
**pulmonary
artery** and **aorta**.

TRICUSPID
VALVE

MITRAL
VALVE

Annulus
fibrosus

The great veins do not have valves guarding their entrance to the heart.
Thickening and contraction of the muscle around their mouths prevent **backflow** of blood
from heart.

HEART

The human heart is really a DOUBLE PUMP i.e. two pumps in series – each pump quite separate from the other.

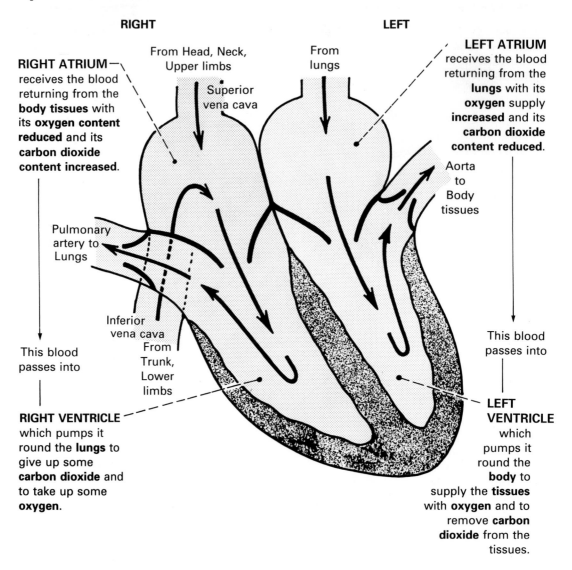

RIGHT

LEFT

RIGHT ATRIUM— receives the blood returning from the **body tissues** with its **oxygen content reduced** and its **carbon dioxide content increased**.

From Head, Neck, Upper limbs

Superior vena cava

From lungs

LEFT ATRIUM receives the blood returning from the **lungs** with its **oxygen** supply **increased** and its **carbon dioxide content reduced**.

Aorta to Body tissues

Pulmonary artery to Lungs

Inferior vena cava From Trunk, Lower limbs

This blood passes into

This blood passes into

RIGHT VENTRICLE which pumps it round the **lungs** to give up some **carbon dioxide** and to take up some **oxygen**.

LEFT VENTRICLE which pumps it round the **body** to supply the **tissues** with **oxygen** and to remove **carbon dioxide** from the tissues.

This diagram simplifies the structure of the heart to make it easier to understand the function of its various parts.

HEART SOUNDS

During each **cardiac cycle** *2 heart sounds* can be heard through a **stethoscope** applied to the **chest wall**.

1st HEART SOUND
Valve flaps, blood and ventricular walls vibrate when **atrio-ventricular valve flaps** close at the beginning of **ventricular systole**

2nd HEART SOUND
Valve flaps, blood and vessel walls vibrate when **semilunar valves** close at the beginning of **ventricular diastole**

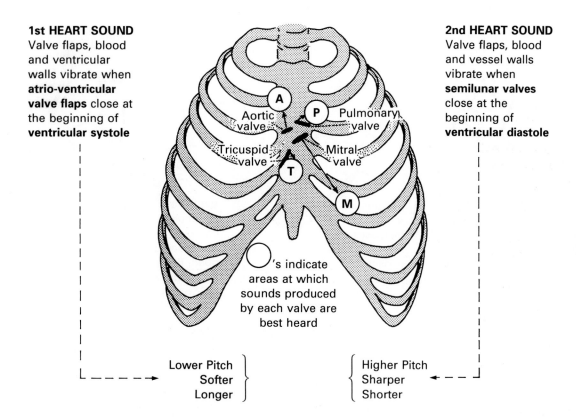

Aortic valve — A

Pulmonary valve — P

Tricuspid valve — T

Mitral valve — M

○'s indicate areas at which sounds produced by each valve are best heard

Lower Pitch
Softer
Longer

Higher Pitch
Sharper
Shorter

The sounds may be represented phonetically:-

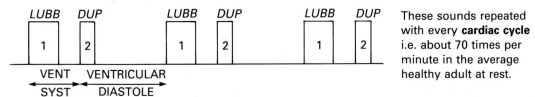

LUBB DUP   LUBB DUP   LUBB DUP
1   2   1   2   1   2

VENT VENTRICULAR
SYST DIASTOLE

These sounds repeated with every **cardiac cycle** i.e. about 70 times per minute in the average healthy adult at rest.

If the valves have been damaged by disease additional sounds (**murmurs**) can be heard as the blood flows forwards through narrowed valves or leaks backwards through incompetent valves. *Systolic* murmurs occur *between* LUBB and DUP. *Diastolic* murmurs occur between DUP and the *next* LUBB.

If the sounds of the heart are amplified, a third and a fourth heart sound can be detected. They are occasionally heard with a stethoscope over normal hearts.

CARDIAC CYCLE – 1

Diagrammatic representation of the sequence of events in the heart during *one* heart beat.

SYSTOLE [Period of Contraction]

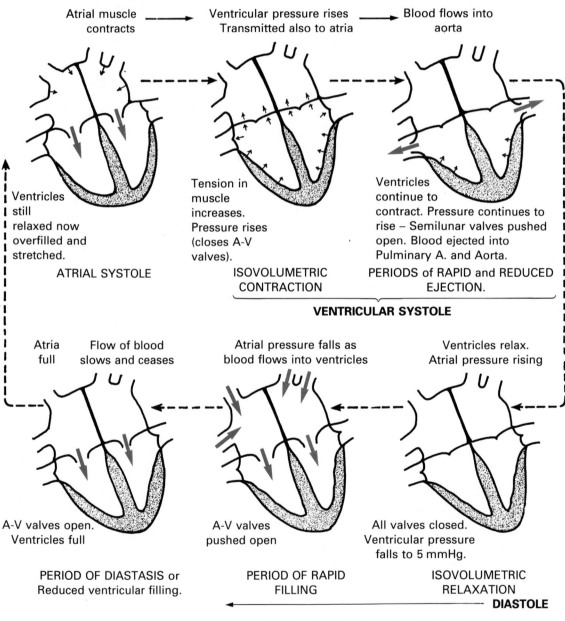

Atrial muscle contracts ——→ Ventricular pressure rises Transmitted also to atria ——→ Blood flows into aorta

Ventricles still relaxed now overfilled and stretched.

ATRIAL SYSTOLE

Tension in muscle increases. Pressure rises (closes A-V valves).

ISOVOLUMETRIC CONTRACTION

Ventricles continue to contract. Pressure continues to rise – Semilunar valves pushed open. Blood ejected into Pulminary A. and Aorta.

PERIODS of RAPID and REDUCED EJECTION.

VENTRICULAR SYSTOLE

Atria full   Flow of blood slows and ceases

Atrial pressure falls as blood flows into ventricles

Ventricles relax. Atrial pressure rising

A-V valves open. Ventricles full

PERIOD OF DIASTASIS or Reduced ventricular filling.

A-V valves pushed open

PERIOD OF RAPID FILLING

All valves closed. Ventricular pressure falls to 5 mmHg.

ISOVOLUMETRIC RELAXATION

DIASTOLE

[Period of Relaxation – i.e. when heart is resting.]

The total cycle of events takes about 0.8 second when heart is beating 75 times per minute.

CARDIAC CYCLE – 2

Shown below are the pressure changes during one cardiac cycle which occur in the **aorta**, the **left** ventricle and the **left** atrium, along with the changes in the left ventricular volume. An ECG and the heart sounds are also shown. These should be studied and correlated with the events which occur during the cardiac cycle described opposite.

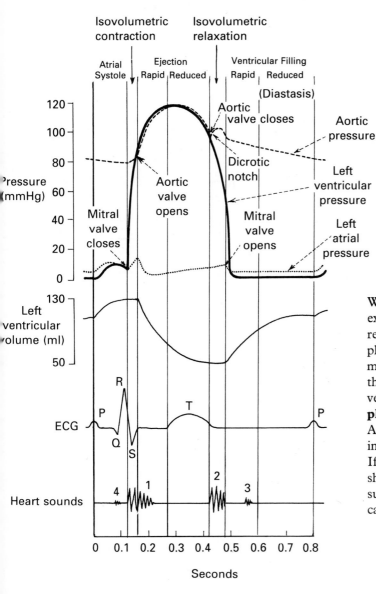

On the **right** side of the heart pressures change at about the same time as on the left, but R. **systolic** pressure is only 25 mmHg. **Diastolic** pressure in the **pulmonary artery** is about 10 mmHg and in the **R. ventricle** about 2 mmHg.

When the ventricle ejects its stroke volume, about 50 ml of blood **remains** in the ventricle. This **residual** volume becomes **less** with increased contractility during exercise. It **increases** in severe heart failure.

With the increase in heart rate in exercise, the time of **diastasis** is reduced more than the other phases of the cardiac cycle. The more the heart rate increases, the shorter diastasis becomes. At very rapid rates the **rapid filling phase** can be encroached on. Atrial contraction is then important for ventricular filling. If the filling phase becomes too short, cardiac output drops suddenly and unconsciousness can occur.

CARDIAC MUSCLE CELLS

Cardiac cells are striated and consist of sarcomeres just like skeletal muscle (p.314). Unlike skeletal muscle cardiac fibres branch and interdigitate. Adjacent cells are attached end to end. At the attachments, which are always at Z-lines, the cell membranes parallel each other and form an **intercalated disk** which runs in step-like fashion through the muscle tissue.

Desmosomes (p.24) hold adjacent cells together and allow the pull of the contractile units to be transmitted in the longitudinal axis of the cells. Where the disks run longitudinally to adjacent cells, gap junctions (p.24) are found which allow electrical excitation to spread from cell to cell throughout the muscle. Cardiac muscle contains actin, myosin, troponin C and tropomysin filaments and a T system located at the Z-lines (cf. p314).

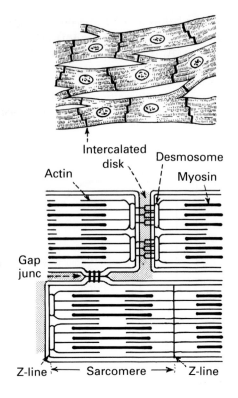

Cardiac Excitation – Contraction and Calcium. Like skeletal muscle, the link between electrical excitation and cardiac muscle contraction is Ca^{2+} ions.

Ca^{2+} entry during the action potential plateau triggers Ca^{2+} release into the cytosol. It combines with troponin C to produce contraction. It is then rapidly taken up by the SR, the mitochondria and pumped out through the membrane causing relaxation of the muscle. Ca^{2+} taken into the SR recirculates to the quick release site.

Adrenaline increases Ca^{2+} influx; digitalis reduces Ca^{2+} efflux; so both increase the contractile force of the heart.

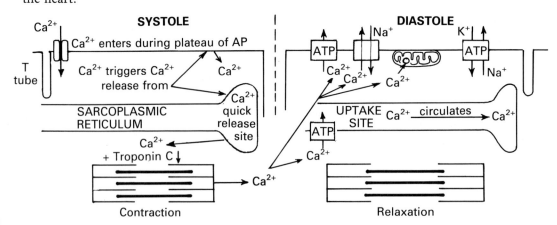

ORIGIN AND CONDUCTION OF THE HEART BEAT

The rhythmic contraction of the heart is called the heart beat. The electrical activity which produces contraction of the cardiac muscle originates in special cells called 'pacemaker' cells in the **sino-atrial node** which lies in the wall of the right atrium.

Inherent, spontaneous impulses are discharged rhythmically from 'pacemaker' cells in the
SINO-ATRIAL (SA) NODE

The wave of excitation spreads through three bundles of Purkinje-like tissue and the muscle of both ATRIA which are excited to contract.

The impulse is then conducted more slowly through another mass of NODAL TISSUE – the
ATRIO-VENTRICULAR (AV) NODE and then through the fibrous ring by the BUNDLE of HIS (AV BUNDLE) which in the interventricular septum splits into a left and right BUNDLE BRANCH. The left branch divides into a left anterior and left posterior. These three bundle branches continue down either side of the interventricular septum and then divide into PURKINJE FIBRES which spread under all parts of the endocardium of both ventricles. The impulse thus very rapidly reaches the whole ventricular muscle so that all parts contract almost simultaneously.

The right atrium starts contracting before left atrium.

A ring of fibrous tissue separates atria from ventricles. The heart beat is not transmitted from atria to ventricles directly by ordinary **cardiac** muscle.

Purkinje fibres

Left and Right bundle branches

× 200

CARDIAC ACTION POTENTIALS

Two types of action potential (p.66) occur in the heart. The **fast response** is found in heart *muscle* and Purkinje fibres. The **slow response** is found in SA and AV nodes. The fast response has *5 phases*, numbered 0-4. Each phase is the result of *changes* in membrane *permeability* to Na^+, K^+ or Ca^{2+} by opening or closing *ion channels*.

FAST RESPONSE

Phase 0
Rapid depolarization due to opening of fast Na^+ channels, controlled by m activation and h inactivation gates (p.60).

NB: Resting membrane potential is about -90mV, decreases to +20mV.

Phase 1
Closure of Na^+ channels. Efflux of K^+.

Phase 2
Plateau. K^+ efflux is balanced by slow influx of Ca^{2+} plus a little Na^+. Potential stays about 0.

Phase 3
Ca^{2+} influx declines. K^+ efflux increases rate of repolarization.

Phase 4
Resting potential is restored.

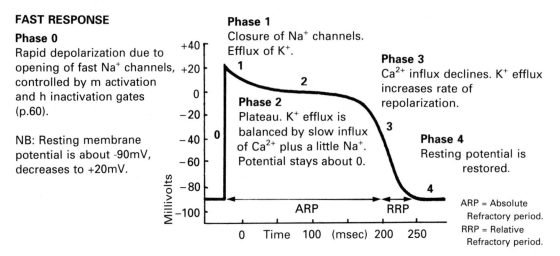

ARP = Absolute Refractory period.
RRP = Relative Refractory period.

Ca^{2+} moves into the cells during the plateau through two types of channel called L-type (long-lasting), the commonest – blocked by Ca^{2+} channel blocking agents – and T-type (transient) – not blocked by Ca^{2+} channel blockers.

The *duration* of the action potential *decreases* with an increased heart rate. It is shorter also in atrial muscle. *Contraction* of muscle *starts* just after depolarization. Peak contraction coincides approximately with repolarization.

SLOW RESPONSE

Phase 0
The spike of the fast response is absent. Depolarization is caused by Ca^{2+} influx through L-type channels.

Phase 3
No plateau. Repolarization by efflux of K^+ is more gradual

Phase 4
This is called the pacemaker potential. A slow depolarization till threshold is reached, then an action potential is triggered. It has 3 components: K^+ efflux decrease, some Na^+ influx and Ca^{2+} influx via T-type channels. Leads to further Ca^{2+} influx via L-type channels and the upstroke of the action potential.

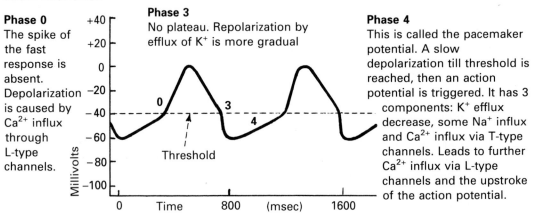

Adrenaline and noradrenaline make the slope of phase 4 *steeper* by increasing Ca^{2+} influx, hence heart *rate* is *increased*. Ca^{2+} influx also increases *force of contraction*.

Acetylcholine makes slope of phase 4 *less steep* by increasing K^+ efflux, hence heart *rate* is *decreased*.

110

ELECTROCARDIOGRAM

The wave of excitation which spreads through the heart wall consists of changes in the electrical activity of the membrane of cardiac muscle cells. Like nerve and skeletal muscle, the outer surface of **active** cardiac muscle is electrically negative relative to the resting cardiac muscle ahead of the zone of excitation. The electrical currents generate lines of force similar to those produced by a magnet and are conducted through the salty water-like body fluids to the surface of the body and can be received, amplified and recorded by electrodes of an instrument – an **electrocardiograph**. The record obtained is an **electrocardiogram** (ECG).

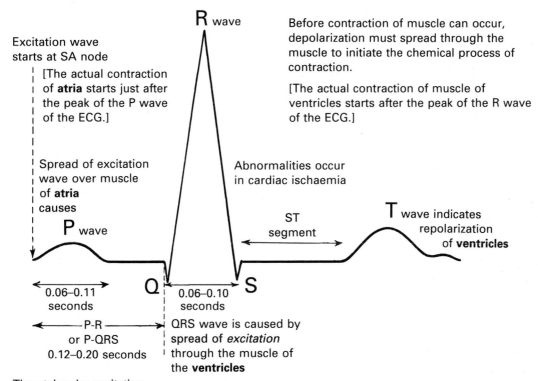

R wave

Excitation wave starts at SA node

[The actual contraction of **atria** starts just after the peak of the P wave of the ECG.]

Spread of excitation wave over muscle of **atria** causes

P wave

0.06–0.11 seconds

P-R or P-QRS 0.12–0.20 seconds

Before contraction of muscle can occur, depolarization must spread through the muscle to initiate the chemical process of contraction.

[The actual contraction of muscle of ventricles starts after the peak of the R wave of the ECG.]

Abnormalities occur in cardiac ischaemia

ST segment

T wave indicates repolarization of **ventricles**

Q

0.06–0.10 seconds

S

QRS wave is caused by spread of *excitation* through the muscle of the **ventricles**

Time taken by excitation wave to travel from the SA node over the **atria** to the AV node and along the conducting tissues to the ventricular muscle.

P-QRS interval is usually called the P-R interval because Q wave is frequently absent. (Lengthening of P-R interval indicates partial blockage of **conduction** usually at the AV node.)

Any disorder affecting the conducting system or the cardiac muscle gives changes in the ECG.

STARLING'S LAW OF THE HEART

Starling's Law of the heart states that the work performed by the ventricle is a function of end-diastolic fibre length. As **Otto Frank** had shown similar effects in the heart of a frog about twenty years earlier, it is commonly called the **Frank-Starling Law** or the **Frank-Starling Mechanism**.

The relationship between end-diastolic fibre length and contraction force in a left ventricle is represented by the two curves in the graph.

The lower curve is constructed by filling the ventricle with increasing quantities of blood and then measuring the diastolic pressure just before contraction, i.e. the end-diastolic pressure. As the ventricle is filled the muscle is stretched, so end-diastolic pressure is proportional to and therefore an index of the initial length of the muscle fibres.

The systolic pressure curve (the upper curve) is constructed by measuring the maximum systolic pressure produced during ventricular contraction at each end-diastolic volume.

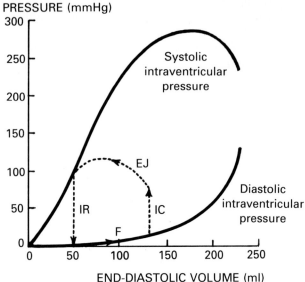

As the end-diastolic volume increases, the sarcomeres in the cardiac muscle are stretched and the systolic pressure developed increases. It reaches a peak when the diastolic volume is 180ml. This is the length at which the actin and myosin filaments are so related that they are producing maximum cross bridge formation (p.315) and the muscle is therefore developing maximum tension. If the fibres are stretched more (i.e. at higher diastolic volumes), less than optimum cross bridge formation occurs and the systolic pressure decreases again. In addition, stretching the fibres increases the sensitivity of the contractile mechanism to Ca^{2+}. This is a contributory factor to the increase in force of contraction with increase in length.

The dashed lines form a loop called a **volume-pressure diagram** of the cardiac cycle in a normal beating heart at rest (see p.107). F shows the end-diastolic pressures during ventricular filling from 50 to 130 ml. IC shows the pressure increase to aortic diastolic pressure (80 mmHg) during **isovolumetric contraction**. EJ shows the changes in volume and systolic pressure during the ejection phase (80 ml ejected) and IR shows the drop in pressure during the normal phase of **isovolumetric relaxation**.

The Frank-Starling mechanism allows the heart to adapt rapidly to a change in venous return. This would occur for instance if you lay down and raised your legs in the air. The increased venous return would stretch the right ventricle, which would then contract more to pump more blood through the heart. If you then stood up again the opposite would occur. The mechanism has a more vital role in maintaining equal output from the right and left ventricles. If the left ventricle pumped even a very small quantity of blood less than the right, blood would soon accumulate in the pulmonary blood vessels leading to an increased pressure in the pulmonary circulation and an effusion of fluid into the small air sacs of the lungs.

NERVOUS REGULATION OF ACTION OF HEART

Although the heart initiates its own beat, its rate and contractility are finely adjusted, to meet the body's constantly changing requirements, by nervous impulses travelling from controlling centres in the brain and spinal cord via parasympathetic and sympathetic nerves.

ACTION of PARASYMPATHETIC –
Stimulation of the vagus (X cranial nerve) reduces (-) the heart's activity:
**slows heart rate,
conduction at AV node delayed,
force of contraction decreased,
excitability decreased.**

[Variation in this 'vagal tone' is chief factor in producing alteration of heart rate. At rest, the parasympathetic influence is dominant. L. vagus affects AV node mainly; R. vagus affects SA node mainly.]

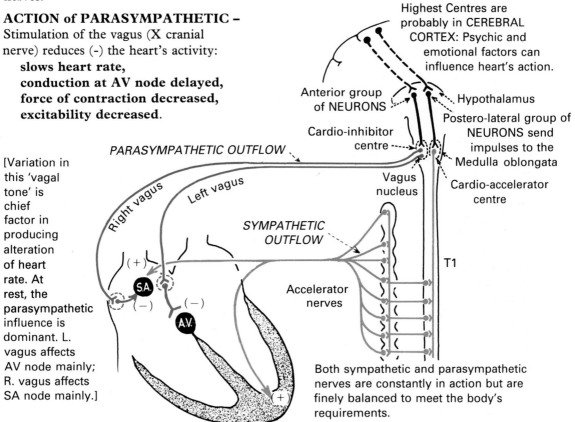

Highest Centres are probably in CEREBRAL CORTEX: Psychic and emotional factors can influence heart's action.

Anterior group of NEURONS

Cardio-inhibitor centre

PARASYMPATHETIC OUTFLOW

Right vagus   Left vagus

Vagus nucleus

Hypothalamus

Postero-lateral group of NEURONS send impulses to the Medulla oblongata

Cardio-accelerator centre

SYMPATHETIC OUTFLOW

SA.   (+)   (−)   (−)   AV.

Accelerator nerves

T1

Both sympathetic and parasympathetic nerves are constantly in action but are finely balanced to meet the body's requirements.

ACTION of SYMPATHETIC –
Stimulation of the sympathetic increases (+) the heart's activity:
**rate of contraction increased,
conductivity increased,
force of contraction increased,
excitability increased.**

Stimulation of symp. and/or inhibition of para. } Increase } of heart's
Stimulation of para. and/or inhibition of symp. } *Inhibition* } activity

[The sympathetic influence is dominant e.g. in stress, exercise, excessive heat, and other conditions requiring greater blood flow.]

CARDIAC REFLEXES

There are **ingoing (sensory)** fibres travelling in the **parasympathetic** nerves which convey information to the **medulla** about events taking place in the heart.

These afferent impulses do not normally reach consciousness. They are important as the **afferent pathways** in **cardiac reflexes** by means of which the heart's action is adjusted to the body's requirements.

One of these reflexes is

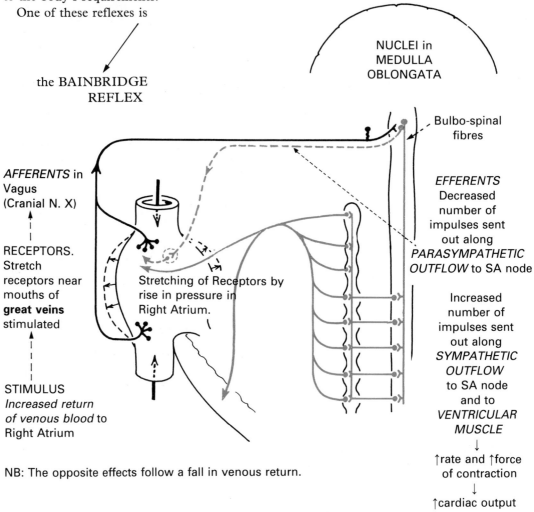

the BAINBRIDGE REFLEX

NUCLEI in MEDULLA OBLONGATA

Bulbo-spinal fibres

AFFERENTS in Vagus (Cranial N. X)

RECEPTORS. Stretch receptors near mouths of **great veins** stimulated

Stretching of Receptors by rise in pressure in Right Atrium.

STIMULUS *Increased return of venous blood* to Right Atrium

EFFERENTS Decreased number of impulses sent out along *PARASYMPATHETIC OUTFLOW* to SA node

Increased number of impulses sent out along *SYMPATHETIC OUTFLOW* to SA node and to *VENTRICULAR MUSCLE*
↓
↑rate and ↑force of contraction
↓
↑cardiac output

NB: The opposite effects follow a fall in venous return.

It is an important adaptive mechanism whereby heart rate and force of contraction are reflexly adjusted to match the quantity of venous blood returning to the heart.

Since 1925, when Bainbridge described this classic reflex, subsequent studies have pointed out that an increased venous return causing stretch of the R. atrium will also increase the cardiac output and stimulate the **baroreceptor reflex** which will **decrease** the heart rate. Hence the change which occurs in the heart rate by increased venous return will be the resultant of both of these antagonistic reflexes.

CARDIAC REFLEXES

Perhaps the most important cardiac reflex is the baroreceptor reflex which controls arterial blood pressure. Heart rate, force of contraction, resistance of arterioles and capacity of veins are involved.

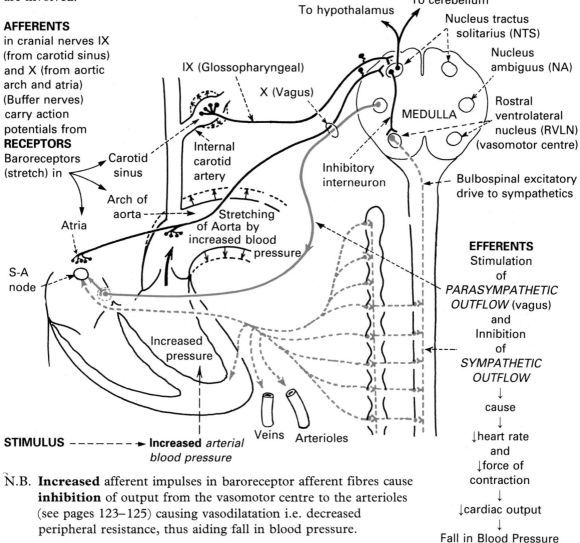

AFFERENTS
in cranial nerves IX
(from carotid sinus)
and X (from aortic
arch and atria)
(Buffer nerves)
carry action
potentials from
RECEPTORS
Baroreceptors
(stretch) in

To hypothalamus

To cerebellum

Nucleus tractus
solitarius (NTS)

Nucleus
ambiguus (NA)

IX (Glossopharyngeal)

X (Vagus)

MEDULLA

Rostral
ventrolateral
nucleus (RVLN)
(vasomotor centre)

Internal
carotid
artery

Carotid
sinus

Inhibitory
interneuron

Bulbospinal excitatory
drive to sympathetics

Arch of
aorta

Atria

Stretching
of Aorta by
increased blood
pressure

S-A
node

EFFERENTS
Stimulation
of
*PARASYMPATHETIC
OUTFLOW* (vagus)
and
Innibition
of
*SYMPATHETIC
OUTFLOW*
↓
cause
↓
↓heart rate
and
↓force of
contraction
↓
↓cardiac output
↓
Fall in Blood Pressure

Increased
pressure

Veins   Arterioles

STIMULUS - - - - - - ► **Increased** *arterial
blood pressure*

N.B. **Increased** afferent impulses in baroreceptor afferent fibres cause
inhibition of output from the vasomotor centre to the arterioles
(see pages 123–125) causing vasodilatation i.e. decreased
peripheral resistance, thus aiding fall in blood pressure.

A **decrease** in arterial blood pressure → ↓ firing in baroreceptor afferents → ↓ in
inhibition of vasomotor centre → ↑ firing via sympathetic nerves to arterioles, heart and
veins → ↑ blood pressure.

The baroreceptor reflex reduces the short-term variation in arterial pressure to about half
that which would occur if there was no baroreceptor reflex present. The long-term control
of blood pressure – over days or weeks – is determined by body fluid balance which is
mainly controlled by the kidneys. The atrial receptors which are low pressure receptors
play a part in this.

CARDIAC OUTPUT

The cardiac output is the volume of blood ejected by one ventricle in one minute and can be measured by the Fick principle as follows:

A cannula (long tube) is inserted into a **vein** and passed into the **right ventricle** or **pulmonary artery** – to obtain a sample of **mixed venous blood** – which has given up some of its oxygen to the tissues. The oxygen content is analysed.

100 ml VENOUS Blood hold 14 ml OXYGEN.

Each 100 ml blood gains 5 ml oxygen as it passes through the lungs. The blood in the lungs takes up 250 ml oxygen from the atmosphere per minute.

Therefore there must be $\left(\dfrac{250 \times 100}{5}\right)$ ml

[i.e. 5000 ml] of blood leaving the right ventricle and passing through the lungs to the left atrium per minute to take up this 250 ml oxygen.

The amount of **oxygen** taken up by the lungs per minute is measured by a **spirometer**.
250 ml OXYGEN are removed from the lungs by blood each minute.

A needle is inserted into an **artery** in the leg and a sample of **arterial blood** – which has received its fresh oxygen supply in the lungs – is obtained. The oxygen content is analysed.

100 ml ARTERIAL Blood hold 19 ml OXYGEN.

(After WISHART)

The same volume of blood must leave the left ventricle and enter the aorta in the same time otherwise blood would soon be dammed back in the lungs; i.e. If heart contracts 72 times per minute

stroke volume = $\dfrac{5000}{72} \approx 70$ ml per beat for each ventricle.

The Fick principle can be applied in general to measure consumption of O_2 and other substances in organs.

A more popular method for measuring cardiac output is the **thermodilution** technique. A bolus of cold saline is injected into the **right atrium**. The temperature change that this causes in the **pulmonary artery** is recorded with a thermister-tipped catheter. This change is proportional to the cardiac output which can be computed. Another technique employs echocardiography to measure stroke volume. Also, blood velocity in the aorta can be measured by a technique involving pulsed waves of ultrasound having their frequency altered by reflection from moving red blood corpuscles – the Doppler effect. This, along with the cross-sectional area of the aorta, measured by echocardiography, allows computation of cardiac output.

In **exercise**, cardiac output can be increased to 20–35 litres per minute (depending on training) mainly by increased **heart rate** but partly by increased stroke volume.

BLOOD VESSELS

The system of tubes through which the heart pumps blood.

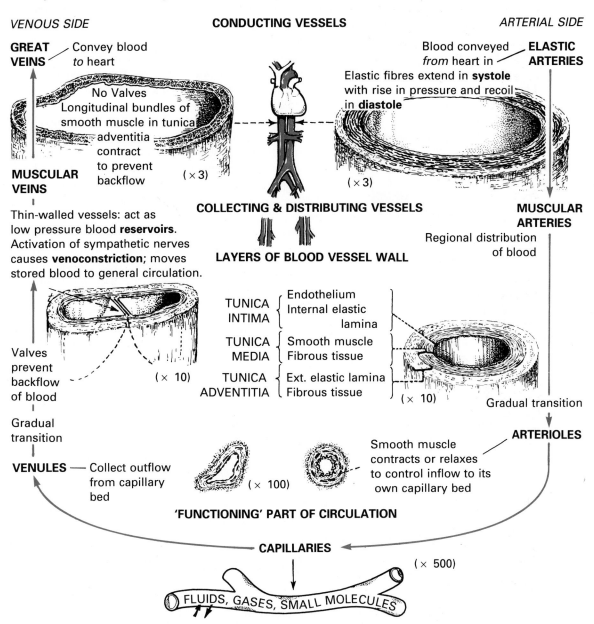

VENOUS SIDE · **CONDUCTING VESSELS** · *ARTERIAL SIDE*

GREAT VEINS — Convey blood *to* heart

Blood conveyed *from* heart in — **ELASTIC ARTERIES**

No Valves Longitudinal bundles of smooth muscle in tunica adventitia contract to prevent backflow (× 3)

Elastic fibres extend in **systole** with rise in pressure and recoil in **diastole** (× 3)

MUSCULAR VEINS

COLLECTING & DISTRIBUTING VESSELS

Thin-walled vessels: act as low pressure blood **reservoirs**. Activation of sympathetic nerves causes **venoconstriction**; moves stored blood to general circulation.

LAYERS OF BLOOD VESSEL WALL

MUSCULAR ARTERIES

Regional distribution of blood

Valves prevent backflow of blood (× 10)

TUNICA INTIMA	{ Endothelium Internal elastic lamina }
TUNICA MEDIA	{ Smooth muscle Fibrous tissue }
TUNICA ADVENTITIA	{ Ext. elastic lamina Fibrous tissue }

(× 10)

Gradual transition

Gradual transition

ARTERIOLES

VENULES — Collect outflow from capillary bed (× 100)

Smooth muscle contracts or relaxes to control inflow to its own capillary bed

'FUNCTIONING' PART OF CIRCULATION

CAPILLARIES (× 500)

FLUIDS, GASES, SMALL MOLECULES

Only from **capillaries** can blood give up food and oxygen to tissues, and receive waste products and carbon dioxide from tissues.

The endothelium releases nitric oxide which relaxes smooth muscle; takes up and metabolises vasoactive substances; synthesizes prostaglandins (see p.31); prevents blood from clotting.

BLOOD PRESSURE MODEL 1

In order to understand the relationship between **arterial blood pressure** (BP), **mean arterial blood pressure** (MABP), **cardiac output** (CO), **stroke volume** (SV), **heart rate** (HR) and **total peripheral resistance** (TPR), it is useful to compare the arterial side of the cardiovascular system to a model consisting of a series of branching **elastic** tubes. These are fed from a reservoir, through a one-way valve, to a **pump** with a **plunger** which can push fluid through a second one-way valve into the tubular system. The **outlet** at the end of each branch can be altered to be either *wide* or *narrow*. The tubular system, like the arterial system, is full of fluid.

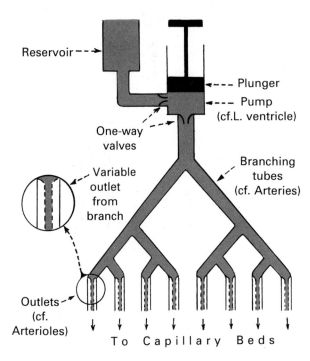

Reservoir --->

Plunger --->
Pump --->
(cf.L. ventricle)

One-way valves

Variable outlet from branch

Branching tubes (cf. Arteries)

Outlets (cf. Arterioles)

To Capillary Beds

The more fluid that is pumped into the system the higher the pressure in the system will be. If we call the pressure in the system 'BP' and the amount of fluid pumped into the system per minute 'CO', then BP will be proportional to CO.

If the amount of fluid pumped into the system (CO) is kept constant for several minutes and the outlets are widened, the pressure (BP) will *drop*. If the outlets are then narrowed again, BP will *rise*. If the outlets are narrow the resistance to outflow will be high and when they are wide the resistance to outflow will be low thus, if we call the resistance to outflow 'TPR' then BP is proportional to TPR. Thus we can say BP = CO × TPR.

The amount of fluid pumped into the system (CO) has 2 components: 1. The number of times the plunger is depressed per minute and 2. The volume of fluid pumped per stroke. If we call these 2 components HR and SV respectively, then CO = HR × SV.

Obviously in such a system the pressure will *rise* as the plunger is pushed down. The pressure will *drop* between strokes since fluid is running out the ends of the branches. If we level out these peaks and troughs we will produce a mean pressure; let's call it 'MABP'. We can now replace BP with MABP.

Relating the features of the model to the cardiovascular system, the equations demonstrate that:

$$MABP = CO \times TPR$$

i.e. Mean Arterial Blood Pressure = Cardiac Output × Total Peripheral Resistance;

$$and\ CO = HR \times SV$$

i.e. Cardiac Output = Heart Rate × Stroke Volume.

BLOOD PRESSURE MODEL 2

Two physical factors affect arterial blood pressure: **blood volume** and **compliance** of the arteries (ability of the arterial walls to stretch).

BLOOD VOLUME

The arterial system is full of blood. Similarly the model is full of fluid. If you increase the **volume** used to fill the model, the tubes, being elastic, will **stretch** to accommodate the extra fluid. At the same time, the **pressure** in the system will increase due to the increased tension in the walls of the tubes. In the same way an increase in the circulating blood volume will increase blood pressure. This is controlled mainly by the kidneys (see p.183).

ARTERIAL COMPLIANCE

Depression of the plunger increases the volume and thus the pressure in the system. The tubes **stretch** to **accommodate** this extra volume. However, the stiffer the tubes are (less elastic or less compliant) the greater the **resistance** to stretch will be and the more the **pressure** will increase. This is why a decrease in the elasticity of arteries (hardening of the arteries) causes an increase in blood pressure in elderly subjects.

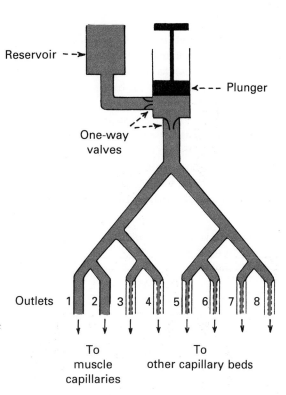

DISTRIBUTION OF BLOOD FLOW

The model can help illustrate how blood can be **redistributed**. Supposing outlets 1 and 2 are **wide** and the rest are **narrow**: as fluid is pumped into the system, **more fluid** will come out of outlets 1 and 2 than the others. Increased pumping will increase the pressure in the system and increase the outflow from 1 and 2 even further. During exercise, the arterioles to skeletal muscle dilate (widen), the heart rate increases and the blood pressure rises and, in the same way as the outflow from 1 and 2 increases, the flow of blood to the capillaries of muscles **increases** supplying them with more O_2, glucose etc. Blood can be redistributed to the skin or other tissues in a similar way.

CONTROL OF BLOOD FLOW

The model illustrates also some aspects about **blood flow**. When the outlets are **narrowed**, 'BP' the pressure behind (nearer the pump) will **rise** but at the same time the volume and pressure of the fluid flowing out (into the capillary beds) will be **reduced**. Flow through the narrowed outlets can be increased, however, if the work of the pump (CO) and hence the pressure in the system is increased further.

BLOOD PRESSURE

The left ventricle ejects about 80 ml of blood with each beat into the arterial system. Not all of this amount of blood can pass immediately through arterioles into capillaries and veins during one systolic contraction of the heart. Roughly 80% of the stroke volume from the left ventricle is accommodated in the arterial system during systole and passed on during diastole.

Conducting arteries are always more or less stretched. The more they stretch (i.e. the greater their compliance) the lower the peak pressure will be.

Peripheral resistance is chiefly due to partial constriction ('tone') of smooth muscle in walls of arterioles. (The calibre is regulated mainly by the sympathetic nervous system – pages 123–125.)

Blood pressure during systole rises because the quantity of blood entering the arterial system from the heart exceeds the run off to the periphery. At peak systolic pressure, inflow and run off are equal. Pressure then declines because run off to the periphery is greater than inflow from the heart to the arterial system. The pressure is highest at the height of the heart's contraction, i.e. **systolic blood pressure**, and lowest when the heart is relaxing, i.e. **diastolic blood pressure**.

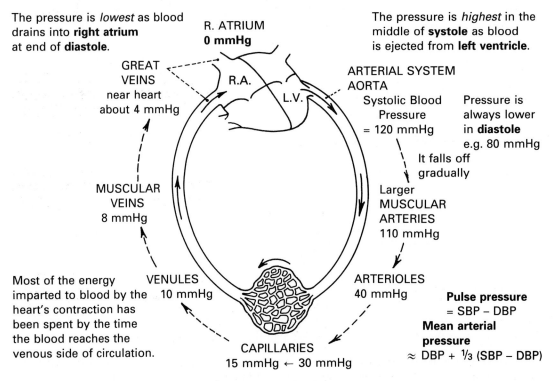

The pressure is *lowest* as blood drains into **right atrium** at end of **diastole**.

R. ATRIUM
0 mmHg

The pressure is *highest* in the middle of **systole** as blood is ejected from **left ventricle**.

GREAT VEINS
near heart
about 4 mmHg

R.A.

L.V.

ARTERIAL SYSTEM
AORTA

Systolic Blood Pressure = 120 mmHg

Pressure is always lower in **diastole** e.g. 80 mmHg

It falls off gradually

MUSCULAR VEINS
8 mmHg

Larger MUSCULAR ARTERIES
110 mmHg

Most of the energy imparted to blood by the heart's contraction has been spent by the time the blood reaches the venous side of circulation.

VENULES
10 mmHg

ARTERIOLES
40 mmHg

Pulse pressure = SBP – DBP

Mean arterial pressure
$\approx$ DBP + $\frac{1}{3}$ (SBP – DBP)

CAPILLARIES
15 mmHg $\leftarrow$ 30 mmHg

NOTE:- Any alteration in the **total amount** or the **viscosity** of blood will also affect **blood pressure**.

When standing still, the effect of **gravity** on the venous blood in the legs increases the pressure in the veins of the feet to 90 mmHg. Muscle movements lower this pressure.

MEASUREMENT OF ARTERIAL BLOOD PRESSURE

The arterial blood pressure is measured in man by means of a **sphygmomanometer**.

This consists of a rubber bag (covered with a cloth or nylon envelope) which is wrapped round the upper arm over the **brachial artery**. One tube connects the inside of the bag with a **manometer** containing **mercury**.

Another tube connects the inside of the bag to a hand operated **pump** with a release **valve**.

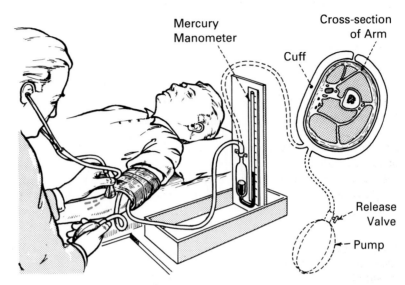

Mercury Manometer

Cross-section of Arm

Cuff

Release Valve

Pump

METHOD

Air is pumped into the rubber bag till the pressure in the cuff is greater than the pressure in the artery even during heart's systole. Artery is then closed down during systole and diastole. (At same time air is holding up mercury column in manometer.)

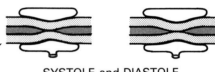

SYSTOLE and DIASTOLE

By releasing the valve on the pump the pressure in the cuff is gradually reduced till maximum pressure in artery just overcomes the pressure in the cuff – some blood begins to spurt through during systole. At this point faint rhythmical **tapping sounds** begin to be heard through **stethoscope** (Korotkow sounds). The height of mercury in millimetres is taken as the systolic blood pressure (e.g. 120 mmHg).

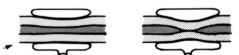

SYSTOLE – Artery still closed during DIASTOLE

Pressure in the cuff is reduced still further till it is just less than the lowest pressure in artery towards the end of diastole (i.e. just before next heart beat). Blood flow is unimpeded during

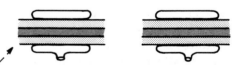

SYSTOLE and DIASTOLE

systole and diastole. The sounds stop. The height of mercury in the manometer at this point is taken as the **diastolic** Blood Pressure (e.g. about 80 mmHg).
These values differ with **sex**, **age exercise**, **sleep**, etc.

When blood is forced through a restriction in a vessel, turbulent flow of blood is produced. This causes vibrations in the auditory frequencies, thus tapping sounds called Korotkow sounds are produced.

ELASTIC ARTERIES

The large **conducting arteries** near the **heart** are **elastic arteries**.

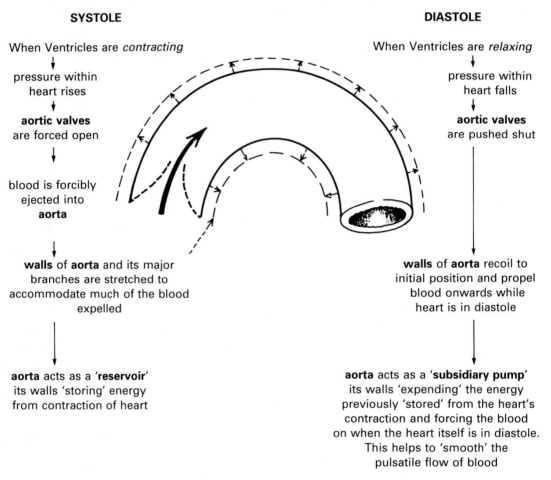

SYSTOLE

When Ventricles are *contracting*
↓
pressure within
heart rises
↓
aortic valves
are forced open
↓
blood is forcibly
ejected into
aorta
↓
walls of **aorta** and its major
branches are stretched to
accommodate much of the blood
expelled
↓
aorta acts as a **'reservoir'**
its walls 'storing' energy
from contraction of heart

DIASTOLE

When Ventricles are *relaxing*
↓
pressure within
heart falls
↓
aortic valves
are pushed shut
↓
walls of **aorta** recoil to
initial position and propel
blood onwards while
heart is in diastole
↓
aorta acts as a **'subsidiary pump'**
its walls 'expending' the energy
previously 'stored' from the heart's
contraction and forcing the blood
on when the heart itself is in diastole.
This helps to 'smooth' the
pulsatile flow of blood

The same changes occur on the right side of the heart but, since the pressures are lower, the forces involved are less.

As blood is pumped from the heart during systole, this distension and increase in pressure which starts in the aorta passes along the whole arterial system as a wave – the **pulse wave**.

The expansion and subsequent relaxation of the wall of the radial artery can be felt as **'the pulse'** at the wrist.

A great increase in blood pressure can result if these walls lose some of their elasticity with age or disease and can no longer stretch readily to accommodate so much of the heart's output during systole: nor recoil so far in diastole. The systolic and diastolic values may both be higher.

REGULATION OF ARTERIOLES

The **diameter** of **arterioles** can be changed by contraction or relaxation of the smooth **muscle** in their walls, hence **onward flow** of blood to the capillary beds which they supply can be controlled. There are **3 levels** of arteriolar control:

1. Many arterioles e.g. in brain react to a sudden rise in blood pressure by **contracting**, so that onward flow and capillary pressure stay constant (the **myogenic** response).
2. Release of **local metabolites** balances blood flow with the **metabolic activity** of the tissue e.g. heart, brain and muscle.
3. Circulating **vasoactive chemicals** and **autonomic nerves** can reduce circulation through e.g. skin and abdominal organs, even by overriding the other control mechanisms, to redirect blood to maintain the circulation of blood to the brain.

ARTERIOLES in SALIVARY GLANDS
An enzyme released from gland cells causes the formation of the vasodilator peptide **bradykinin**. Vasoactive Intestinal Peptide **(VIP)** released along with acetylcholine on stimulation of parasympathetics aids **vasodilatation**.

Stimulation of SYMPATHETIC NERVES gives **vasoconstriction** by **noradrenergic** fibres, **vasodilatation** by **cholinergic** fibres releasing VIP along with acetylcholine. But **vasoconstriction** in i.e. *overall effect* in body is one of **vasoconstriction** → increased blood pressure. (In these vessels vasodilatation occurs passively after reduction of sympathetic vasoconstrictor impulses.)

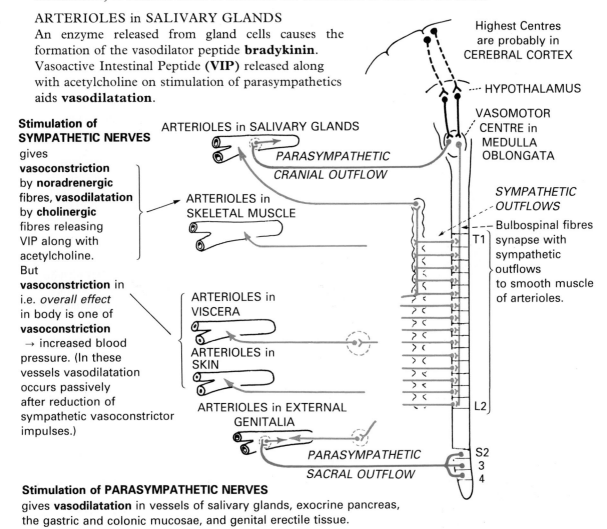

Highest Centres are probably in CEREBRAL CORTEX

···· HYPOTHALAMUS

VASOMOTOR CENTRE in MEDULLA OBLONGATA

SYMPATHETIC OUTFLOWS

--- Bulbospinal fibres synapse with sympathetic outflows to smooth muscle of arterioles.

ARTERIOLES in SALIVARY GLANDS
PARASYMPATHETIC CRANIAL OUTFLOW

ARTERIOLES in SKELETAL MUSCLE

ARTERIOLES in VISCERA

ARTERIOLES in SKIN

ARTERIOLES in EXTERNAL GENITALIA

PARASYMPATHETIC SACRAL OUTFLOW

T1

L2

S2 3 4

Stimulation of PARASYMPATHETIC NERVES
gives **vasodilatation** in vessels of salivary glands, exocrine pancreas, the gastric and colonic mucosae, and genital erectile tissue.

Veins have a sympathetic nerve supply. When activated it reduces capacity of venous system thus increasing return of blood to the heart.

REFLEX AND CHEMICAL REGULATION OF ARTERIOLAR TONE – 1

Afferent impulses are constantly reaching the nucleus of tractus solitarius in the medulla oblongata in ingoing nerves from all parts of the body. These form the afferent pathways for vasomotor reflexes

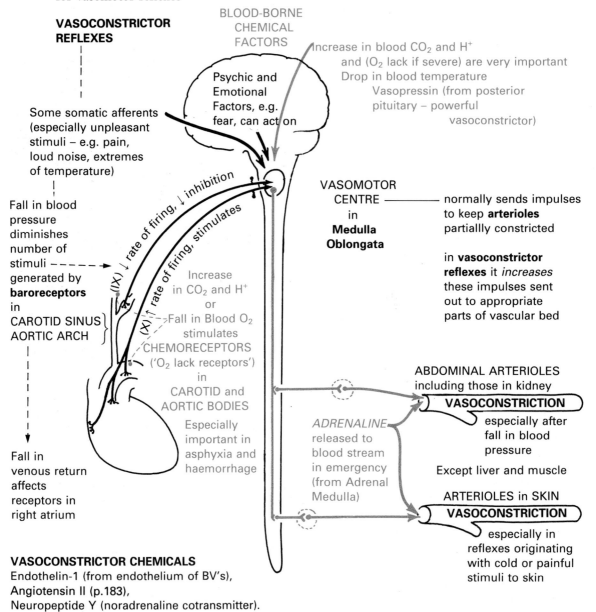

VASOCONSTRICTOR REFLEXES

BLOOD-BORNE CHEMICAL FACTORS

Increase in blood CO_2 and H^+ and (O_2 lack if severe) are very important
Drop in blood temperature
Vasopressin (from posterior pituitary – powerful vasoconstrictor)

Psychic and Emotional Factors, e.g. fear, can act on

Some somatic afferents (especially unpleasant stimuli – e.g. pain, loud noise, extremes of temperature)

Fall in blood pressure diminishes number of stimuli generated by **baroreceptors** in CAROTID SINUS AORTIC ARCH

↓ rate of firing, ↓ inhibition (IX)

↑ rate of firing, stimulates (X)

Increase in CO_2 and H^+ or Fall in Blood O_2 stimulates CHEMORECEPTORS ('O_2 lack receptors') in CAROTID and AORTIC BODIES

Especially important in asphyxia and haemorrhage

VASOMOTOR CENTRE in **Medulla Oblongata** —— normally sends impulses to keep **arterioles** partiallly constricted

in **vasoconstrictor reflexes** it *increases* these impulses sent out to appropriate parts of vascular bed

ADRENALINE released to blood stream in emergency (from Adrenal Medulla)

ABDOMINAL ARTERIOLES including those in kidney
VASOCONSTRICTION
especially after fall in blood pressure

Except liver and muscle

ARTERIOLES in SKIN
VASOCONSTRICTION
especially in reflexes originating with cold or painful stimuli to skin

Fall in venous return affects receptors in right atrium

VASOCONSTRICTOR CHEMICALS
Endothelin-1 (from endothelium of BV's),
Angiotensin II (p.183),
Neuropeptide Y (noradrenaline cotransmitter).

Widespread **vasoconstriction** increases the peripheral resistance and gives a rise in blood pressure.

REFLEX AND CHEMICAL REGULATION OF ARTERIOLAR TONE – 2

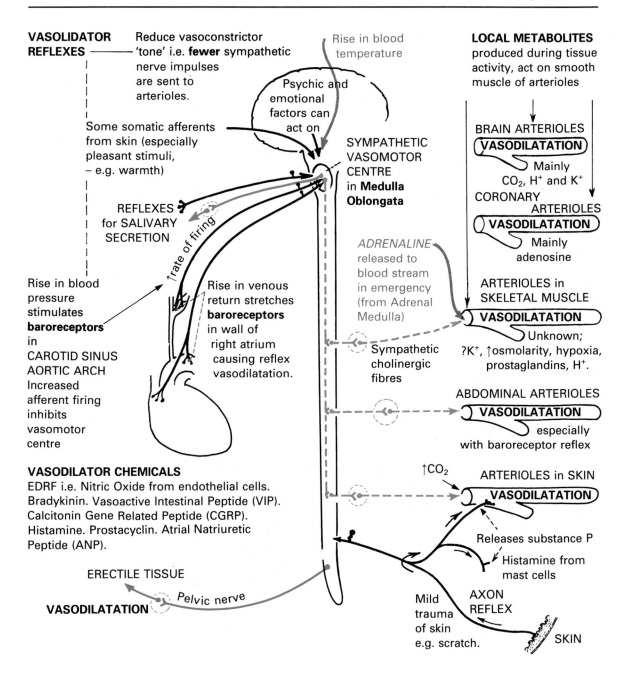

VASOLIDATOR REFLEXES ——— Reduce vasoconstrictor 'tone' i.e. **fewer** sympathetic nerve impulses are sent to arterioles.

Some somatic afferents from skin (especially pleasant stimuli, – e.g. warmth)

REFLEXES for SALIVARY SECRETION

Rise in blood pressure stimulates **baroreceptors** in CAROTID SINUS AORTIC ARCH Increased afferent firing inhibits vasomotor centre

VASODILATOR CHEMICALS
EDRF i.e. Nitric Oxide from endothelial cells. Bradykinin. Vasoactive Intestinal Peptide (VIP). Calcitonin Gene Related Peptide (CGRP). Histamine. Prostacyclin. Atrial Natriuretic Peptide (ANP).

ERECTILE TISSUE

VASODILATATION Pelvic nerve

↑rate of firing

Rise in blood temperature

Psychic and emotional factors can act on

SYMPATHETIC VASOMOTOR CENTRE in Medulla Oblongata

Rise in venous return stretches **baroreceptors** in wall of right atrium causing reflex vasodilatation.

ADRENALINE released to blood stream in emergency (from Adrenal Medulla)

Sympathetic cholinergic fibres

↑CO_2

Mild trauma of skin e.g. scratch.

LOCAL METABOLITES produced during tissue activity, act on smooth muscle of arterioles

BRAIN ARTERIOLES
VASODILATATION Mainly CO_2, H^+ and K^+

CORONARY ARTERIOLES
VASODILATATION Mainly adenosine

ARTERIOLES in SKELETAL MUSCLE
VASODILATATION Unknown; ?K^+, ↑osmolarity, hypoxia, prostaglandins, H^+.

ABDOMINAL ARTERIOLES
VASODILATATION especially with baroreceptor reflex

ARTERIOLES in SKIN
VASODILATATION

Releases substance P
Histamine from mast cells

AXON REFLEX

SKIN

Widespread **vasodilatation** decreases peripheral resistance and produces a fall in blood pressure.

CAPILLARIES

Interstitial fluid forms the immediate environment of all cells. To keep this environment and the supply of nutrients constant, there is a 'continuous movement of fluid through the arteriolar end of the semipermeable walls of capillaries into the interstitial fluid and removal of fluid into capillaries at their venular end.

Exchange of water and electrolytes is determined by forces called Starling forces i.e. sum of opposing hydrostatic and osmotic forces between CAPILLARY BLOOD and INTERSTITIAL FLUID.

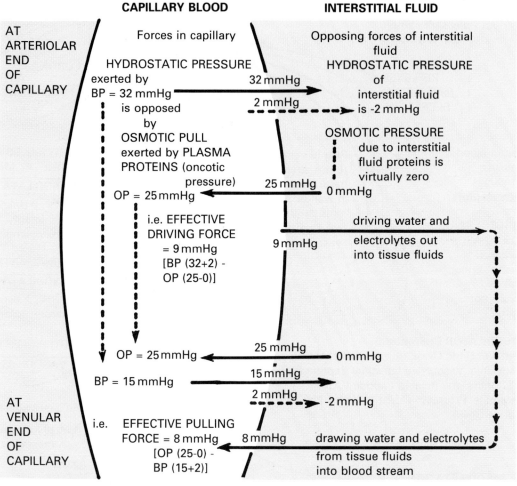

These exchanges in systemic capillaries result in a continuous turnover and renewal of **interstitial fluid**.

Electrolytes (Crystalloids, e.g. Na^+, Cl^-, etc.) in plasma and interstitial fluid also exert an **osmotic pressure** (OP) – this is huge (about 6000 mmHg). As the electrolyte concentration is the same on each side of the capillary membrane the **crystalloid OP** *does not* affect fluid movement. Protein is confined mainly to the plasma hence its OP *does* affect fluid movement.

VEINS: VENOUS RETURN

Capillaries unite to form veins which convey blood back to the heart. By the time blood reaches the veins much of the force imparted to it by the heart's contraction has been spent but some remains.

VENOUS RETURN to the heart depends on various factors: –
  GRAVITY – helps return from head when upright but opposes return from legs.
  'Vis a fronte' – the force from in front i.e. contraction of ventricle moves A-V ring down causing suction effect on blood in great veins.

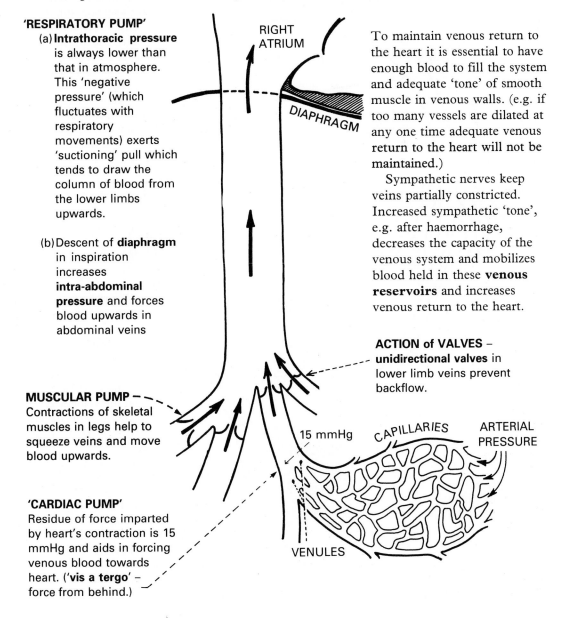

'RESPIRATORY PUMP'
  (a) **Intrathoracic pressure** is always lower than that in atmosphere. This 'negative pressure' (which fluctuates with respiratory movements) exerts 'suctioning' pull which tends to draw the column of blood from the lower limbs upwards.

  (b) Descent of **diaphragm** in inspiration increases **intra-abdominal pressure** and forces blood upwards in abdominal veins

MUSCULAR PUMP – Contractions of skeletal muscles in legs help to squeeze veins and move blood upwards.

'CARDIAC PUMP'
Residue of force imparted by heart's contraction is 15 mmHg and aids in forcing venous blood towards heart. (**'vis a tergo'** – force from behind.)

RIGHT ATRIUM

DIAPHRAGM

To maintain venous return to the heart it is essential to have enough blood to fill the system and adequate 'tone' of smooth muscle in venous walls. (e.g. if too many vessels are dilated at any one time adequate venous return to the heart will not be maintained.)

Sympathetic nerves keep veins partially constricted. Increased sympathetic 'tone', e.g. after haemorrhage, decreases the capacity of the venous system and mobilizes blood held in these **venous reservoirs** and increases venous return to the heart.

ACTION of VALVES – **unidirectional valves** in lower limb veins prevent backflow.

15 mmHg

CAPILLARIES

ARTERIAL PRESSURE

VENULES

127

BLOOD FLOW

The rate of blood flow varies in different parts of the vascular system. It is rapid in large vessels; slower in small vessels. [The larger the *total* cross-sectional area of a particular class of vessel the slower the rate of flow.]

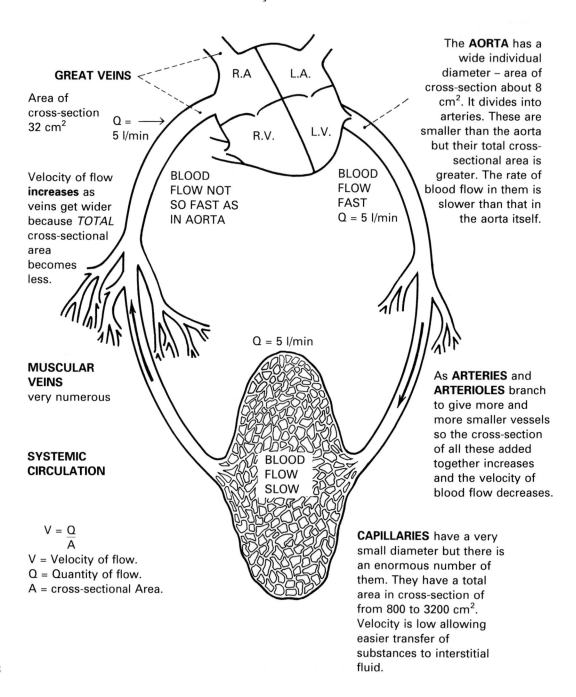

GREAT VEINS

Area of cross-section 32 cm²

$Q = 5 \text{ l/min}$

Velocity of flow **increases** as veins get wider because *TOTAL* cross-sectional area becomes less.

R.A   L.A.

R.V.   L.V.

BLOOD FLOW NOT SO FAST AS IN AORTA

BLOOD FLOW FAST $Q = 5 \text{ l/min}$

The **AORTA** has a wide individual diameter – area of cross-section about 8 cm². It divides into arteries. These are smaller than the aorta but their total cross-sectional area is greater. The rate of blood flow in them is slower than that in the aorta itself.

MUSCULAR VEINS very numerous

SYSTEMIC CIRCULATION

$Q = 5 \text{ l/min}$

BLOOD FLOW SLOW

As **ARTERIES** and **ARTERIOLES** branch to give more and more smaller vessels so the cross-section of all these added together increases and the velocity of blood flow decreases.

$$V = \frac{Q}{A}$$

V = Velocity of flow.
Q = Quantity of flow.
A = cross-sectional Area.

CAPILLARIES have a very small diameter but there is an enormous number of them. They have a total area in cross-section of from 800 to 3200 cm². Velocity is low allowing easier transfer of substances to interstitial fluid.

PULMONARY CIRCULATION 1

PULMONARY CAPILLARIES have a much lower hydrostatic pressure than systemic capillaries. Hence the osmotic 'pull' of the plasma proteins (25 mmHg), the oncotic pressure, exceeds the driving force of the BP (5–10 mmHg) along the whole length of the pulmonary capillary. This fact, along with efficient lymphatic drainage of the interstitial spaces, keeps alveoli normally free of fluid.

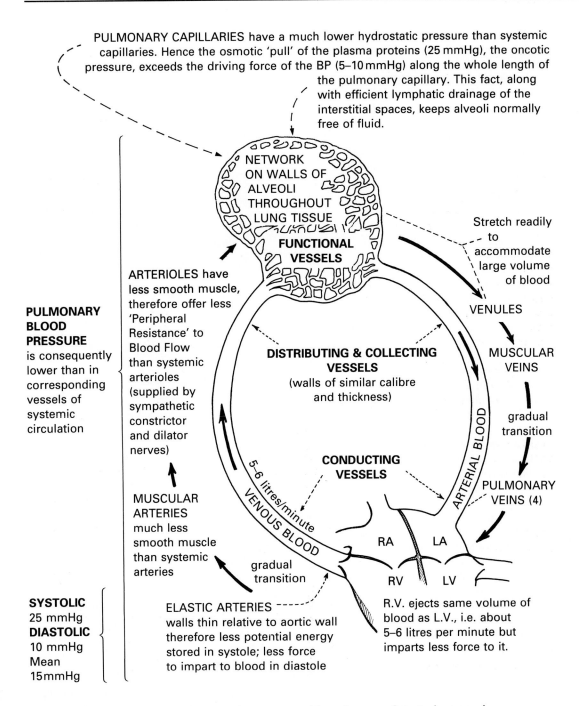

NETWORK ON WALLS OF ALVEOLI THROUGHOUT LUNG TISSUE
FUNCTIONAL VESSELS

Stretch readily to accommodate large volume of blood

VENULES

MUSCULAR VEINS

gradual transition

PULMONARY VEINS (4)

ARTERIOLES have less smooth muscle, therefore offer less 'Peripheral Resistance' to Blood Flow than systemic arterioles (supplied by sympathetic constrictor and dilator nerves)

DISTRIBUTING & COLLECTING VESSELS
(walls of similar calibre and thickness)

CONDUCTING VESSELS

ARTERIAL BLOOD

5–6 litres/minute
VENOUS BLOOD

RA LA
RV LV

PULMONARY BLOOD PRESSURE is consequently lower than in corresponding vessels of systemic circulation

MUSCULAR ARTERIES much less smooth muscle than systemic arteries

gradual transition

ELASTIC ARTERIES walls thin relative to aortic wall therefore less potential energy stored in systole; less force to impart to blood in diastole

R.V. ejects same volume of blood as L.V., i.e. about 5–6 litres per minute but imparts less force to it.

SYSTOLIC 25 mmHg
DIASTOLIC 10 mmHg
Mean 15mmHg

Increased cardiac output in **exercise** occurs with only a **moderate** increase in **pressure**. Reduced resistance occurs mainly by the opening of closed capillaries. Decreased activity in sympathetic constrictor nerves may contribute.

PULMONARY CIRCULATION 2

Gravity has an important effect on **pulmonary circulation**. When standing erect, the **apex** of the lung is about 20 cm **above** the pulmonary artery valve (PAV) and the **base** of the lung about 20 cm **below**. Since a column of **blood 13 cm** in height exerts the **same** pressure as a **10 mm** column of **mercury (Hg)** the pressure of blood at the **apex** of the lung will be about 15 mmHg **below** the pressure at the pulmonary artery valve and the pressure at the **base** about 15mmHg **above** (see scale at left of diagram).

The lungs can be divided into 3 zones, 1, 2 and 3. The systolic and diastolic pressures in the pulmonary **artery** (PA) at the middle of each zone will be about 15/0, 25/10 and 35/20 mmHg respectively, and the mean pressures in the pulmonary **veins** (PV) will be -3, 7 and 17mmHg respectively. The alveolar air pressure throughout the lung and surrounding all the capillary groups A, B and C will be about **atmospheric pressure**. Hence, in **zone 1**, some of the capillaries will be **collapsed** during diastole. In fact, the mean apical flow is about one tenth the basal flow at rest. In **zone 2** the capillaries will be **continuously open**. In **zone 3** the capillaries will be **distended**.

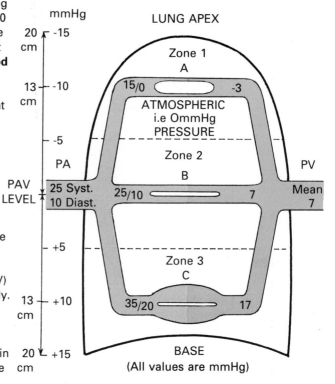

(All values are mmHg)

These effects of gravity are **abolished** when the subject **lies down** and the capacity of the pulmonary vessels then increases from about 500 ml to about 700 ml.

Expiration against a closed glottis (the **Valsalva manoeuvre) raises** intra-alveolar and intra-pleural pressures; venous return to the right heart is **reduced** and output from right and then left ventricles declines slowly. An **intra-pleural** pressure of **+20 mmHg** can be attained and, if maintained, results in fainting.

Local vasoconstriction is brought on by low O_2 or high CO_2, thus directing blood to other, **better ventilated** alveoli. Chronic hypoxia and acidosis produce pulmonary hypertension.

Endothelial cells of **pulmonary** vessels have important **functions**: they produce angiotensin converting enzyme which converts angiotensin I to the active angiotensin II. They remove bradykinin from and reduce noradrenaline and serotonin in the circulation and synthesize prostaglandins and thromboxanes.

Sympathetic nerves can cause **vasoconstriction** via α adrenergic receptors and **dilatation** via β receptors. Some vagal fibres which release VIP may be vasodilator.

DISTRIBUTION OF WATER AND ELECTROLYTES IN BODY FLUIDS

Water makes up about 60% of the adult human body, i.e. about 42 litres in a 70 kg man.

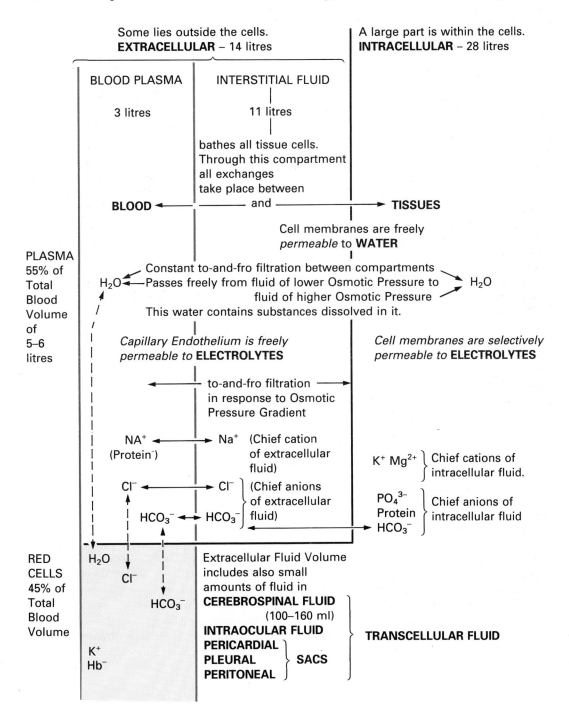

Some lies outside the cells.
EXTRACELLULAR – 14 litres

A large part is within the cells.
INTRACELLULAR – 28 litres

BLOOD PLASMA

3 litres

INTERSTITIAL FLUID

11 litres

bathes all tissue cells. Through this compartment all exchanges take place between

BLOOD ◄──────── and ────────► **TISSUES**

Cell membranes are freely *permeable* to **WATER**

PLASMA 55% of Total Blood Volume of 5–6 litres

Constant to-and-fro filtration between compartments
H_2O ◄── Passes freely from fluid of lower Osmotic Pressure to ──► H_2O
fluid of higher Osmotic Pressure
This water contains substances dissolved in it.

Capillary Endothelium is freely permeable to **ELECTROLYTES**

Cell membranes are selectively permeable to **ELECTROLYTES**

◄── to-and-fro filtration ──►
in response to Osmotic Pressure Gradient

NA^+ ◄──────► Na^+ (Chief cation
(Protein⁻)   of extracellular
                       fluid)

K^+ Mg^{2+} } Chief cations of intracellular fluid.

Cl^- ◄──────── Cl^- } (Chief anions
                         of extracellular
HCO_3^- ◄──► HCO_3^- } fluid)

PO_4^{3-}
Protein } Chief anions of intracellular fluid
HCO_3^-

RED CELLS 45% of Total Blood Volume

H_2O

Cl^-

HCO_3^-

K^+
Hb^-

Extracellular Fluid Volume includes also small amounts of fluid in
CEREBROSPINAL FLUID
(100–160 ml)
INTRAOCULAR FLUID
PERICARDIAL
PLEURAL } **SACS**
PERITONEAL

} **TRANSCELLULAR FLUID**

WATER BALANCE

In health the total amount of body water (and salt) is kept reasonably constant in spite of wide fluctuations in daily intake which is made up of ingested fluids, water in food and water of metabolism. Approximately 2,500 ml are taken in and put out per day. In the gastro-intestinal tract a lot of fluid is secreted and reabsorbed. In the kidneys a lot of fluid is filtered and reabsorbed.

A **balance** is struck between

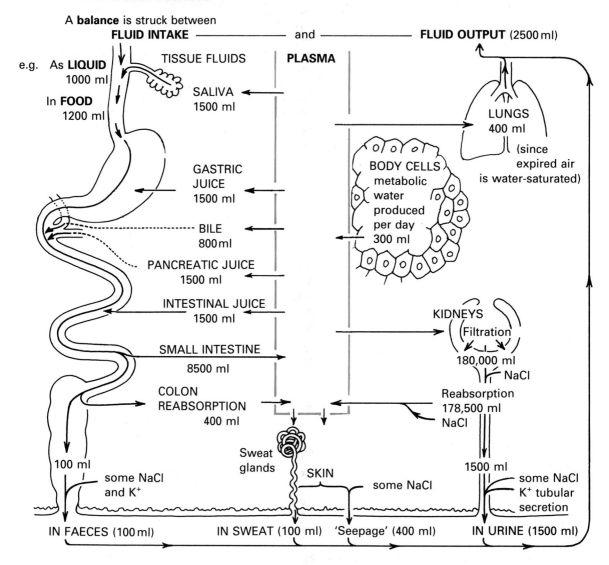

Except in growth, convalescence or pregnancy, when new tissue is being formed, an *increase* or *decrease* in **intake** leads to an appropriate *increase* or *decrease* in **output** to maintain the **balance**. Sweating is variable and can increase to over 2 litres/hour.

BLOOD

Blood is the specialized fluid tissue of the transport system. (Specific Gravity, 1.05–1.06; pH, 7.35–7.45; average amount, 5.6 litres, about 8% or 50–80 ml/kg of body weight.)

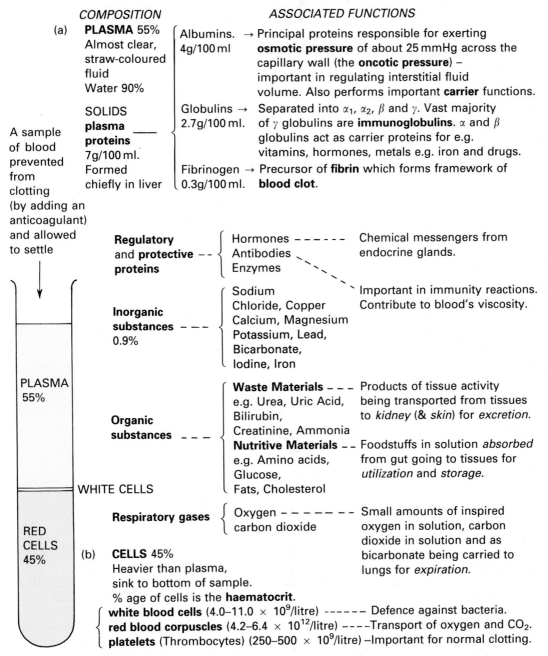

COMPOSITION

ASSOCIATED FUNCTIONS

(a) **PLASMA** 55%
Almost clear,
straw-coloured
fluid
Water 90%

Albumins.
4g/100 ml

→ Principal proteins responsible for exerting
osmotic pressure of about 25 mmHg across the
capillary wall (the **oncotic pressure**) –
important in regulating interstitial fluid
volume. Also performs important **carrier** functions.

SOLIDS
plasma
proteins
7g/100 ml.
Formed
chiefly in liver

A sample
of blood
prevented
from
clotting
(by adding an
anticoagulant)
and allowed
to settle

Globulins →
2.7g/100 ml.

Separated into α_1, α_2, β and γ. Vast majority
of γ globulins are **immunoglobulins**. α and β
globulins act as carrier proteins for e.g.
vitamins, hormones, metals e.g. iron and drugs.

Fibrinogen →
0.3g/100 ml.

Precursor of **fibrin** which forms framework of
blood clot.

Regulatory
and **protective**
proteins

Hormones ------
Antibodies
Enzymes

Chemical messengers from
endocrine glands.

Important in immunity reactions.
Contribute to blood's viscosity.

Inorganic
substances
0.9%

Sodium
Chloride, Copper
Calcium, Magnesium
Potassium, Lead,
Bicarbonate,
Iodine, Iron

PLASMA
55%

Organic
substances

Waste Materials – –
e.g. Urea, Uric Acid,
Bilirubin,
Creatinine, Ammonia

Products of tissue activity
being transported from tissues
to *kidney* (& *skin*) for *excretion.*

Nutritive Materials – –
e.g. Amino acids,
Glucose,
Fats, Cholesterol

Foodstuffs in solution *absorbed*
from gut going to tissues for
utilization and *storage.*

WHITE CELLS

Respiratory gases

Oxygen – – – – – –
carbon dioxide

Small amounts of inspired
oxygen in solution, carbon
dioxide in solution and as
bicarbonate being carried to
lungs for *expiration.*

RED
CELLS
45%

(b) **CELLS** 45%
Heavier than plasma,
sink to bottom of sample.
% age of cells is the **haematocrit.**

white blood cells ($4.0–11.0 \times 10^9$/litre) ------ Defence against bacteria.
red blood corpuscles ($4.2–6.4 \times 10^{12}$/litre) ----Transport of oxygen and CO_2.
platelets (Thrombocytes) ($250–500 \times 10^9$/litre) –Important for normal clotting.

If blood is allowed to clot and the clot removed, the remaining fluid is SERUM. It is like plasma without fibrinogen and clotting factors.

HAEMOSTASIS AND BLOOD COAGULATION

When blood vessels are ruptured, **3 mechanisms** arrest bleeding (haemostasis):
1. **Constriction of blood vessels** – spasm of smooth muscle in their walls.
2. **Platelets plug** the **gap**; adhere to exposed collagen; release growth factors to increase endothelial, smooth muscle and fibroblast cells and release serotonin and thromboxane A2 to constrict blood vessels.
3. **Blood coagulation** (clotting) involving enzymes and chemicals called clotting factors (f) which ultimately result in THROMBIN catalysing the formation of FIBRIN.

BLOOD COAGULATION is initiated when plasma contacts **damaged endothelium** of blood vessels.

(The Roman numerals are clotting factors. **Activation** is indicated by **'a'**.)

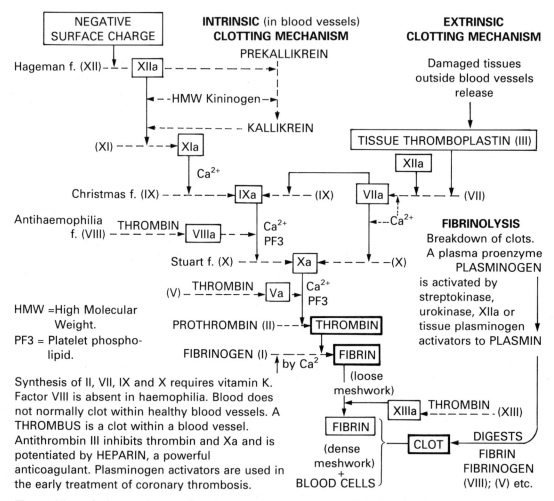

HMW = High Molecular Weight.
PF3 = Platelet phospholipid.

Synthesis of II, VII, IX and X requires vitamin K. Factor VIII is absent in haemophilia. Blood does not normally clot within healthy blood vessels. A THROMBUS is a clot within a blood vessel. Antithrombin III inhibits thrombin and Xa and is potentiated by HEPARIN, a powerful anticoagulant. Plasminogen activators are used in the early treatment of coronary thrombosis.

To avoid confusion an international agreement was responsible for the Roman numerals given to the clotting factors but since some original names are still used they have been included.

FACTORS REQUIRED FOR NORMAL HAEMATOPOIESIS

Haematopoiesis, also called Haemopoiesis – formation of normal blood cells.
Erythropoiesis – formation of red blood cells (RBC).

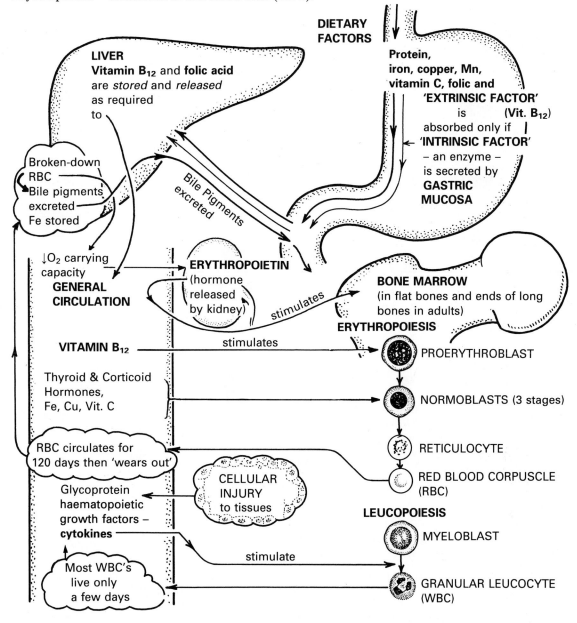

In health the number of RBC and the amount of Hb in them remain fairly constant.
Destruction of old cells is balanced by formation of new. Anoxia stimulates production of erythropoietin. Colony stimulating factors (CSF) and interleukins are cytokines and stimulate haematopoiesis.

135

HAEMATOPOIESIS

In the adult the formed elements of the blood stream develop from primitive **reticular cells**, chiefly in **red bone marrow** of flat bones, ribs, sternum, pelvis, vertebrae, skull and also upper humerus and femur.

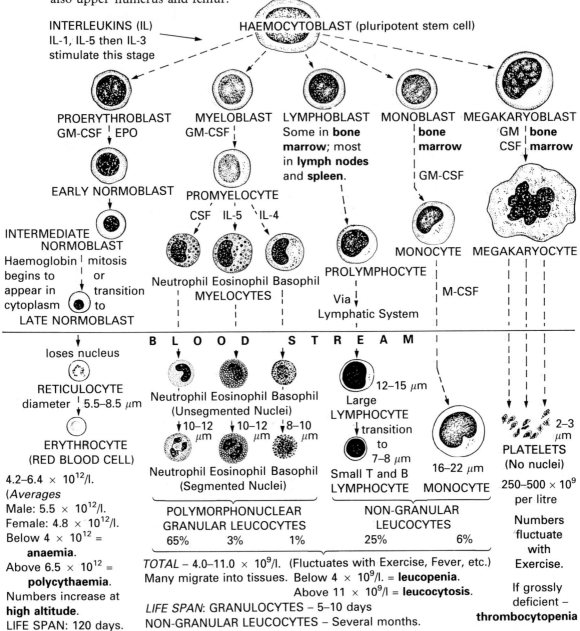

Basophils release histamine and heparin. **Eosinophils** attack parasites. **Neutrophils** kill bacteria. **Monocytes** migrate into tissues and become **tissue macrophages**. CSF = colony stimulating factor; G = granulocyte; M = macrophage; EPO = erythropoietin.

BLOOD GROUPS

There are present in the **plasma** of some individuals, substances which can cause the **agglutination** (clumping together) and subsequent **haemolysis** (breakdown) of the **red blood cells** of some other individuals.

If such reactions follow **blood transfusion** the two bloods are said to be **incompatible**.

Human red cell membranes contain a variety of blood group **antigens** which are also called **agglutinogens**. A and B antigens are the most important although there are many more.

Two **factors** *are involved in an* **agglutination** *reaction*: –
An **agglutinogen** present in **donor's** Red Blood Cell e.g. A or B
A specific **agglutinin** present in **recipient's** Plasma e.g. α or β

Obviously no such combination occurs naturally otherwise auto-agglutination would result.

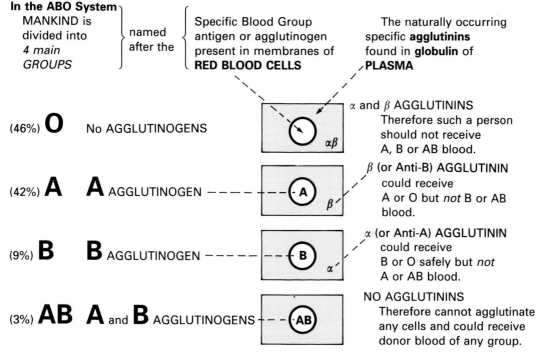

In the ABO System
MANKIND is divided into *4 main* GROUPS } *named after the* { Specific Blood Group antigen or agglutinogen present in membranes of **RED BLOOD CELLS**

The naturally occurring specific **agglutinins** found in **globulin** of **PLASMA**

(46%) **O**   No AGGLUTINOGENS

α and β AGGLUTININS
Therefore such a person should not receive A, B or AB blood.

(42%) **A**   **A** AGGLUTINOGEN

β (or Anti-B) AGGLUTININ could receive A or O but *not* B or AB blood.

(9%) **B**   **B** AGGLUTINOGEN

α (or Anti-A) AGGLUTININ could receive B or O safely but *not* A or AB blood.

(3%) **AB**   **A** and **B** AGGLUTINOGENS

NO AGGLUTININS
Therefore cannot agglutinate any cells and could receive donor blood of any group.

In practice it is important that the **donor's cells** should not be agglutinated by the **recipient's plasma**. Agglutination of recipient's cells by donor agglutinins is less likely to occur since the plasma in the transfusion is so diluted in the recipient that it rarely causes agglutination.

Some individuals with A agglutinogen have an additional agglutinogen called A_1. Thus the A group is subdivided into types A_1 (those with both agglutinogens: 80%) and A_2 (those with only the A agglutinogen: 20%). Therefore there are really 6 ABO groups: O, A_1, A_2, B, A_1B and A_2B.

A and B antigens are present also in other tissues e.g. salivary glands, liver, kidney, semen, amniotic fluid, testes, lungs and pancreas.

137

BLOOD GROUPS

To determine the blood group to which an individual belongs **two test sera** only are required and the **red blood cells** to be grouped.

DROP of GROUP **A** SERUM & GROUP **B** SERUM
(on   [N.B. These droplets are of **plasma**
glass   – **NOT** red blood cells.
slide)   i.e. only **agglutinins** are present.]

To each test serum a saline suspension of **red blood cells** is added, i.e. only **agglutinogens** are added.

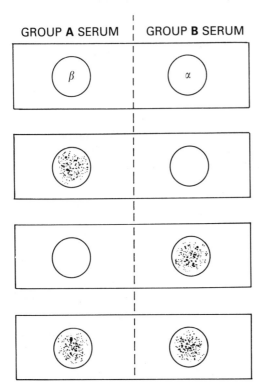

GROUP **A** SERUM   GROUP **B** SERUM

GROUP O blood cells give **no** agglutination since **no** agglutinogens are present in these cells to be clumped by test sera agglutinins.

GROUP B blood cells (B agglutinogen present) give agglutination with (GROUP A serum – since the specific Anti-B (β) agglutinin is present in the first test serum.

GROUP A blood cells give agglutination with GROUP B serum – since the specific Anti-A (α) agglutinin is present in this serum.

GROUP AB blood cells give agglutination with both test sera.

As well as determining blood group in this way, the blood of donor is always matched directly with blood of patient to avoid sub-group incompatibility.

Agglutination is usually visible under the microscope within a few minutes. The clumped cells look like grains of cayenne pepper in a clear liquid. If no agglutination occurs the fluid remains uniformly pink.

If the wrong blood is given to a patient, clumps of red blood cells may block small blood vessels in vital organs, e.g. lung or brain. The subsequent haemolysis (breakdown) of agglutinated cells may lead to severe jaundice, damage to the renal tubules, anuria and death.

1 to 1.5 litres of one's own blood can be removed over a 3 week period prior to surgery. This avoids the risk of transfusion reactions and the transmission of AIDS.

RHESUS FACTOR

In addition to the antigens of the **ABO** blood group system there **are innumerable** other agglutinogens in red cells. Those of the **Rhesus (Rh) system** are clinically important. The 'Rh factor' actually contains the C, D, E and many more antigens. By far the most important is the D agglutinogen.

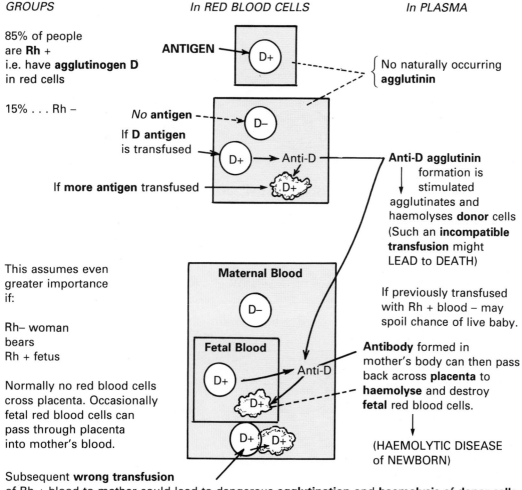

GROUPS   *In RED BLOOD CELLS*   *In PLASMA*

85% of people
are **Rh +**
i.e. have **agglutinogen D**
in red cells

ANTIGEN → D+

No naturally occurring **agglutinin**

15% . . . Rh –

No antigen ⟶ D–

If **D antigen** is transfused ⟶ D+ → Anti-D

If **more antigen** transfused ⟶ D+

Anti-D agglutinin formation is stimulated agglutinates and haemolyses **donor** cells (Such an **incompatible transfusion** might LEAD to DEATH)

This assumes even greater importance if:

Rh– woman bears Rh + fetus

Normally no red blood cells cross placenta. Occasionally fetal red blood cells can pass through placenta into mother's blood.

Maternal Blood

D–

Fetal Blood

D+ → Anti-D

D+

D+ D+

If previously transfused with Rh + blood – may spoil chance of live baby.

Antibody formed in mother's body can then pass back across **placenta** to **haemolyse** and destroy **fetal** red blood cells.

↓

(HAEMOLYTIC DISEASE of NEWBORN)

Subsequent **wrong transfusion** of Rh + blood to mother could lead to dangerous **agglutination** and **haemolysis** of **donor cells** within mother's own body.

An **Rh-ve** mother carrying an **Rh + ve** fetus is given a single dose of **anti-D** antibodies during her pregnancy and immediately after delivery of the child. This passive immunization prevents the mother forming her own anti-D antibodies and has considerably reduced the incidence of haemolytic disease.

INHERITANCE OF RHESUS FACTOR

The Rh BLOOD GROUP FACTOR is inherited on Mendelian principles, the presence of Rh factor being dominant.

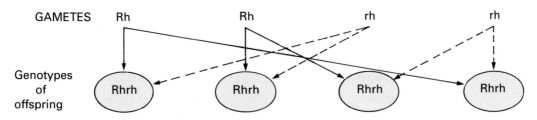

All children will be heterozygous-Rhrh; since all carry the FACTOR they are Rh Positive; i.e during pregnancy the rh negative woman will have an Rh Positive fetus.

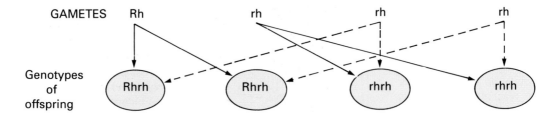

Some children will be heterozygous Rhrh Positive, like the father; others homozygous rhrh negative like the mother.

LYMPHATIC SYSTEM

ALL CELLS
are bathed by TISSUE FLUID.
This diffuses from CAPILLARIES.
Some returns to CAPILLARIES.
Some drains into blind-ended,
thin-walled LYMPHATICS.
It is then known as **lymph** (similar to
plasma but less protein).

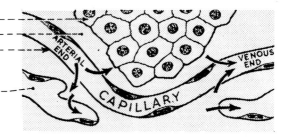

A network of **lymphatic vessels** drains about 3 litres of lymph per day from tissue spaces throughout the body (except in central nervous system). They unite to form larger and larger vessels → **right lymphatic duct** and **thoracic (left lymphatic) duct** → **innominate veins** (i.e. lymph is returned to the blood stream here). In the course of larger vessels, lymph is filtered through **lymph nodes**.

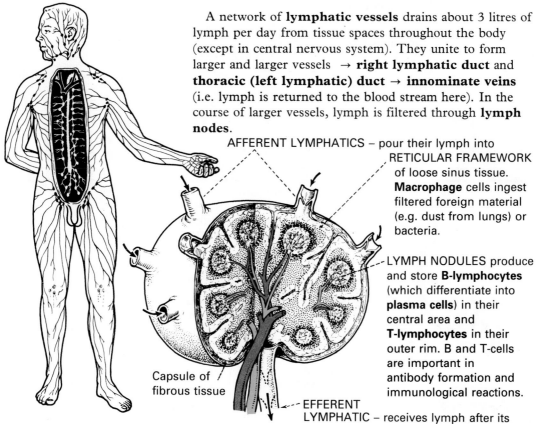

AFFERENT LYMPHATICS – pour their lymph into RETICULAR FRAMEWORK of loose sinus tissue. **Macrophage** cells ingest filtered foreign material (e.g. dust from lungs) or bacteria.

LYMPH NODULES produce and store **B-lymphocytes** (which differentiate into **plasma cells**) in their central area and **T-lymphocytes** in their outer rim. B and T-cells are important in antibody formation and immunological reactions.

Capsule of fibrous tissue

EFFERENT LYMPHATIC – receives lymph after its slow passage through node

Movement of **lymph** towards **heart** depends partly on compression of lymphatic vessels by muscles of limbs and partly on 'suction' created by movements of respiration. Valves within the vessels prevent backflow. The lymphoid tissue of the body which includes lymph nodes, spleen, thymus, tonsils, etc., forms an important part of the body's defence against invading agents such as **protozoa, bacteria, viruses**, or other poisonous **toxins**. These act as **antigens** stimulating **antibody formation** – which can subsequently destroy or neutralize the antigen.

SPLEEN

The spleen is a vascular organ, weighing about 200 grams. It is situated in the left side of the abdomen behind the stomach and above the kidney.

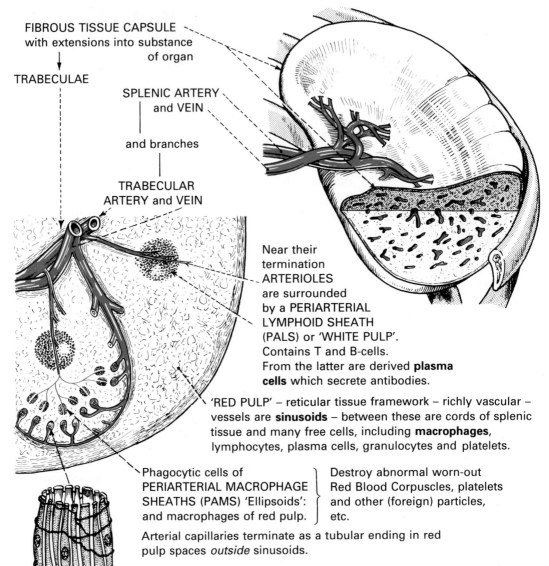

FIBROUS TISSUE CAPSULE with extensions into substance of organ

↓

TRABECULAE

SPLENIC ARTERY and **VEIN**

and branches

TRABECULAR ARTERY and VEIN

Near their termination ARTERIOLES are surrounded by a PERIARTERIAL LYMPHOID SHEATH (PALS) or 'WHITE PULP'. Contains T and B-cells. From the latter are derived **plasma cells** which secrete antibodies.

'RED PULP' – reticular tissue framework – richly vascular – vessels are **sinusoids** – between these are cords of splenic tissue and many free cells, including **macrophages**, lymphocytes, plasma cells, granulocytes and platelets.

Phagocytic cells of PERIARTERIAL MACROPHAGE SHEATHS (PAMS) 'Ellipsoids': and macrophages of red pulp.

} Destroy abnormal worn-out Red Blood Corpuscles, platelets and other (foreign) particles, etc.

Arterial capillaries terminate as a tubular ending in red pulp spaces *outside* sinusoids.

SINUSOID

Blood is filtered in red pulp. Normal, flexible red cells squeeze their way back into sinusoids which lead to the splenic venous system. Less flexible abnormal RBCs are removed. During fetal life the spleen forms red and white blood cells. After splenectomy (removal of spleen) the process of removal of worn-out cells is taken over by liver and bone marrow. Splenectomy increases risk of bacterial infection as antibody production is reduced also. Malaria has an increased mortality rate as RBCs containing the parasite are not removed.

THYMUS

The thymus is an irregularly-shaped organ lying behind the breast bone. It is relatively large in the child and reaches its maximum size at puberty. It closely resembles a lymph node.

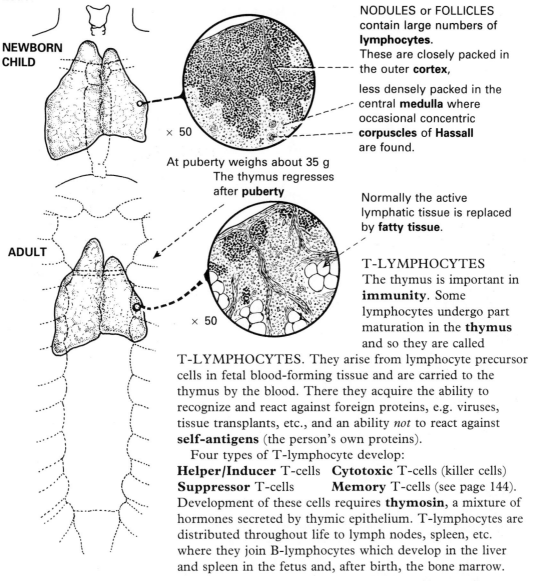

NEWBORN CHILD

× 50

At puberty weighs about 35 g
The thymus regresses
after **puberty**

ADULT

× 50

NODULES or FOLLICLES contain large numbers of **lymphocytes**.
These are closely packed in the outer **cortex**,

less densely packed in the central **medulla** where occasional concentric **corpuscles** of **Hassall** are found.

Normally the active lymphatic tissue is replaced by **fatty tissue**.

T-LYMPHOCYTES
The thymus is important in **immunity**. Some lymphocytes undergo part maturation in the **thymus** and so they are called T-LYMPHOCYTES. They arise from lymphocyte precursor cells in fetal blood-forming tissue and are carried to the thymus by the blood. There they acquire the ability to recognize and react against foreign proteins, e.g. viruses, tissue transplants, etc., and an ability *not* to react against **self-antigens** (the person's own proteins).

Four types of T-lymphocyte develop:
Helper/Inducer T-cells   **Cytotoxic** T-cells (killer cells)
Suppressor T-cells   **Memory** T-cells (see page 144).
Development of these cells requires **thymosin**, a mixture of hormones secreted by thymic epithelium. T-lymphocytes are distributed throughout life to lymph nodes, spleen, etc. where they join B-lymphocytes which develop in the liver and spleen in the fetus and, after birth, the bone marrow.

Acquired immune deficiency syndrome (AIDS) is a disease caused by destruction of **helper T**-cells (T_4) by the virus **HTLV-III** or **HIV** (human immunodeficiency virus). Antibody formation is thus destroyed and the patient becomes vulnerable to infection and cancer.

IMMUNE SYSTEM (NATURAL IMMUNITY)

The body is protected from invading microorganisms by the **immune system**, which can be divided into two categories – NATURAL immunity and ACQUIRED immunity. **Natural** immunity provides the basic means for the destruction of organisms. **Acquired** immunity improves and enhances the **efficiency** of the natural mechanisms and remembers the infection the next time it is encountered. **Antigens** (foreign agents) induce **specific** immune responses.

NATURAL DEFENCES

Skin
Its horny layer provides a physical barrier.

Competition for nutrients
Growth of disease – causing organisms is inhibited by the growth of **non-pathogenic** bacteria in the gastro-intestinal and urogenital tracts which successfully compete with them for nutrients.
Urine washes organisms from the urethra.

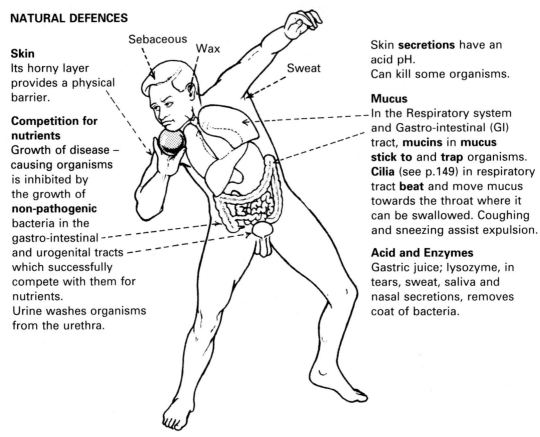

Sebaceous   Wax   Sweat

Skin **secretions** have an acid pH.
Can kill some organisms.

Mucus
In the Respiratory system and Gastro-intestinal (GI) tract, **mucins** in **mucus stick to** and **trap** organisms. **Cilia** (see p.149) in respiratory tract **beat** and move mucus towards the throat where it can be swallowed. Coughing and sneezing assist expulsion.

Acid and Enzymes
Gastric juice; lysozyme, in tears, sweat, saliva and nasal secretions, removes coat of bacteria.

If invasion of tissues occurs:

Interferons protect host from viral infection and stimulate Natural killer (NK) cells.

Complement system – plasma proteins which enhance phagocytosis – makes holes in membrane of organisms and activates inflammation.

Natural killer (NK) cells – large granular lymphocytes – kill virus infected cells and some types of cancer cells.

Phagocytosis: Neutrophil leucocytes migrate into the tissues and they, along with monocytes of the blood which become **macrophages** of the tissues (the tissue or monocyte-macrophage system - formerly the reticuloendothelial system), **engulf** and **eat** foreign particulate matter in the same way that amoebae eat food particles (see p.7).

Inflammation, a response to damaged tissue characterised by redness, pain, heat and swelling, 'walls off' the injured site, destroys organisms and repairs tissues.

IMMUNE SYSTEM 2 (ACQUIRED IMMUNITY)

The **immune system** recognizes, remembers and produces **antibodies** against many millions of **antigens** (foreign agents) that invade the body. There are two types of immune response: (a) **humoral** – protection is by **antibodies** – major defence against bacteria, and (b) **cell mediated** – protection is by **T-lymphocytes** which react directly with foreign cells, e.g. tissue transplants, cells infected by organisms and cancer cells.

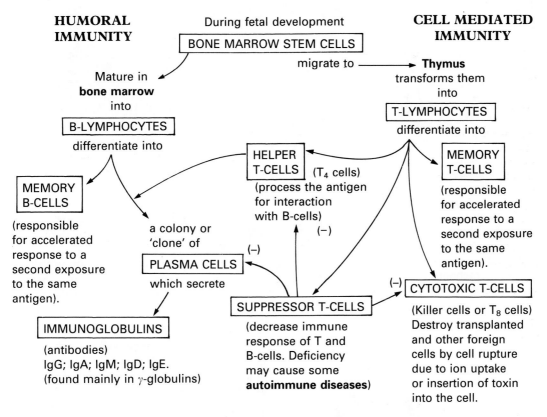

The **complement system**: A system of plasma enzymes identified by the numbers C1-C9. They complement or enhance immune, allergic and inflammatory reactions. They cause release of histamine which increases permeability of capillaries. They attract phagocytes to the site of injury. Bacteria are opsonized (made ready for eating). They punch holes in the membrane of microorganisms causing them to rupture.

   Interleukins: Hormone substances produced by lymphocytes. **Interleukin-1** (IL-1) affects hypothalamus and produces fever. **Interleukin-2** (IL-2) stimulates clones of activated T and B-cells. Secreted by helper T-cells. **Interleukin-4** (IL-4) is also secreted by helper T-cells. Causes plasma cells to secrete IgE. **Interleukin-5** (IL-5) causes plasma cells to secrete IgA.

   Interferons: α and β – produced by virus infected cells. Inhibit viral replication in unaffected cells; stimulate T-cell growth; activate NK cells. γ – secreted by helper, cytotoxic T-cells and NK cells – strongly stimulates phagocytosis. Activates NK cells. Enhances immune responses.

CEREBROSPINAL FLUID

Cerebrospinal fluid (CSF) is like blood plasma but has very little protein, less K^+, glucose and $HCO3^-$, but more Na^+, Cl^- and Mg^2. These differences indicate that active secretion is involved in its formation.
VOLUME: 150 ml, in man. *SPECIFIC GRAVITY*: 1.005–1.008.

FORMATION

Capillary plexus

Secretory epithelium

BRAIN is covered by 4 membranes

DURA MATER
{ Periosteal layer
{ Meningeal layer
ARACHNOID MATER
PIA MATER

ARACHNOID VILLI project into VENOUS SINUSES containing blood

CSF from lateral ventricles via foramen of Munro

×100

CHOROID PLEXUSES in ventricles secrete CSF continuously (500 ml/day).

The **subarachnoid space** contains CSF (which links with CSF in ventricles of the brain), blood vessels, nerve roots and fine fibrous strands – **arachnoid trabeculae** – which support the brain.

III ventricle

Aqueduct of Sylvius

IV ventricle

Medial foramen of Magendie, two lateral foramena of Luschka

CIRCULATION
CSF formed in lateral ventricles joins that from IIIrd & IVth ventricles to circulate over surface of brain and spinal cord in subarachnoid space.

REABSORPTION through vascular tufts – **arachnoid villi** – into blood stream. [Effective forces:- **hydrostatic pressure** of CSF – 120 mm H_2O – is greater than venous pressure in sinuses: it is aided by osmotic pull of plasma proteins within plasma in returning CSF to blood stream.]

SPINAL CORD

DURA MATER
ARACHNOID MATER
PIA MATER

FUNCTIONS OF CSF
1. Forms a protective water jacket which cushions the brain.
2. Alteration of volume can compensate for fluctuations in amount of blood within skull and thus keep total volume of cranial contents constant.
3. Low K^+ concentration allows neurons to generate very high electrical potentials.
   Endothelial cells of brain capillaries and choroid epithelial cells have tight junctions which prevent e.g. some drugs and transmitters passing from blood to brain interstitial fluid and CSF. They cannot cross this **blood-brain barrier**.

RESPIRATORY SYSTEM

RESPIRATORY SYSTEM

All living cells require to get **oxygen** from the fluid around them and to get rid of **carbon dioxide** to it.

Internal respiration is the exchange of these gases between tissue cells and their fluid environment.

External respiration is the exchange of these gases (oxygen and carbon dioxide) between the body and the external environment.

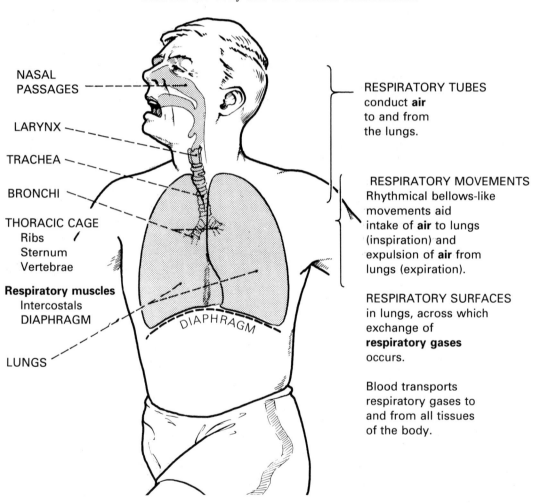

NASAL PASSAGES

LARYNX

TRACHEA

BRONCHI

THORACIC CAGE
Ribs
Sternum
Vertebrae

Respiratory muscles
Intercostals
DIAPHRAGM

LUNGS

DIAPHRAGM

RESPIRATORY TUBES
conduct **air**
to and from
the lungs.

RESPIRATORY MOVEMENTS
Rhythmical bellows-like
movements aid
intake of **air** to lungs
(inspiration) and
expulsion of **air** from
lungs (expiration).

RESPIRATORY SURFACES
in lungs, across which
exchange of
respiratory gases
occurs.

Blood transports
respiratory gases to
and from all tissues
of the body.

AIR CONDUCTING PASSAGES

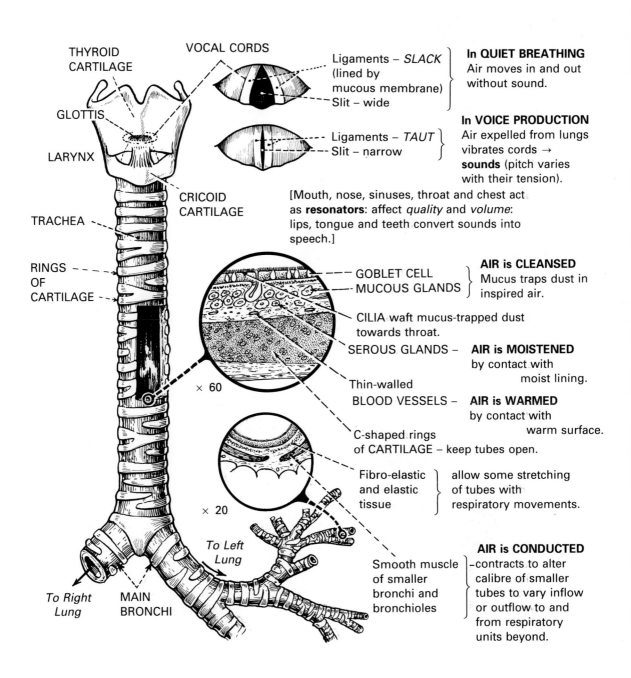

THYROID CARTILAGE

VOCAL CORDS

GLOTTIS

LARYNX

CRICOID CARTILAGE

TRACHEA

RINGS OF CARTILAGE

Ligaments – *SLACK* (lined by mucous membrane)

Slit – wide

In QUIET BREATHING Air moves in and out without sound.

Ligaments – *TAUT*

Slit – narrow

In VOICE PRODUCTION Air expelled from lungs vibrates cords → **sounds** (pitch varies with their tension).

[Mouth, nose, sinuses, throat and chest act as **resonators**: affect *quality* and *volume*: lips, tongue and teeth convert sounds into speech.]

GOBLET CELL

MUCOUS GLANDS

AIR is CLEANSED Mucus traps dust in inspired air.

CILIA waft mucus-trapped dust towards throat.

SEROUS GLANDS –

× 60

AIR is MOISTENED by contact with moist lining.

Thin-walled BLOOD VESSELS –

AIR is WARMED by contact with warm surface.

C-shaped rings of CARTILAGE – keep tubes open.

Fibro-elastic and elastic tissue

allow some stretching of tubes with respiratory movements.

× 20

To Left Lung

Smooth muscle of smaller bronchi and bronchioles

AIR is CONDUCTED –contracts to alter calibre of smaller tubes to vary inflow or outflow to and from respiratory units beyond.

To Right Lung

MAIN BRONCHI

LUNGS: RESPIRATORY SURFACES

The trachea and the bronchial 'tree' conduct air down to the **respiratory surfaces**. There is no exchange of gases in these tubes.

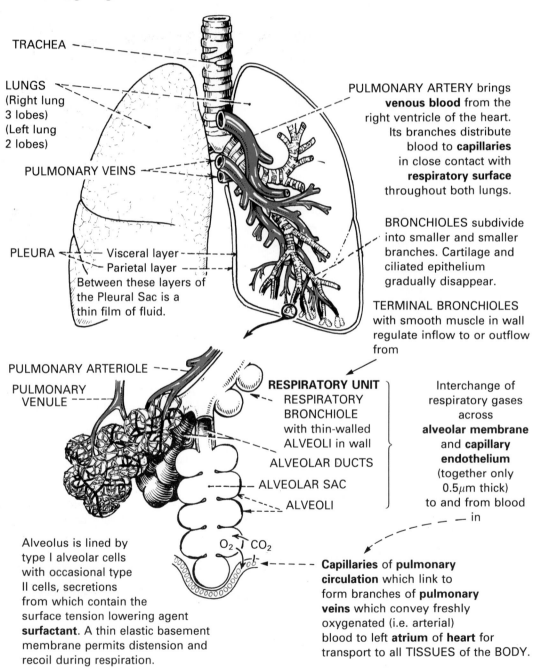

TRACHEA

LUNGS
(Right lung
3 lobes)
(Left lung
2 lobes)

PULMONARY VEINS

PLEURA — Visceral layer
— Parietal layer
Between these layers of
the Pleural Sac is a
thin film of fluid.

PULMONARY ARTERIOLE

PULMONARY VENULE

Alveolus is lined by
type I alveolar cells
with occasional type
II cells, secretions
from which contain the
surface tension lowering agent
surfactant. A thin elastic basement
membrane permits distension and
recoil during respiration.

O_2 CO_2

PULMONARY ARTERY brings venous blood from the right ventricle of the heart. Its branches distribute blood to **capillaries** in close contact with **respiratory surface** throughout both lungs.

BRONCHIOLES subdivide into smaller and smaller branches. Cartilage and ciliated epithelium gradually disappear.

TERMINAL BRONCHIOLES with smooth muscle in wall regulate inflow to or outflow from

RESPIRATORY UNIT
RESPIRATORY
BRONCHIOLE
with thin-walled
ALVEOLI in wall

ALVEOLAR DUCTS

ALVEOLAR SAC

ALVEOLI

Interchange of respiratory gases across **alveolar membrane** and **capillary endothelium** (together only $0.5\mu m$ thick) to and from blood in

Capillaries of **pulmonary circulation** which link to form branches of **pulmonary veins** which convey freshly oxygenated (i.e. arterial) blood to left **atrium** of **heart** for transport to all TISSUES of the BODY.

THORAX

The thorax (or chest) is the closed cavity which contains the **lungs, heart** and great vessels.

It is enclosed and bounded:
ABOVE by the upper RIBS and tissues of the neck;
AT THE SIDES by the RIBS and INTERCOSTAL MUSCLES;
AT THE BACK by the RIBS and VERTEBRAL COLUMN (or back bone);
IN FRONT by the RIBS, COSTAL CARTILAGES and STERNUM (or breast bone);
BELOW by the DIAPHRAGM (a strong dome-shaped sheet of skeletal muscle with a central tendon which separates the thoracic cavity from the abdominal cavity.

Lung

Pleura: parietal, visceral layers

Crura

Vertebral column

The thorax is lined by two thin layers of membrane – the PLEURA – the inner (visceral) layer of which covers the LUNGS. The outer (parietal) layer covers the inner wall of the thorax. In health there is a thin film of fluid between these two pleural layers which causes adhesion but allows them to slip (like two glass sheets with fluid between). Elastic recoil of lungs *tends* to pull visceral layer away from parietal layer. This creates sub-atmospheric or negative intrapleural pressure (about -2 mmHg). In **quiet inspiration**, the chest wall is *tending* to pull away from lungs and the intra-pleural pressure becomes about -6 mmHg. With **forced inspiration**, it can become -30 mmHg.

NB: A negative pressure is a pressure *below* atmospheric pressure (approx. 760 mmHg). A positive pressure is *above* atmospheric pressure.

Capacity of thoracic cage and the **pressure** between pleural surfaces change rhythmically about 12–14 times a minute with the **movements** of **respiration** – air movement in and out of the lungs follows the dimension changes.

MECHANISM OF BREATHING

The rhythmical changes in the capacity of the thorax are brought about by the action of skeletal muscles. The changes in lung volume, with intake or expulsion of air, follow.

In NORMAL QUIET BREATHING

INSPIRATION

external intercostal muscles actively contract
– ribs and sternum move
  upwards and outwards
  because first rib is fixed
– width of chest increases
  from side to side and depth
  from front to back increases.

diaphragm contracts
– descends
– length of chest increases.
capacity of **thorax** is
  increased
↓
pressure between **pleural surfaces** (already negative) becomes more negative: from -2 to -6 mmHg (i.e. an increased 'suction pull' is exerted on **lung tissue**)
↓
elastic tissue of lungs is *stretched*
↓
lungs *expand* to fill **thoracic cavity**
↓
air pressure in alveoli is now -1.5 mmHg, i.e. *less* than atmospheric pressure
↓
air is sucked into **alveoli** from atmosphere because of pressure difference.

EXPIRATION

external intercostal muscles relax
– ribs and sternum move
downwards and inwards
– width and depth of
chest diminishes.
diaphragm relaxes –
ascends – length of chest
diminishes.
capacity of **thorax** is
decreased
↓
pressure between **pleural** surfaces becomes less negative: from -6 to -2 mmHg (i.e. less pull is exerted on **lung tissue**)
↓
elastic tissue of lungs
recoils
↓
air pressure in alveoli is now + 1.5 mmHg.
i.e. *greater* than atmospheric pressure
↓
air is forced out of **alveoli** to atmosphere

In FORCED BREATHING

Muscles of nostrils and round glottis may contract to aid entrance of air to lungs.
Extensors of vertebral column may aid inspiration.
Muscles of neck contract – move 1st rib upwards (and sternum upwards and forwards).

Internal intercostal may contract – move ribs downwards more actively.
Abdominal muscles contract – actively aid ascent of diaphragm.

ARTIFICIAL RESPIRATION

If breathing has ceased in cases of drowning, electrocution, gas poisoning, etc., a life may be saved if artificial respiration is applied promptly. Respiration always ceases before the heart stops beating.

Mouth-to-mouth breathing is superior to all other methods.

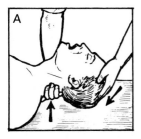

Applicator clears patient's mouth and throat of obstruction, then lays him on his back and positions himself at the side of the patient. He places one hand under his neck and the other on his forehead.

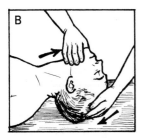

Applicator tilts the patient's head right back, raising his chin up. This causes the tongue to lift away from the back of the patient's throat and opens up airway.

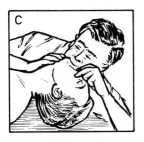

The applicator pinches shut the patient's nostrils, seals his lips round the patient's mouth and 12–14 times per minute blows in air until about twice the normal chest movement is observed.

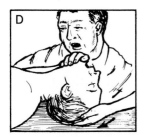

When he removes his mouth the patient breathes out passively. The applicator takes another breath. There is enough residual oxygen in the applicator's own expired air for the patient's needs.

VOLUMES AND CAPACITIES OF LUNGS

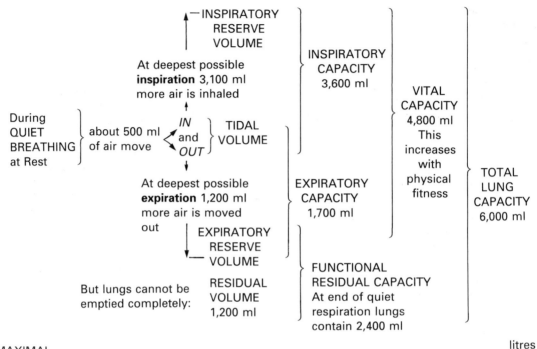

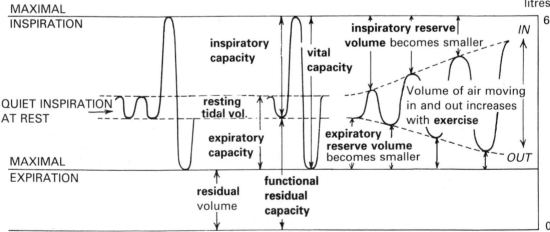

(after Pappenheimer, J.R., et al (1950) Fed. Proc., **9**,602). *Not to scale*

Values for volumes and capacities are typical values but will vary with the subject's size and weight. Values are usually about 25% less in women.

At rest a normal male adult breathes in and out about 12 times per minute. The amount of air breathed in per minute is therefore 500 ml × 12 i.e. 6000 ml or 6 litres – this is the **respiratory minute volume** or **pulmonary ventilation**. In exercise it may go up to as much as 200 litres.

In deep breathing the volume of **atmospheric air inspired** with each inspiration and the amount which reaches the **alveoli** increase.

COMPOSITION OF RESPIRED AIR

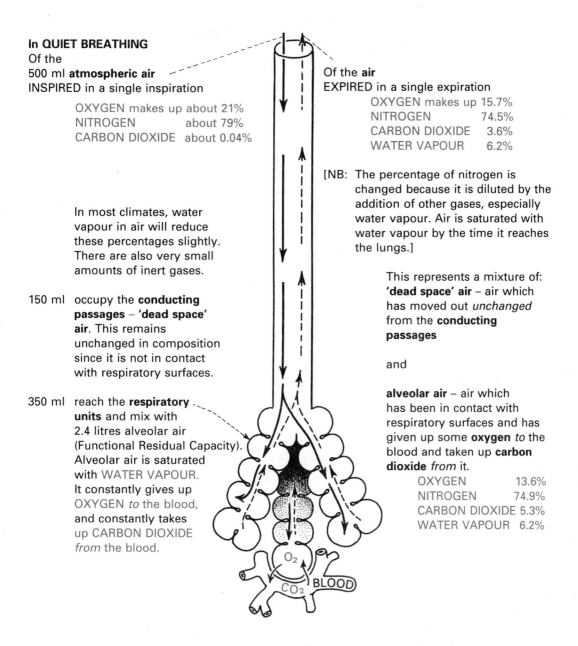

In QUIET BREATHING
Of the
500 ml **atmospheric air**
INSPIRED in a single inspiration

>OXYGEN makes up about 21%
>NITROGEN about 79%
>CARBON DIOXIDE about 0.04%

In most climates, water vapour in air will reduce these percentages slightly. There are also very small amounts of inert gases.

150 ml occupy the **conducting passages** – 'dead space' **air**. This remains unchanged in composition since it is not in contact with respiratory surfaces.

350 ml reach the **respiratory units** and mix with 2.4 litres alveolar air (Functional Residual Capacity). Alveolar air is saturated with WATER VAPOUR. It constantly gives up OXYGEN to the blood, and constantly takes up CARBON DIOXIDE from the blood.

Of the **air**
EXPIRED in a single expiration

>OXYGEN makes up 15.7%
>NITROGEN 74.5%
>CARBON DIOXIDE 3.6%
>WATER VAPOUR 6.2%

[NB: The percentage of nitrogen is changed because it is diluted by the addition of other gases, especially water vapour. Air is saturated with water vapour by the time it reaches the lungs.]

This represents a mixture of:
'dead space' air – air which has moved out *unchanged* from the **conducting passages**

and

alveolar air – air which has been in contact with respiratory surfaces and has given up some **oxygen** *to* the blood and taken up **carbon dioxide** *from* it.

>OXYGEN 13.6%
>NITROGEN 74.9%
>CARBON DIOXIDE 5.3%
>WATER VAPOUR 6.2%

In **VOLUNTARY DEEP BREATHING** at rest (hyperventilating) more new air exchanges with the alveolar air. Thus O_2 content of alveolar air will increase and the CO_2 content will decrease.

MOVEMENT OF RESPIRATORY GASES

A gas moves from an area where it is present at higher pressure to an area where it is present at lower pressure. The movement of gas molecules continues till the pressure exerted by them is the same throughout both areas. *Dry* atmospheric air (at sea level) has a pressure of 1 atmosphere = 760 mmHg = 101.3 kilopascals (kPa).

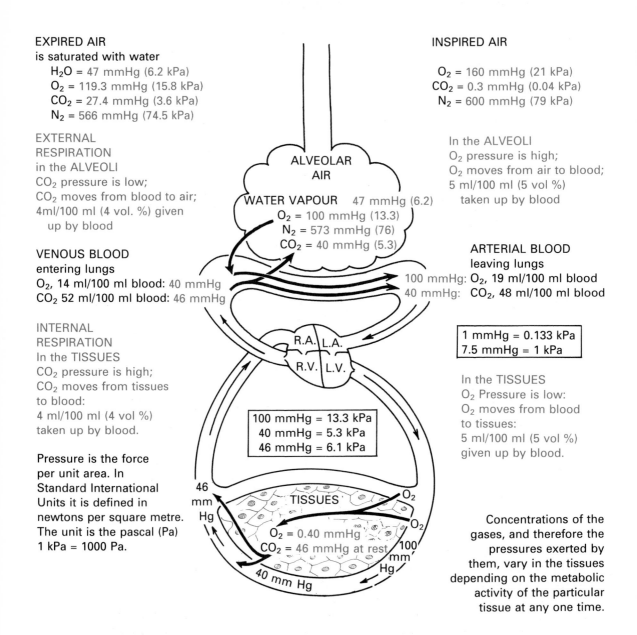

EXPIRED AIR
is saturated with water
H_2O = 47 mmHg (6.2 kPa)
O_2 = 119.3 mmHg (15.8 kPa)
CO_2 = 27.4 mmHg (3.6 kPa)
N_2 = 566 mmHg (74.5 kPa)

EXTERNAL RESPIRATION
in the ALVEOLI
CO_2 pressure is low;
CO_2 moves from blood to air;
4ml/100 ml (4 vol. %) given up by blood

VENOUS BLOOD
entering lungs
O_2, 14 ml/100 ml blood: 40 mmHg
CO_2 52 ml/100 ml blood: 46 mmHg

INTERNAL RESPIRATION
In the TISSUES
CO_2 pressure is high;
CO_2 moves from tissues to blood:
4 ml/100 ml (4 vol %) taken up by blood.

Pressure is the force per unit area. In Standard International Units it is defined in newtons per square metre. The unit is the pascal (Pa) 1 kPa = 1000 Pa.

INSPIRED AIR

O_2 = 160 mmHg (21 kPa)
CO_2 = 0.3 mmHg (0.04 kPa)
N_2 = 600 mmHg (79 kPa)

In the ALVEOLI
O_2 pressure is high;
O_2 moves from air to blood;
5 ml/100 ml (5 vol %) taken up by blood

ALVEOLAR AIR
WATER VAPOUR   47 mmHg (6.2)
O_2 = 100 mmHg (13.3)
N_2 = 573 mmHg (76)
CO_2 = 40 mmHg (5.3)

ARTERIAL BLOOD
leaving lungs
100 mmHg: O_2, 19 ml/100 ml blood
40 mmHg: CO_2, 48 ml/100 ml blood

1 mmHg = 0.133 kPa
7.5 mmHg = 1 kPa

In the TISSUES
O_2 Pressure is low:
O_2 moves from blood to tissues:
5 ml/100 ml (5 vol %) given up by blood.

R.A. L.A.
R.V. L.V.

100 mmHg = 13.3 kPa
40 mmHg = 5.3 kPa
46 mmHg = 6.1 kPa

46 mm Hg

TISSUES O_2
O_2
O_2 = 0.40 mmHg
CO_2 = 46 mmHg at rest
100 mm Hg
40 mm Hg

Concentrations of the gases, and therefore the pressures exerted by them, vary in the tissues depending on the metabolic activity of the particular tissue at any one time.

ALVEOLAR VENTILATION AND DEAD SPACE

At rest, with each breath, we breathe in about 500 ml of fresh *atmospheric air* (the TIDAL volume). Of this volume 350 ml mix with air already in the lung alveoli and 150 ml occupy the air passages (anatomical dead space) and do not take part in exchange with gases in the blood. It is instructive to consider the fate of one breath of dry air at rest. Fot simplicity, consider the rate of breathing to be 10 breaths per minute.

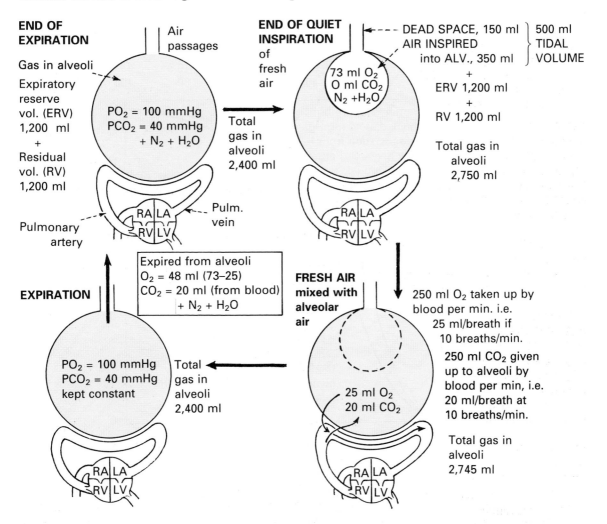

END OF EXPIRATION

Gas in alveoli

Expiratory reserve vol. (ERV) 1,200 ml
+
Residual vol. (RV) 1,200 ml

$PO_2 = 100$ mmHg
$PCO_2 = 40$ mmHg
$+ N_2 + H_2O$

Air passages

Total gas in alveoli 2,400 ml

Pulmonary artery

Pulm. vein

END OF QUIET INSPIRATION of fresh air

73 ml O_2
0 ml CO_2
$N_2 + H_2O$

DEAD SPACE, 150 ml ⎫ 500 ml
AIR INSPIRED ⎬ TIDAL
into ALV., 350 ml ⎭ VOLUME
+
ERV 1,200 ml
+
RV 1,200 ml

Total gas in alveoli 2,750 ml

EXPIRATION

Expired from alveoli
$O_2 = 48$ ml (73–25)
$CO_2 = 20$ ml (from blood)
$+ N_2 + H_2O$

$PO_2 = 100$ mmHg
$PCO_2 = 40$ mmHg
kept constant

Total gas in alveoli 2,400 ml

FRESH AIR mixed with alveolar air

25 ml O_2
20 ml CO_2

250 ml O_2 taken up by blood per min. i.e. 25 ml/breath if 10 breaths/min.

250 ml CO_2 given up to alveoli by blood per min, i.e. 20 ml/breath at 10 breaths/min.

Total gas in alveoli 2,745 ml

Although shown in stages, the process is continuous.
In this case, **dead space ventilation** $= 150 \times 10 = 1,500$ ml/minute.
Alveolar ventilation $= 350 \times 10 = 3,500$ ml/minute.
Total ventilation $= 500 \times 10 = 5,000$ ml/minute.
For simplicity, the CO_2 in 350 ml of *atmospheric air* which would be 0.14 ml has been called 0 ml and the N_2 which would be approximately 276 ml has not been quantified, nor has the water output.

DISSOCIATION OF OXYGEN FROM HAEMOGLOBIN

The amount of O_2 taken up by **haemoglobin** in the **lungs** or given up by **oxyhaemoglobin** in the **tissues** depends on the **partial pressure** of the O_2 in the immediate environment.

It is also influenced by the **partial pressure** of **CO_2,** by **temperature**, by **acidity** and by the concentration of 2,3-diphosphoglycerate (DPG) [or 2,3-biphosphoglycerate (BPG)].

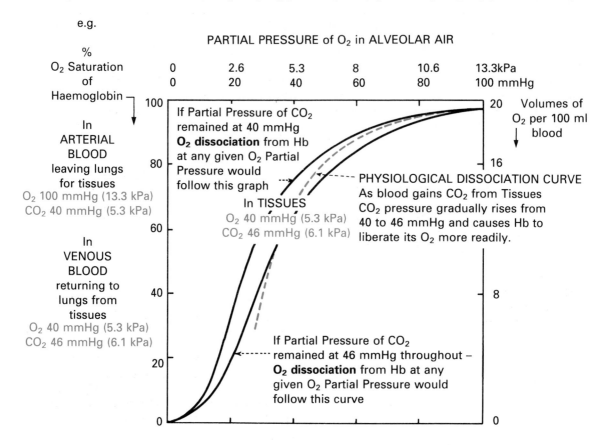

This effect of CO_2 partial pressure on dissociation of O_2 from Hb (the Böhr effect) is advantageous, e.g. an increase in CO_2 partial pressure locally during tissue activity causes Hb to part more readily with its O_2 to the active tissues.

Similarly, an increase in temperature, H^+ and DPG move the curve to the right. DPG is formed when glucose is broken down for energy (glycolysis) in RBCs. Its presence favours the dissociation of oxygen from HbO_2. Thyroxine, human growth hormone and testosterone increase DPG formation. It is higher also in people living at high altitude. Fetal haemoglobin has a higher affinity for O_2 than maternal haemoglobin because it binds DPG less strongly.

UPTAKE AND RELEASE OF CARBON DIOXIDE

CO_2 is carried by the blood in 3 forms: (a) about 90% is carried as **bicarbonate formed** chiefly in the RBCs and **carried** largely by plasma, (b) about 5% is carried **dissolved** in blood water, and (c) about 5% is carried combined to the terminal amino groups of blood proteins as carbamino compounds. Especially important is the globin of haemoglobin.

The Haldane effect

The presence of reduced Hb in the peripheral blood helps with the loading of CO_2 into the blood from the tissues. The oxygenation which occurs in the pulmonary capillaries helps with the off-loading of CO_2 from the blood into the alveoli. The fact that the deoxygenation of the blood increases its ability to carry CO_2 is known as the Haldane effect. The explanation for this is that reduced Hb has a better ability to mop up H^+ produced when carbonic acid dissociates in the reaction $CO_2 + H_2O \rightleftharpoons H_2CO_3 \rightleftharpoons H^+ + HCO_3^-$, hence driving the reaction to the right. In addition, reduced Hb can bind much more CO_2 than HbO_2.

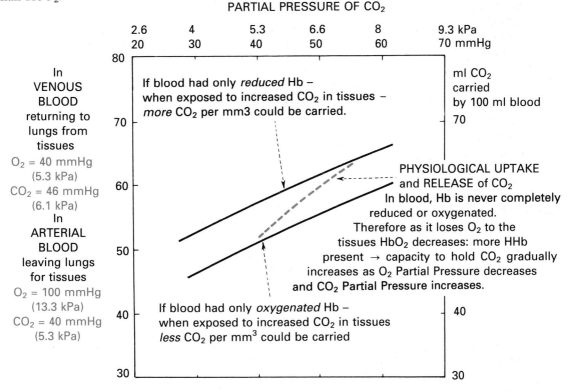

i.e the more **oxygen** the blood holds the less **CO_2** it can hold and vice versa. This facilitates uptake of CO_2 in tissues and release of CO_2 in the lungs.

159

CARRIAGE AND TRANSFER OF OXYGEN AND CARBON DIOXIDE

When **arterial blood** is delivered by **systemic capillaries** to the tissues it is exposed to:–

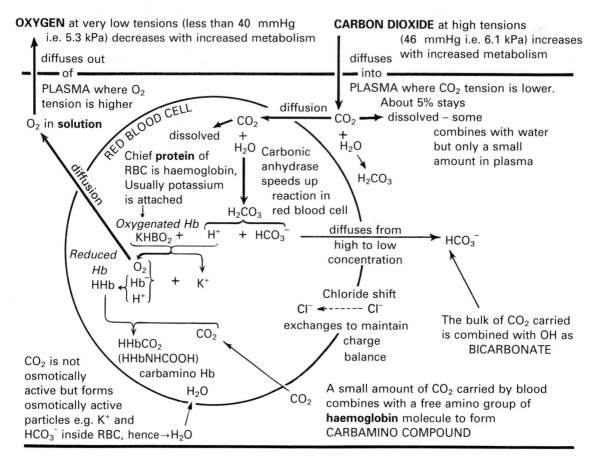

OXYGEN at very low tensions (less than 40 mmHg i.e. 5.3 kPa) decreases with increased metabolism

diffuses out of PLASMA where O_2 tension is higher

O_2 in **solution**

RED BLOOD CELL

diffusion

Chief **protein** of RBC is haemoglobin, Usually potassium is attached

↓

Oxygenated Hb
KHBO$_2$ +   H$^+$ + HCO$_3^-$

Reduced Hb
HHb ← $\begin{cases} Hb^- \\ H^+ \end{cases}$ + K$^+$

O$_2$

HHbCO$_2$
(HHbNHCOOH)
carbamino Hb

H$_2$O

CO$_2$

CO$_2$ is not osmotically active but forms osmotically active particles e.g. K$^+$ and HCO$_3^-$ inside RBC, hence→H$_2$O

dissolved
+
H$_2$O Carbonic anhydrase speeds up reaction in red blood cell

H$_2$CO$_3$

diffuses from high to low concentration

Chloride shift
Cl$^-$ ←------ Cl$^-$
exchanges to maintain charge balance

CARBON DIOXIDE at high tensions (46 mmHg i.e. 6.1 kPa) increases with increased metabolism

diffuses into PLASMA where CO$_2$ tension is lower. About 5% stays dissolved – some combines with water but only a small amount in plasma

CO$_2$ ←
+
H$_2$O

H$_2$CO$_3$

HCO$_3^-$

The bulk of CO$_2$ carried is combined with OH as
BICARBONATE

A small amount of CO$_2$ carried by blood combines with a free amino group of **haemoglobin** molecule to form CARBAMINO COMPOUND

During its passage through the tissues, each 100 ml of blood gives up about 5 ml of oxygen, i.e. its Hb is still up to 70% O$_2$ saturated.

The release of O$_2$ to tissues is speeded up by an increase in temperature, acidity or DPG such as occurs when tissues are active.

During its passage through the tissues, each 100 ml of blood takes up about 4 ml CO$_2$.

CO$_2$ is carried, 5% in solution, 5% as carbamino compounds and 90% as HCO$_3^-$.

Carbonic anhydrase causes rapid formation of HCO$_3^-$ inside the RBC and it then diffuses down a concentration gradient into the plasma.

CARRIAGE AND TRANSFER OF OXYGEN AND CARBON DIOXIDE

When **venous blood** flows through the **pulmonary capillaries** it is exposed to:–

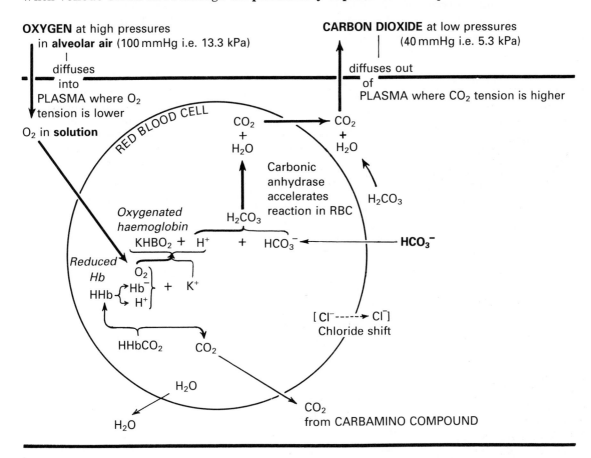

OXYGEN at high pressures in **alveolar air** (100 mmHg i.e. 13.3 kPa)

diffuses into PLASMA where O_2 tension is lower

O_2 in **solution**

CARBON DIOXIDE at low pressures (40 mmHg i.e. 5.3 kPa)

diffuses out of PLASMA where CO_2 tension is higher

RED BLOOD CELL

$CO_2 + H_2O \longrightarrow CO_2 + H_2O$

Carbonic anhydrase accelerates reaction in RBC

H_2CO_3

Oxygenated haemoglobin H_2CO_3

$KHBO_2 + H^+ + HCO_3^- \longleftarrow HCO_3^-$

Reduced Hb

$HHb \begin{cases} Hb^- \\ H^+ \end{cases} \begin{matrix} O_2^- \end{matrix} + K^+$

$[\,Cl^- \dashrightarrow Cl^-\,]$ Chloride shift

$HHbCO_2 \qquad CO_2$

H_2O

CO_2 from CARBAMINO COMPOUND

H_2O

As blood passes through capillaries of lungs, 100 ml take up approximately 5 ml of **oxygen**. O_2 combines with haemoglobin (Hb) molecule. It becomes about 95–97% saturated with oxygen.

As blood passes through capillaries of lungs, each 100 ml blood gives up approximately 4 ml of carbon dioxide. A small amount is released from combination with the free amino group in haemoglobin molecule – carbamino compound. Most comes from bicarbonate in RBC and plasma by processes indicated in diagram.

NERVOUS CONTROL OF RESPIRATORY MOVEMENTS

Normal respiratory movements are involuntary. They are carried out automatically (i.e. without conscious control) through the rhythmical discharge of nerve impulses from **controlling centres** in the medulla oblongata and pons. Respiratory neurons in the brainstem are of two types: **I neurons** discharge during **inspiration**; **E neurons** discharge during **expiration**.

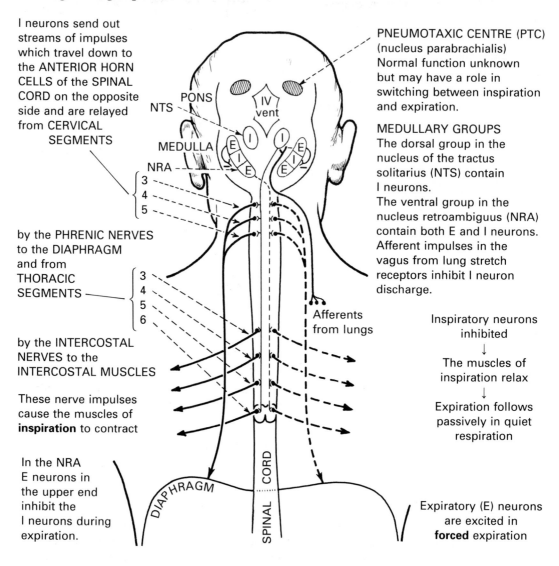

I neurons send out streams of impulses which travel down to the ANTERIOR HORN CELLS of the SPINAL CORD on the opposite side and are relayed from CERVICAL SEGMENTS

PONS
NTS
IV vent

MEDULLA
NRA
E I I E
I E
3
4
5

by the PHRENIC NERVES to the DIAPHRAGM and from THORACIC SEGMENTS
3
4
5
6

by the INTERCOSTAL NERVES to the INTERCOSTAL MUSCLES

These nerve impulses cause the muscles of **inspiration** to contract

In the NRA E neurons in the upper end inhibit the I neurons during expiration.

DIAPHRAGM   SPINAL CORD

Afferents from lungs

PNEUMOTAXIC CENTRE (PTC) (nucleus parabrachialis) Normal function unknown but may have a role in switching between inspiration and expiration.

MEDULLARY GROUPS
The dorsal group in the nucleus of the tractus solitarius (NTS) contain I neurons.
The ventral group in the nucleus retroambiguus (NRA) contain both E and I neurons. Afferent impulses in the vagus from lung stretch receptors inhibit I neuron discharge.

Inspiratory neurons inhibited
↓
The muscles of inspiration relax
↓
Expiration follows passively in quiet respiration

Expiratory (E) neurons are excited in **forced** expiration

Despite intensive research, the mechanism responsible for rhythmic respiratory discharge remains unsettled. The main components are in the medulla where there may be a group of pacemaker neurons situated.

CHEMICAL REGULATION OF RESPIRATION

The activity of the respiratory centres is regulated by the O_2, CO_2 and H^+ content of the blood. **Carbon dioxide** and $\mathbf{H^+}$ are the most important. CO_2 dissolves in cerebrospinal fluid (CSF) which bathes receptors sensitive to H^+ on the ventral aspect of the medulla. Stimulation of these receptors is responsible for about 70% of the increase in the rate and depth of respiration in response to increased CO_2. Carotid and aortic bodies are responsible for the other 30% of the response to raised CO_2. They also increase ventilation in response to a rise in H^+ or a large drop in PaO_2 (to below 60 mmHg).

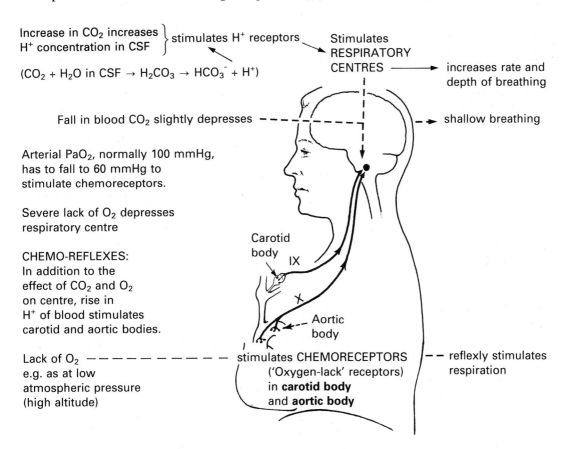

Increase in CO_2 increases H^+ concentration in CSF } stimulates H^+ receptors

$(CO_2 + H_2O$ in CSF $\rightarrow H_2CO_3 \rightarrow HCO_3^- + H^+)$

Stimulates RESPIRATORY CENTRES → increases rate and depth of breathing

Fall in blood CO_2 slightly depresses − − − → shallow breathing

Arterial PaO_2, normally 100 mmHg, has to fall to 60 mmHg to stimulate chemoreceptors.

Severe lack of O_2 depresses respiratory centre

CHEMO-REFLEXES:
In addition to the effect of CO_2 and O_2 on centre, rise in H^+ of blood stimulates carotid and aortic bodies.

Carotid body   IX

Aortic body

Lack of O_2 − − − − − − − − − stimulates CHEMORECEPTORS ('Oxygen-lack' receptors) in **carotid body** and **aortic body** − − reflexly stimulates respiration
e.g. as at low atmospheric pressure (high altitude)

Note:– These reflexes are usually powerful enough to override the direct depressant action of lack of O_2 on respiratory centres themselves

The **chemical** and **nervous** means of regulating the activity of **respiratory centres** act together to adjust rate and depth of breathing to keep the $PaCO_2$ close to 40 mmHg. This automatically sets the PaO_2 to an appropriate value depending on the partial pressure of O_2. For example, exercise causes increased requirement for O_2 and the production of more CO_2. Ventilation is increased to get rid of the extra CO_2 and keep the alveolar $PaCO_2$ at 40 mmHg. More oxygen is used by the tissues. The alveolar PO_2 and PCO_2 both remain constant

VOLUNTARY AND REFLEX FACTORS IN THE REGULATION OF RESPIRATION

Although fundamentally automatic and regulated by chemical factors in the blood there is a separate voluntary system for the regulation of ventilation. It originates in the cerebral cortex and sends impulses to the nerves of the respiratory muscles via the corticospinal tracts. In addition, ingoing impulses from many parts of the body modify the activity of the **respiratory centres** and consequently alter the outgoing impulses to the respiratory muscles to coordinate **rhythm, rate** or **depth** of breathing with other activities of the body.

Impulses from HIGHER CENTRES – PSYCHIC and EMOTIONAL INFLUENCES

{
Voluntary alterations in breathing.
Interruptions of expiration in **speech** and **singing**.
Deep inspiration then short spasmodic expirations in **laughter** and **weeping**.
Prolonged expiration in **sighing**.
Deep inspiration with mouth open in **yawning**.
Slow shallow breathing in **suspense** and **concentration**.
Rapid breathing in **fear** and **excitement**.
}

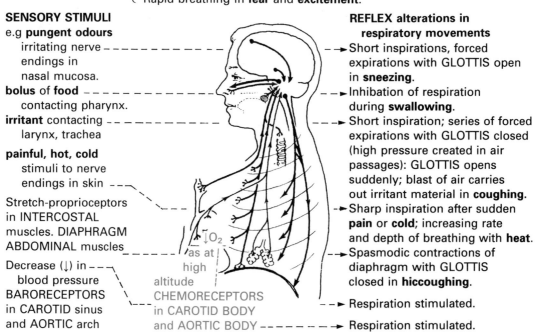

SENSORY STIMULI
e.g **pungent odours**
  irritating nerve endings in nasal mucosa.
bolus of **food** contacting pharynx.
irritant contacting larynx, trachea
painful, hot, cold stimuli to nerve endings in skin
Stretch-proprioceptors in INTERCOSTAL muscles. DIAPHRAGM ABDOMINAL muscles
Decrease (↓) in blood pressure BARORECEPTORS in CAROTID sinus and AORTIC arch

↓O₂ as at high altitude CHEMORECEPTORS in CAROTID BODY and AORTIC BODY

REFLEX alterations in respiratory movements
Short inspirations, forced expirations with GLOTTIS open in **sneezing**.
Inhibation of respiration during **swallowing**.
Short inspiration; series of forced expirations with GLOTTIS closed (high pressure created in air passages): GLOTTIS opens suddenly; blast of air carries out irritant material in **coughing**.
Sharp inspiration after sudden **pain** or **cold**; increasing rate and depth of breathing with **heat**.
Spasmodic contractions of diaphragm with GLOTTIS closed in **hiccoughing**.
Respiration stimulated.
Respiration stimulated.

Proprioceptors stimulated during muscle movements send impulses to respiratory centre → ↑ rate and depth of breathing. (NB: This occurs with active or passive movements of limbs.)

In normal breathing respiratory rate and rhythm are thought to be influenced rhythmically by the **Hering-Breuer reflex**.

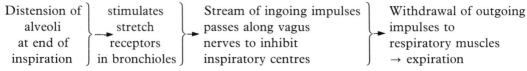

Distension of alveoli at end of inspiration } → stimulates stretch receptors in bronchioles } → Stream of ingoing impulses passes along vagus nerves to inhibit inspiratory centres } → Withdrawal of outgoing impulses to respiratory muscles → expiration

EXCRETORY SYSTEM

EXCRETORY SYSTEM

The respiratory system, the skin and the **kidneys** are the chief excretory organs of the body.

Function of the Kidneys

The kidneys adjust loss of water and electrolytes from the body to keep body fluids constant in amount and composition. They excrete waste products of metabolism, foreign chemicals such as drugs and food additives, secrete the hormones renin and erythropoietin and they activate vitamin D.

They are involved in blood pressure regulation since, in controlling sodium balance, they also control total body water and extracellular volume. The renin-angiotensin system is similarly involved. They produce such vasoactive substances as prostaglandins which can be constrictor or dilator, and bradykinin the vasodilator peptide.

To understand the way in which the kidney carries out these functions, it is essential to understand first the way in which it is supplied with blood. About 25% of the left ventricle's output of blood in each cardiac cycle is distributed to the kidneys for filtration.

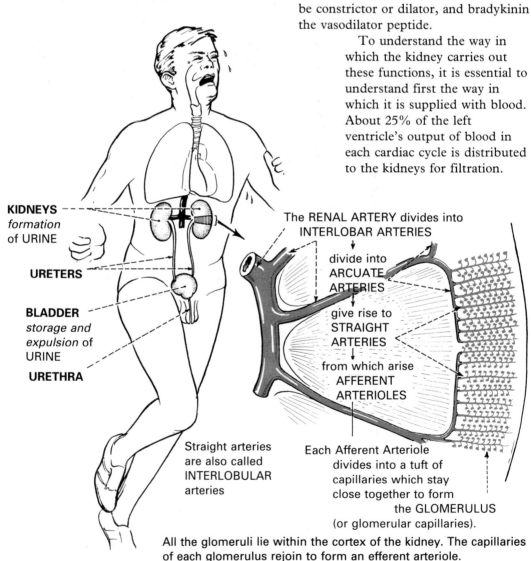

KIDNEYS
formation
of URINE

URETERS

BLADDER
*storage and
expulsion of*
URINE

URETHRA

The RENAL ARTERY divides into
INTERLOBAR ARTERIES
↓
divide into
ARCUATE
ARTERIES
↓
give rise to
STRAIGHT
ARTERIES
↓
from which arise
AFFERENT
ARTERIOLES

Straight arteries
are also called
INTERLOBULAR
arteries

Each Afferent Arteriole
divides into a tuft of
capillaries which stay
close together to form
the GLOMERULUS
(or glomerular capillaries).

All the glomeruli lie within the cortex of the kidney. The capillaries of each glomerulus rejoin to form an efferent arteriole.

KIDNEY BLOOD VESSELS

The route taken by the blood after it passes through the efferent arterioles depends on whether the efferent arterioles are from a juxta-medullary (next to the medulla) glomerulus or an outer cortical glomerulus.

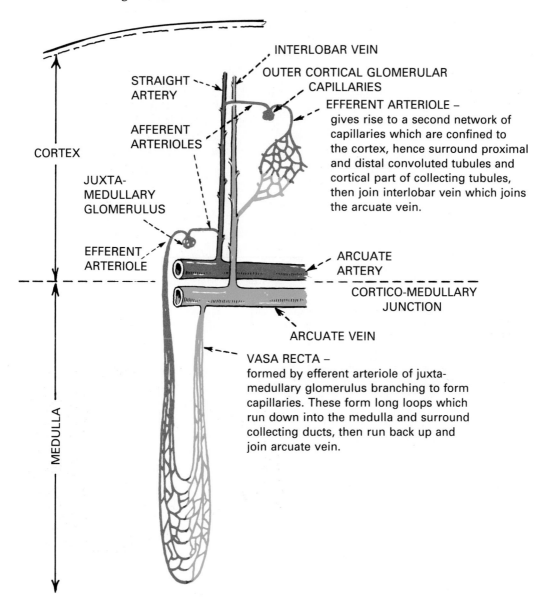

INTERLOBAR VEIN

OUTER CORTICAL GLOMERULAR CAPILLARIES

STRAIGHT ARTERY

EFFERENT ARTERIOLE – gives rise to a second network of capillaries which are confined to the cortex, hence surround proximal and distal convoluted tubules and cortical part of collecting tubules, then join interlobar vein which joins the arcuate vein.

AFFERENT ARTERIOLES

CORTEX

JUXTA-MEDULLARY GLOMERULUS

EFFERENT ARTERIOLE

ARCUATE ARTERY

CORTICO-MEDULLARY JUNCTION

ARCUATE VEIN

VASA RECTA – formed by efferent arteriole of juxta-medullary glomerulus branching to form capillaries. These form long loops which run down into the medulla and surround collecting ducts, then run back up and join arcuate vein.

MEDULLA

The efferent arterioles are narrower than the afferent which causes a higher pressure in the glomerular capillaries than in capillaries in other parts of the body.

Arcuate veins join to form interlobar veins which then join to form renal vein.

KIDNEY-STRUCTURE

Each kidney contains approximately one million functional units – **nephrons** – which form urine.

In the renal corpuscle urine formation starts with *filtration* of the blood

Each AFFERENT ARTERIOLE leads to a tuft of GLOMERULAR capillaries. Surrounding this tuft is the closed end – BOWMAN'S CAPSULE – of a long tortuous RENAL TUBULE which has various parts –

Ascending limb of loop of Henle contacts afferent and efferent arterioles and becomes the distal convoluted tubule.

In the tubules urine formation is completed by *REABSORPTION* across the tubule walls into the blood stream of some substances and by *SECRETION* from the blood into the tubule of others; and *SYNTHESIS* in tubular cells of other substances. COLLECTING TUBULES empty formed urine into the pelvis of the kidney at the tip of the pyramid (papilla).

FIBROUS TISSUE CAPSULE

PROXIMAL CONVOLUTED TUBULE

DIST. CONVOL. TUBULE

ARCUATE VEIN

CORTEX

MEDULLA

RENAL ARTERY and VEIN

PELVIS

PYRAMID

DESCENDING AND ASCENDING LIMBS OF LOOP OF HENLE

CALYX

URETER

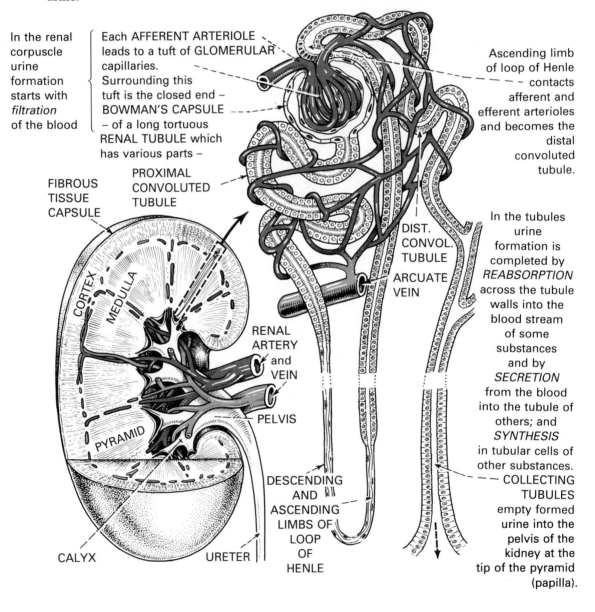

JUXTAGLOMERULAR APPARATUS

As the ascending limb of the loop of Henle passes between the afferent and efferent arterioles to become the distal convoluted tubule, the cells in this part of the nephron are different and form what is called the **macula densa**. These cells, nearest the glomerular tuft, are smaller than the rest of the convoluted tubule cells and form one part of the juxtaglomerular apparatus (JGA). The two other parts of the JGA are the granular or juxtaglomerular cells and the **lacis** or **extraglomerular mesangial cells**.

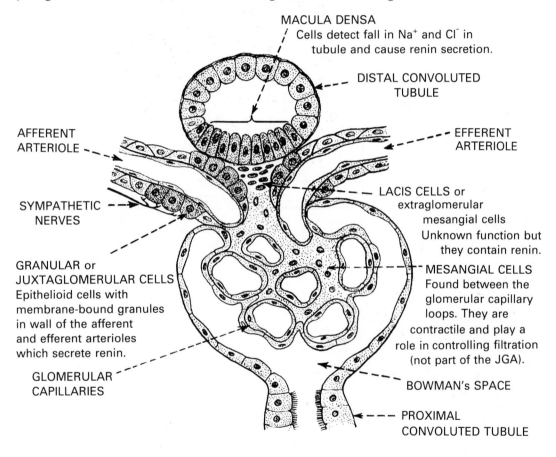

MACULA DENSA
Cells detect fall in Na^+ and Cl^- in tubule and cause renin secretion.

DISTAL CONVOLUTED TUBULE

AFFERENT ARTERIOLE

EFFERENT ARTERIOLE

SYMPATHETIC NERVES

LACIS CELLS or extraglomerular mesangial cells Unknown function but they contain renin.

GRANULAR or JUXTAGLOMERULAR CELLS Epithelioid cells with membrane-bound granules in wall of the afferent and efferent arterioles which secrete renin.

MESANGIAL CELLS Found between the glomerular capillary loops. They are contractile and play a role in controlling filtration (not part of the JGA).

GLOMERULAR CAPILLARIES

BOWMAN's SPACE

PROXIMAL CONVOLUTED TUBULE

Renin is secreted by the juxtaglomerular cells in response to a decrease in extracellular fluid volume and blood pressure or an increase in sympathetic nerve activity. In addition, a fall in tubular Na^+ and Cl^- is detected by the macula densa and causes an increased renin secretion.

URINE FORMATION

Urine formation begins with the filtration of essentially protein free plasma through the glomerular capillaries into Bowman's space. 20% of the water and crystalloid constituents (solute molecules of small size) of the plasma which enters the kidney via the renal artery is filtered through the glomerular membrane.

There are over one million excretory units called nephrons in each kidney. We can represent all the nephrons together in one simple diagram.

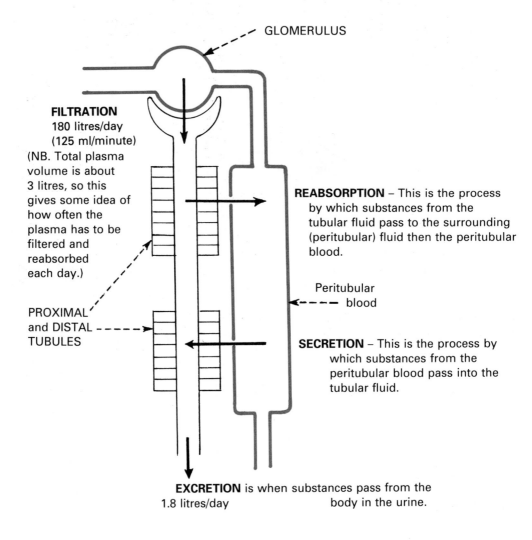

GLOMERULUS

FILTRATION
180 litres/day
(125 ml/minute)
(NB. Total plasma
volume is about
3 litres, so this
gives some idea of
how often the
plasma has to be
filtered and
reabsorbed
each day.)

PROXIMAL
and DISTAL
TUBULES

REABSORPTION – This is the process
by which substances from the
tubular fluid pass to the surrounding
(peritubular) fluid then the peritubular
blood.

Peritubular
blood

SECRETION – This is the process by
which substances from the
peritubular blood pass into the
tubular fluid.

EXCRETION is when substances pass from the
1.8 litres/day   body in the urine.

Note that there are 2 routes for a substance in the blood to be excreted in the urine. 1. It can be filtered and not reabsorbed or 2. it can be secreted and not reabsorbed. In both cases the substances will then be excreted in the urine.

The transport mechanisms for reabsorption and secretion are the same as the transport mechanisms in other cells (see pages 60, 61).

FORCES INVOLVED IN FILTRATION

About 25% of the left ventricle's total output of blood is distributed through the renal arteries to the kidneys where **filtration** of 20% of its plasma takes place.

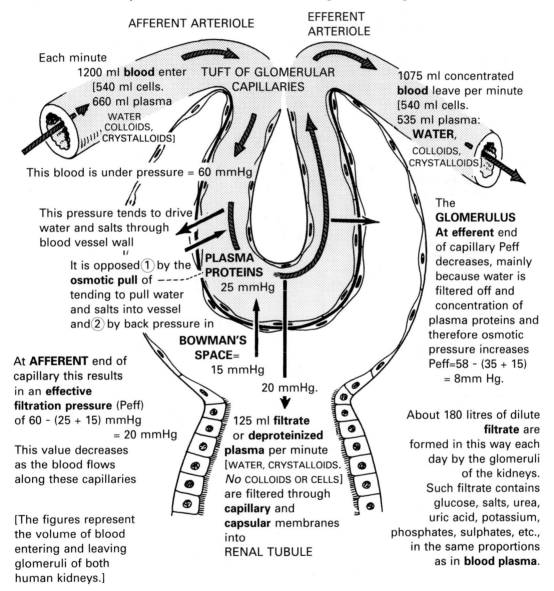

AFFERENT ARTERIOLE

EFFERENT ARTERIOLE

Each minute
1200 ml **blood** enter
[540 ml cells.
660 ml plasma
WATER
COLLOIDS,
CRYSTALLOIDS]

TUFT OF GLOMERULAR CAPILLARIES

1075 ml concentrated **blood** leave per minute
[540 ml cells.
535 ml plasma:
WATER,
COLLOIDS,
CRYSTALLOIDS].

This blood is under pressure = 60 mmHg

This pressure tends to drive water and salts through blood vessel wall

It is opposed ① by the **osmotic pull** of ‑ ‑ ‑ ‑ tending to pull water and salts into vessel and ② by back pressure in

PLASMA PROTEINS
25 mmHg

BOWMAN'S SPACE =
15 mmHg

20 mmHg.

The
GLOMERULUS
At efferent end of capillary Peff decreases, mainly because water is filtered off and concentration of plasma proteins and therefore osmotic pressure increases
Peff = 58 - (35 + 15)
= 8 mm Hg.

At **AFFERENT** end of capillary this results in an **effective filtration pressure** (Peff) of 60 - (25 + 15) mmHg
= 20 mmHg

This value decreases as the blood flows along these capillaries

[The figures represent the volume of blood entering and leaving glomeruli of both human kidneys.]

125 ml **filtrate** or **deproteinized plasma** per minute [WATER, CRYSTALLOIDS. *No* COLLOIDS OR CELLS] are filtered through **capillary** and **capsular** membranes into RENAL TUBULE

About 180 litres of dilute **filtrate** are formed in this way each day by the glomeruli of the kidneys. Such filtrate contains glucose, salts, urea, uric acid, potassium, phosphates, sulphates, etc., in the same proportions as in **blood plasma**.

The glomerular membrane acts as a simple **filter** – i.e. no energy is used up by the cells in filtration. It has 3 layers: capillary endothelial cells with large pores; a basement membrane; epithelial cells of Bowman's capsule called podocytes which have octopus-like extensions or foot processes embedded in the basement membrane.

171

WATER REABSORPTION – PROXIMAL TUBULE

Water is **not actively** reabsorbed by the tubular cells. Its movement is determined passively by the **osmotic gradient** set up by solutes, chiefly by **sodium**.

65% of the **water** and **sodium** filtered into Bowman's capsule from the glomerular capillaries is reabsorbed in the **proximal convoluted tubule.**

Na^+ moves into the epithelial cells of the proximal tubule, see p. 182. It is then actively transported into the **lateral intercellular spaces** by a Na^+, K^+ ATPase pump.

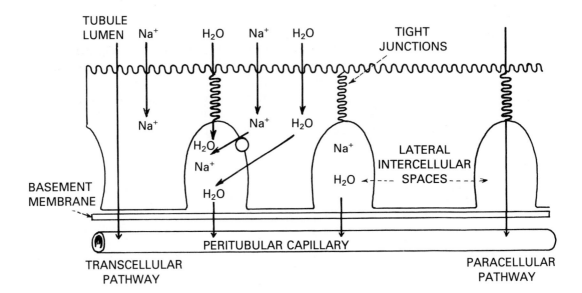

Accumulation of Na^+ in the lateral intercellular spaces creates an osmotic gradient across the epithelium. This osmotic gradient moves **water** into the lateral intercellular spaces either *through* the cells (i.e. via the **transcellular pathway**) or *across* the so-called **tight junctions** (i.e. via the **paracellular pathway**).

As fluid accumulates in the intercellular spaces the hydrostatic pressure increases and forces fluid across the basement membrane into the peritubular capillaries.

A similar mechanism exists for concentrating **bile** in the gall bladder by water reabsorption and for the reabsorption of water and electrolytes in the intestines.

This method of fluid absorption coupling water movement to sodium transport across tight-junctioned epithelia is called the **standing gradient mechanism**.

WATER REABSORPTION – DISTAL AND COLLECTING TUBULES – 1.

Water reabsorption in the distal convoluted tubules and the collecting ducts depends on (1) the permeability of the tubules to water, and (2) the osmotic pressure of the interstitial fluid surrounding the tubules.

The function of the EARLY distal convoluted tubule (first two thirds) differs from that of the last third, called the LATE distal tubule.

The **late** distal tubule and the collecting tubules are **made permeable** to water by the presence in the circulation of antidiuretic hormone (ADH) released from the posterior pituitary gland (p. 212). The **early** distal tubule is **not permeable** to water and its permeability is not changed by ADH.

The osmotic pressure of the **interstitial fluid** which surrounds the tubules throughout the **cortex** is **isosmotic** or the clinical term **isotonic** (300 mosmol/kg H_2O, the same as inside the cells). In the **medulla** there is a **gradient** of osmotic pressure in the interstitial fluid. It increases from 300 mosmol/kg H_2O at the cortico-medullary junction to 1400 mosmol/kg H_2O at the tip of the papilla. The gradient is formed by the counter-current mechanism in the loops of Henle (pp. 175, 176).

When **ADH** is **PRESENT** in circulation:

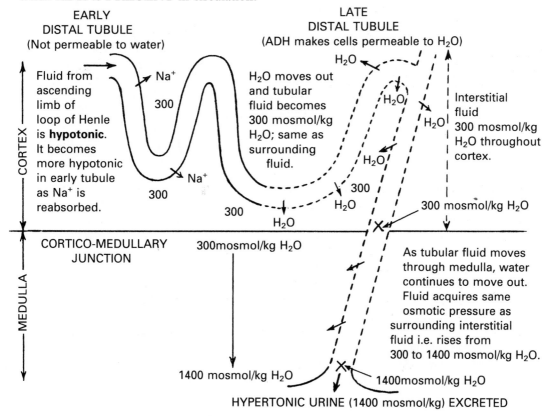

EARLY DISTAL TUBULE (Not permeable to water)

LATE DISTAL TUBULE (ADH makes cells permeable to H_2O)

Fluid from ascending limb of loop of Henle is **hypotonic**. It becomes more hypotonic in early tubule as Na^+ is reabsorbed.

Na^+ 300

Na^+ 300

300

H_2O moves out and tubular fluid becomes 300 mosmol/kg H_2O; same as surrounding fluid.

H_2O

H_2O

H_2O

H_2O

H_2O

300

H_2O

Interstitial fluid 300 mosmol/kg H_2O throughout cortex.

300 mosmol/kg H_2O

CORTEX

MEDULLA

CORTICO-MEDULLARY JUNCTION

300mosmol/kg H_2O

As tubular fluid moves through medulla, water continues to move out. Fluid acquires same osmotic pressure as surrounding interstitial fluid i.e. rises from 300 to 1400 mosmol/kg H_2O.

1400 mosmol/kg H_2O

1400mosmol/kg H_2O

HYPERTONIC URINE (1400 mosmol/kg) EXCRETED

ADH increases intracellular cAMP which causes the insertion of water channels into the membrane of the cells, making them permeable to water.

WATER REABSORPTION – DISTAL AND COLLECTING TUBULES – 2.

Secretion of antidiuretic hormone is **inhibited** by a **decrease** in the osmotic pressure of the plasma or an **increase** in circulating blood volume. These are detected respectively by osmoreceptors in the hypothalamus and low pressure receptors in the left atrium.

Inhibition of ADH secretion results in the excretion of a greater volume of dilute urine, thus decreasing the body fluid volume and increasing its osmotic pressure.

When **ADH** is **ABSENT** from the circulation:

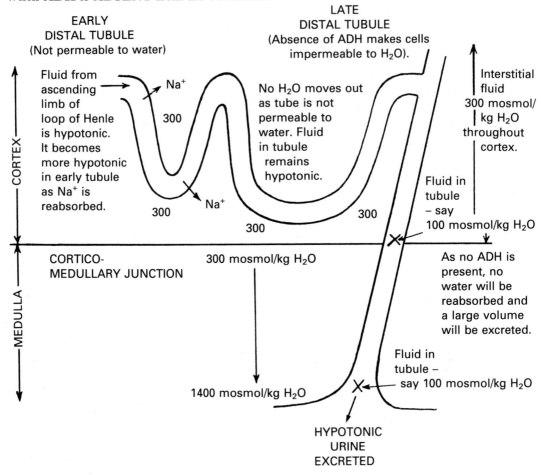

EARLY
DISTAL TUBULE
(Not permeable to water)

LATE
DISTAL TUBULE
(Absence of ADH makes cells
impermeable to H₂O).

Fluid from ascending limb of loop of Henle is hypotonic. It becomes more hypotonic in early tubule as Na⁺ is reabsorbed.

Na⁺

300

300

Na⁺

No H₂O moves out as tube is not permeable to water. Fluid in tubule remains hypotonic.

300

300

Interstitial fluid
300 mosmol/ kg H₂O throughout cortex.

Fluid in tubule – say 100 mosmol/kg H₂O

CORTEX

MEDULLA

CORTICO-MEDULLARY JUNCTION

300 mosmol/kg H₂O

As no ADH is present, no water will be reabsorbed and a large volume will be excreted.

1400 mosmol/kg H₂O

Fluid in tubule – say 100 mosmol/kg H₂O

HYPOTONIC URINE EXCRETED

The degree of inhibition of ADH secretion will depend on the osmotic pressure of the plasma or the volume of the plasma. The amount of ADH secreted will be adjusted so that the osmotic pressure of the plasma and the blood volume are returned to normal values.

FUNCTION OF THE LOOP OF HENLE – 1.

The function of the loop of Henle is to form a **gradient of osmotic pressure** in the **interstitial fluid** of the **medulla** of the kidney. This enables the fluid in the **collecting** tubules to be concentrated as the tubules run through the medulla, and urine, which is hypertonic to plasma, to be excreted.

Fluid in the descending limb of the loop of Henle runs in the opposite direction to (i.e. counter to) the fluid in the ascending limb, hence the mechanism is known as the **counter-current mechanism** for the **concentration** of urine.

The different characteristics of the two limbs are very important and must be remembered in order to understand the mechanism.

The descending limb is **permeable** to water but **not permeable** to solute (especially Na^+ and Cl^-). The ascending limb is **impermeable** to water but **permeable** to solute. In addition, the fluid is continuously flowing round the loop.

It is instructive to imagine that this continuous process can occur in separate stages and, to help to understand how the gradient is formed, consider what changes in osmotic pressure would occur in each separate stage.

Imagine that we can start with all tubular fluid and interstitial fluid (ISF) at 300 mosmol/kg H_2O.

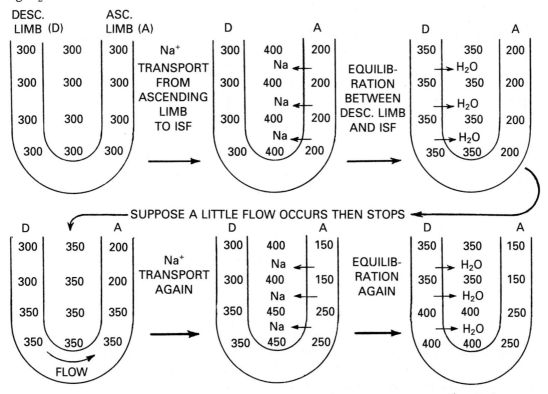

Further flow would increase the osmotic pressure at the tip to 400 mosmol/kg H_2O. The gradient in the interstitial fluid has started to form. If more values were used in each limb and the processes repeated many times over, the steady state shown on page 176 would be reached.

FUNCTION OF THE LOOP OF HENLE – 2.

As fluid moves down the **descending** limb of the loop of Henle, **water** moves **out** because the surrounding interstitial fluid is at a higher osmotic pressure. With maximum concentration the osmotic pressure of the fluid at the bend of the loop can reach 1400 mosmol/kg H_2O. As fluid flows up the **ascending** limb, **solute**, especially Na^+ and Cl^-, **moves out** into the interstitial fluid and, since the ascending limb is **impermeable** to water, water does *not* follow the solute and the fluid passing on to the distal convoluted tubule is **hypotonic**.

Values of the osmotic pressure, with maximum concentration, when the steady state is reached:

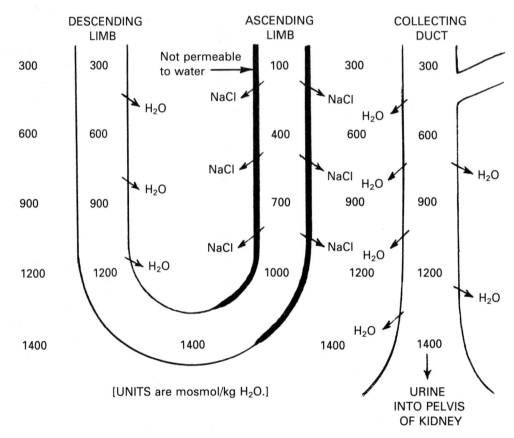

[UNITS are mosmol/kg H_2O.]

The site of **final concentration** is in the **collecting ducts** which run through the medulla to the tips of the papillae. If ADH is present, water diffuses out of the collecting duct fluid into the interstitial fluid. The result is that the fluid at the end of the collecting duct is equilibrated with the interstitial fluid at the tip of the papillae and is **hypertonic**. It passes into the pelvis of the kidney as **hypertonic urine**.

ROLE OF UREA IN THE COUNTER-CURRENT MECHANISM

The gradient of osmotic pressure in the **interstitial fluid** of the medulla of the kidney is not due solely to Na^+ and Cl^-. At the tips of the papillae about 50% of the osmotic pressure is due to **urea**.

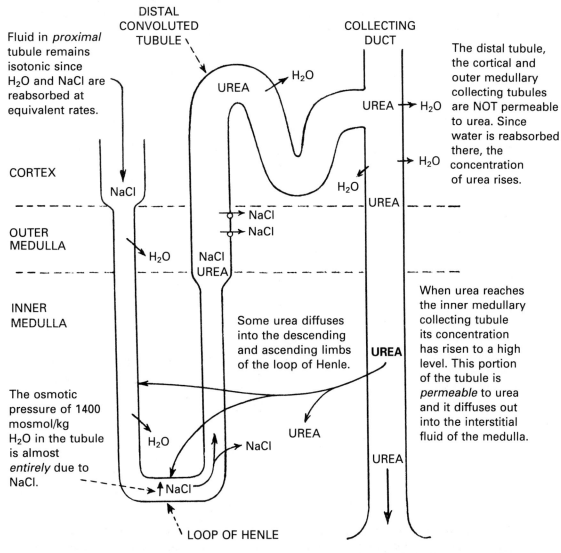

Fluid in *proximal* tubule remains isotonic since H_2O and NaCl are reabsorbed at equivalent rates.

DISTAL CONVOLUTED TUBULE

COLLECTING DUCT

The distal tubule, the cortical and outer medullary collecting tubules are NOT permeable to urea. Since water is reabsorbed there, the concentration of urea rises.

CORTEX

OUTER MEDULLA

INNER MEDULLA

Some urea diffuses into the descending and ascending limbs of the loop of Henle.

When urea reaches the inner medullary collecting tubule its concentration has risen to a high level. This portion of the tubule is *permeable* to urea and it diffuses out into the interstitial fluid of the medulla.

The osmotic pressure of 1400 mosmol/kg H_2O in the tubule is almost *entirely* due to NaCl.

LOOP OF HENLE

At the bend of the loop of Henle the osmotic pressure in the tubule is the same as that of the surrounding interstitial fluid, 1400 mosmol/kg H_2O. But, since *inside* the tubule the osmotic pressure is practically all due to NaCl and in the surrounding interstitial fluid it is only 50% due to NaCl, there is a large NaCl concentration gradient. Hence, as the tubular fluid goes up the thin ascending limb, which is permeable to NaCl, NaCl diffuses *passively* out of the tubule into the interstitial fluid and contributes to the osmotic pressure of the interstitial fluid in the inner medulla.

FUNCTION OF THE VASA RECTA

Creating the osmotic gradient in the medulla of the kidney and producing urine hypertonic to plasma involve the reabsorption into the medullary interstitial fluid of sodium, chloride, urea and water. Accumulation of excess quantities of these substances in the medulla is prevented by their removal into the blood stream by the **vasa recta**. These capillaries from the efferent arteriole of the juxtamedullary glomeruli have an ascending limb, a descending limb and a hairpin bend.

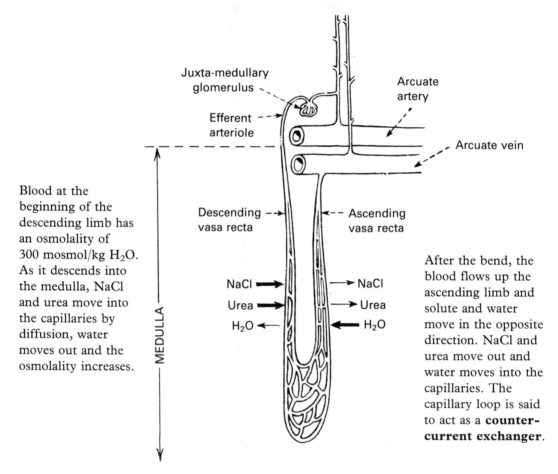

Blood at the beginning of the descending limb has an osmolality of 300 mosmol/kg H_2O. As it descends into the medulla, NaCl and urea move into the capillaries by diffusion, water moves out and the osmolality increases.

After the bend, the blood flows up the ascending limb and solute and water move in the opposite direction. NaCl and urea move out and water moves into the capillaries. The capillary loop is said to act as a **counter-current exchanger**.

In fact, not all the NaCl and urea that enters the descending limb comes out the ascending limb and more water goes into the ascending limb than leaves the descending limb. The blood that empties into the arcuate vein is slightly hypertonic and its volume is greater than that of the blood which comes into the descending limb from the efferent arteriole. About 10 ml of blood per minute with an osmolality of 300 mosmol/kg H_2O enter the descending capillary and 11 ml of blood per minute with an osmolality of 325 mosmol/kg H_2O flow from the ascending limb into the arcuate veins. The solute and water reabsorbed into the medullary interstitial fluid are thus returned to the circulation and a steady state is maintained in the medulla of the kidney.

MAINTENANCE OF ACID-BASE BALANCE – 1

An acid is a substance which liberates H^+ ions (proton donor). A base is a substance which can accept a H^+ ion (proton acceptor). Acids are formed in the body during the breakdown of food, during cell metabolism and, especially, by the production of CO_2 and its combination with water. However the concentration of free H^+ in the body fluids is kept relatively constant at about pH 7.4 (pH 7.4 = 4×10^{-8} mol/litre of $\mathbf{H^+}$).

This equilibrium is maintained by **buffer systems** binding free H^+; by the **lungs** eliminating CO_2 and finally by the **kidneys** excreting H^+ and conserving base (mainly HCO_3^-).

The main extracellular fluid buffer system is the **bicarbonate buffer** system $CO_2 + H_2O \rightleftharpoons H_2CO_3 \rightleftharpoons H^+ + HCO_3^-$. Thus if H^+ is liberated it combines with HCO_3^-, forming carbonic acid which breaks down to $CO_2 + H_2O$. *NB*: HCO_3^- is 'used up' in this reaction.

The Henderson-Hasselbalch equation shows the relationship between pH, CO_2 and HCO_3^-

$$pH \propto \frac{\text{Concentration of } HCO_3^-}{\text{Dissolved } CO_2}$$

The lungs decrease H^+ (increase pH) by eliminating CO_2 in expired air.
The kidneys decrease H^+ (increase pH) by **reabsorption** of HCO_3^- and by **excretion** of H^+.

CONSERVATION OF BASE

NB: brush border

REABSORPTION OF BICARBONATE
Bicarbonate is in a concentration of about 24 mmol/l in filtrate. Most is reabsorbed in the proximal tubule by this mechanism

Secretion of free hydrogen ions counter-transported with sodium ions (secondary active transport)

Secreted hydrogen ions react with bicarbonate to form carbon acid.

This carbonic acid breaks down to form CO_2 and H_2O. Reaction is facilitated by carbonic anhydrase in cell membrane of proximal tubule.

This mechanism reabsorbs base (HCO_3^-)

MAINTENANCE OF ACID-BASE BALANCE – 2

To maintain the body fluids at a **constant pH,** the same quantity of hydrogen ion that is **ingested** in the diet must be **excreted.** In addition, the body must be capable of altering the H^+ **excretion** in response to changes in H^+ **production** and to compensate for any gastrointestinal loss or gain resulting from disease e.g. by vomiting.

The cells of the proximal, late distal convoluted tubule and cortical collecting tubules of the kidney all secrete H^+ into the tubules. There are 2 mechanisms:

In the PROXIMAL TUBULE

H^+ is made available by the speedy combination of H_2O and CO_2 in the presence of the enzyme carbonic anhydrase. The H_2CO_3 so formed dissociates into H^+ and HCO_3^-. The latter is reabsorbed. H^+ ions are counter-transported with Na^+ and secreted into the tubular lumen.

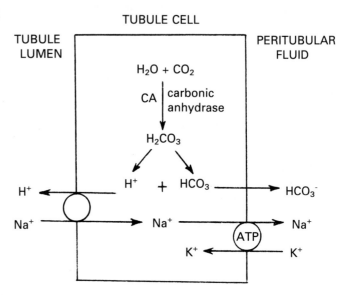

In the LATE DISTAL TUBULE AND CORTICAL COLLECTING DUCTS

H^+ ions are made available in a similar way and are then secreted into the lumen of the tubules by active, ATP driven pumps called proton pumps.

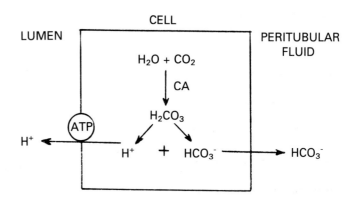

The epithelium of the collecting ducts is made up of **principal cells** (P cells) and **intercalated cells** (I cells). I cells are also present in the late distal tubules. The proton pumps are located in the I cells which also contain abundant carbonic anhydrase.

In acidosis (excess H^+ in the body) the number of proton pumps in the membrane increases.

MAINTENANCE OF ACID-BASE BALANCE – 3

A large increase in concentration of free H^+ in the tubular filtrate (to pH 4.5) would prevent the secretion of H^+ ions from the tubular cells. Two mechanisms bind free H^+ in the filtrate and allow continued **secretion** of H^+.

PHOSPHATE MECHANISM

Dibasic phosphate in filtrate - - - - - - - - - -

Hydrogen ion is **secreted** either counter-transported with Na^+ - - - - - or by primary active transport (proton pump).

Secreted hydrogen ion is bound and **excreted** as - - - - - **monobasic phosphate**.

This mechanism excretes H^+ and **reabsorbs** some base (HCO_3^-).

AMMONIA MECHANISM

This is the most important mechanism for buffering H^+ in tubule.

Hydrogen ion is **secreted** by a proton pump:
Secreted H^+ combines with ammonia (NH_3) which diffuses from the tubular cell - - - - -

Thus an ammonium ion (NH_4^+) is formed.
Cell membrane is permeable to NH_3 but not to NH_4^+ so NH_4^+ containing secreted H^+ is **excreted**.

This mechanism excretes H^+ and **reabsorbs** some base (HCO_3^-).

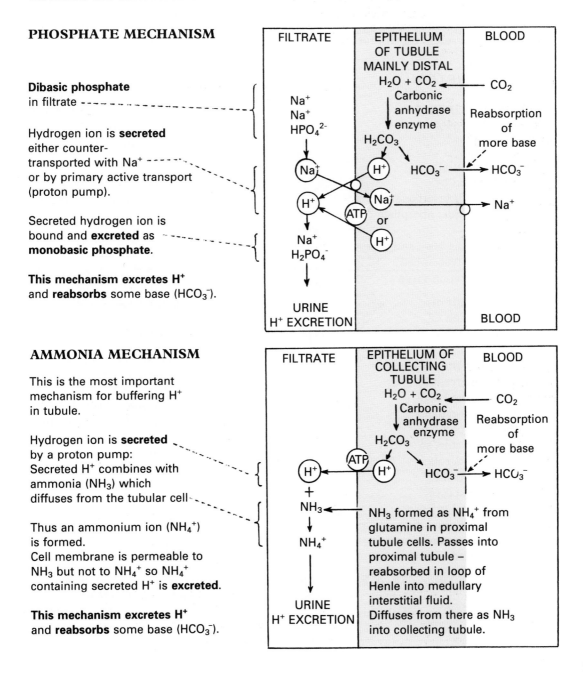

PHOSPHATE MECHANISM

FILTRATE	EPITHELIUM OF TUBULE MAINLY DISTAL	BLOOD

$H_2O + CO_2$ ← CO_2
Carbonic anhydrase enzyme
Reabsorption of more base
H_2CO_3

Na^+
Na^+
HPO_4^{2-}

Na^+ H^+ HCO_3^- → HCO_3^-

H^+ Na^+ (ATP) or → Na^+

Na^+
$H_2PO_4^-$

H^+

URINE
H^+ EXCRETION

BLOOD

AMMONIA MECHANISM

FILTRATE	EPITHELIUM OF COLLECTING TUBULE	BLOOD

$H_2O + CO_2$ ← CO_2
Carbonic anhydrase enzyme
Reabsorption of more base
H_2CO_3

(ATP)
H^+ ← H^+ HCO_3^- → HCO_3^-
+
NH_3 ← NH_3 formed as NH_4^+ from glutamine in proximal tubule cells. Passes into proximal tubule – reabsorbed in loop of Henle into medullary interstitial fluid. Diffuses from there as NH_3 into collecting tubule.
NH_4^+

URINE
H^+ EXCRETION

SODIUM REABSORPTION

More than 99% of the sodium filtered from the glomerular capillaries of the kidneys is **reabsorbed** as the tubular fluid passes along the nephron. Its reabsorption is **dependent** on the active transport by a Na^+, K^+ ATPase mechanism which pumps Na^+ from the basolateral membrane of the tubular cells into the peritubular fluid. The intracellular concentration of sodium is thus kept *low*. Since, in the tubular fluid, its concentration is *high*, Na^+ moves across the **apical** membrane into the cell down the electrochemical gradient.

Na^+ REABSORPTION

PROXIMAL TUBULE
Reabsorbs about 65% of the filtered Na^+.

In **first half** of tubule, Na^+ is reabsorbed by **cotransport** with bicarbonate, glucose, amino acids, phosphate and lactate.
Water follows the Na^+ and, since little Cl^- is reabsorbed here, its concentration **rises**.

In the **second half** of the tubule, the high Cl^- concentration enables it to diffuse passively **through tight junctions** to the lateral intercellular spaces, making the basal side of the cell negatively charged with respect to the tubular fluid side, so Na^+ follows Cl^- across the tight junctions into the intracellular spaces along the electrical gradient. Na^+ is also reabsorbed by the **transcellular route**, countertransported with H^+.

DISTAL TUBULES AND COLLECTING DUCTS
Reabsorb about 10% of the filtered Na^+.

The **early** distal tubule cotransports Na^+ with Cl^-.

The **late** distal tubule and collecting ducts reabsorb Na^+ by its diffusion through water-filled channels of the **principal** cells, driven by their internal negative potential.

LOOP OF HENLE
Reabsorbs about 25% of the filtered Na^+. The **thick ascending** limb of Henle's loop is particularly **important** for Na^+ reabsorption which occurs by cotransport with $2Cl^-$ and $1K^+$ (a $1Na^+$, $2Cl^-$, $1K^+$ symporter). It is also countertransported with H^+.

In the *proximal tubule*, 65% of both the filtered Na^+ and water are reabsorbed, hence the osmolality of the fluid leaving the proximal tubule to enter the loop of Henle is virtually the *same* as that of plasma.

DEFENCE OF BODY FLUID VOLUME

The **volume** of the extracellular fluid (ECF) is determined mainly by the amount of osmotically active solute it contains. Na^+ is the most important active solute in the body, hence mechanisms that control Na^+ balance will also control ECF volume.

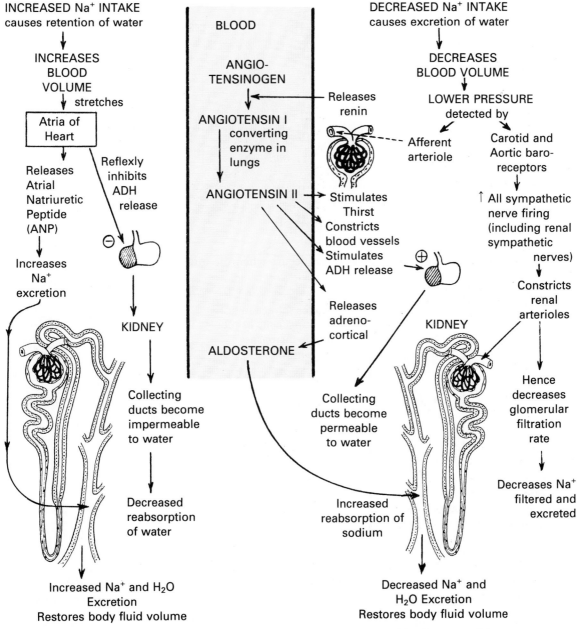

INCREASED Na^+ INTAKE
causes retention of water

↓

INCREASES
BLOOD
VOLUME

↓ stretches

Atria of
Heart

Releases
Atrial
Natriuretic
Peptide
(ANP)

Reflexly
inhibits
ADH
release

⊖

Increases
Na^+
excretion

KIDNEY

Collecting
ducts become
impermeable
to water

↓

Decreased
reabsorption
of water

↓

Increased Na^+ and H_2O
Excretion
Restores body fluid volume

BLOOD

ANGIO-
TENSINOGEN

↓

ANGIOTENSIN I
converting
enzyme in
lungs

ANGIOTENSIN II → Stimulates
Thirst
Constricts
blood vessels
Stimulates
ADH release

Releases
adreno-
cortical

ALDOSTERONE

Releases
renin

Afferent
arteriole

⊕

Collecting
ducts become
permeable
to water

KIDNEY

Increased
reabsorption of
sodium

DECREASED Na^+ INTAKE
causes excretion of water

↓

DECREASES
BLOOD VOLUME

↓

LOWER PRESSURE
detected by

Carotid and
Aortic baro-
receptors

↓

↑ All sympathetic
nerve firing
(including renal
sympathetic
nerves)

↓

Constricts
renal
arterioles

↓

Hence
decreases
glomerular
filtration
rate

↓

Decreases Na^+
filtered and
excreted

Decreased Na^+ and
H_2O Excretion
Restores body fluid volume

Control of vasopressin (ADH) release by changes in volume overrides its control by osmotic changes.

RENAL REGULATION OF POTASSIUM EXCRETION

About 85% of the potassium that is **filtered** by the kidney nephron is **reabsorbed** regardless of the state of potassium balance of the subject. Regulation of **excretion** is mainly controlled by altering potassium **secretion** by the distal tubules and collecting ducts.

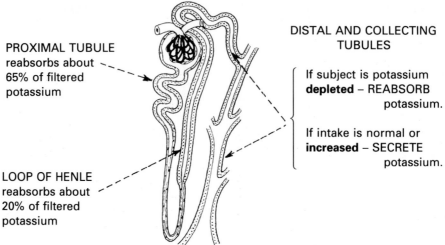

PROXIMAL TUBULE reabsorbs about 65% of filtered potassium

DISTAL AND COLLECTING TUBULES

If subject is potassium **depleted** – REABSORB potassium.

If intake is normal or **increased** – SECRETE potassium.

LOOP OF HENLE reabsorbs about 20% of filtered potassium

The commonest regulatory mechanism occurs when the intake is normal.

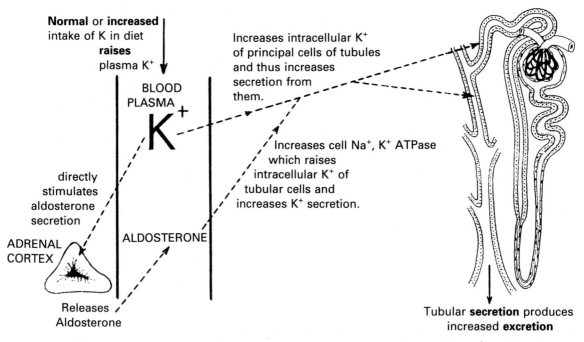

Normal or **increased** intake of K in diet **raises** plasma K^+

BLOOD PLASMA K^+

Increases intracellular K^+ of principal cells of tubules and thus increases secretion from them.

Increases cell Na^+, K^+ ATPase which raises intracellular K^+ of tubular cells and increases K^+ secretion.

directly stimulates aldosterone secretion

ADRENAL CORTEX

ALDOSTERONE

Releases Aldosterone

Tubular **secretion** produces increased **excretion**

ADH, flow rate of tubular fluid, acid-base balance, and tubular fluid Na^+ concentration also modify K^+ secretion but are much less important than **aldosterone** and **plasma K^+ concentration**.

DEFENCE OF BODY FLUID TONICITY

The **tonicity** or **osmolality** of body fluids is controlled by *THIRST* which alters water intake, and *VASOPRESSIN (antidiuretic hormone, ADH)* released from the posterior pituitary gland (page 214) which alters water output by the kidney.

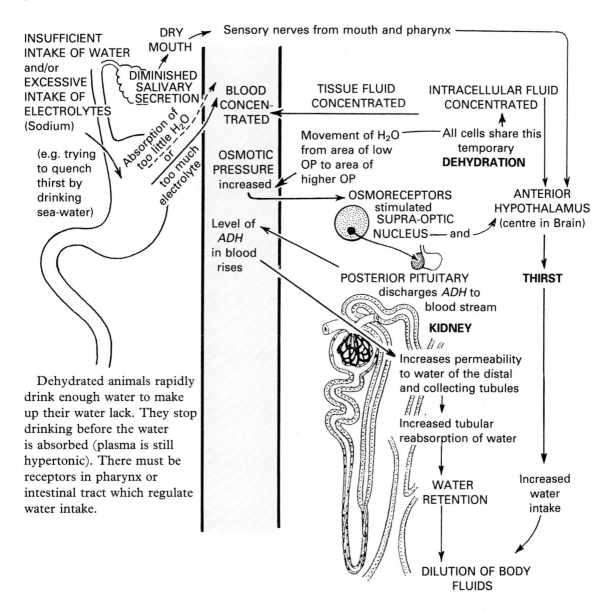

An *EXCESS* intake of water or *INSUFFICIENT* electrolytes will produce mainly decreased osmoreceptor stimulation and hence decreased ADH release leading to increased tonicity of body fluids.

185

PLASMA CLEARANCE

The **plasma clearance** of a substance can be defined in 2 ways. (1) It is the **volume** of plasma (in ml) **cleared** of a given substance per minute by the kidney or (2) it is the **volume** of plasma (in ml) which **contained** the amount of the substance which is **excreted** in the urine in one minute.

Consider three hypothetical substances, **all** of which are **filtered**. 'A' is a substance which is **neither reabsorbed** nor **secreted** by the kidney tubules, 'B' is a substance **some** of which is **reabsorbed** but **none secreted**, and 'C' is a substance **none** of which is **reabsorbed** but some is **secreted** by the tubules.

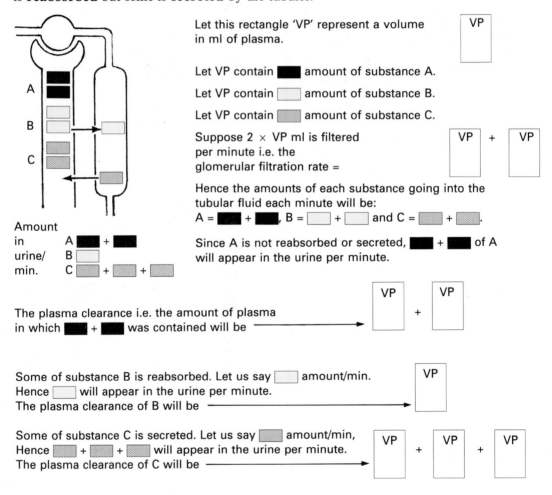

Let this rectangle 'VP' represent a volume in ml of plasma.

Let VP contain ■ amount of substance A.

Let VP contain ☐ amount of substance B.

Let VP contain ▨ amount of substance C.

Suppose 2 × VP ml is filtered per minute i.e. the glomerular filtration rate =

Hence the amounts of each substance going into the tubular fluid each minute will be:
A = ■ + ■, B = ☐ + ☐ and C = ▨ + ▨.

Since A is not reabsorbed or secreted, ■ + ■ of A will appear in the urine per minute.

Amount in urine/min. A ■ + ■ B ☐ C ▨ + ▨ + ▨

The plasma clearance i.e. the amount of plasma in which ■ + ■ was contained will be ⟶ VP + VP

Some of substance B is reabsorbed. Let us say ☐ amount/min. Hence ☐ will appear in the urine per minute. The plasma clearance of B will be ⟶ VP

Some of substance C is secreted. Let us say ▨ amount/min, Hence ▨ + ▨ + ▨ will appear in the urine per minute. The plasma clearance of C will be ⟶ VP + VP + VP

A substance which is neither reabsorbed from nor secreted into the tubules, like inulin, will have a clearance value *equal* to the glomerular filtration rate.

A substance which is reabsorbed into the blood again, like urea, will have a clearance value *less* than the glomerular filtration rate.

A substance which is secreted into the tubular fluid from the peritubular blood, like PAH, will have a clearance value *greater* than the glomerular filtration rate.

186

THE 'CLEARANCE' OF INULIN IN THE NEPHRON

The rate of glomerular filtration (GFR) can be found by measuring the 'plasma clearance' of a substance like substance 'A' on page 186 which is filtered by the renal corpuscle but neither reabsorbed nor secreted by the tubular epithelium. Inulin and creatinine are such substances. The use of inulin is more accurate but the technique using creatinine is simpler.

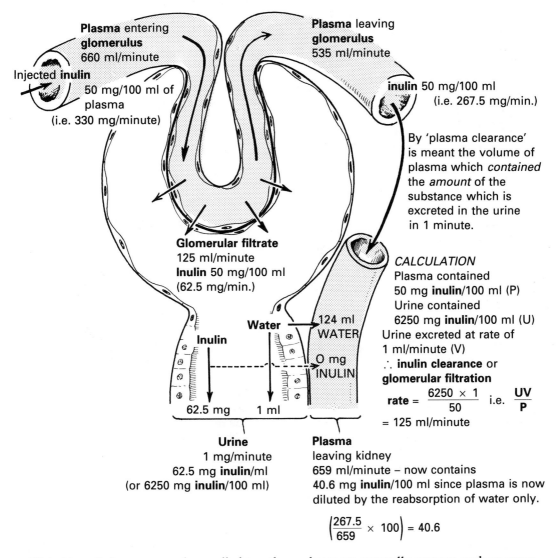

Plasma entering
glomerulus
660 ml/minute

Injected **inulin**
50 mg/100 ml of plasma
(i.e. 330 mg/minute)

Plasma leaving
glomerulus
535 ml/minute

inulin 50 mg/100 ml
(i.e. 267.5 mg/min.)

By 'plasma clearance' is meant the volume of plasma which *contained* the *amount* of the substance which is excreted in the urine in 1 minute.

Glomerular filtrate
125 ml/minute
Inulin 50 mg/100 ml
(62.5 mg/min.)

Water

124 ml
WATER

Inulin

0 mg
INULIN

62.5 mg   1 ml

Urine
1 mg/minute
62.5 mg **inulin**/ml
(or 6250 mg **inulin**/100 ml)

Plasma
leaving kidney
659 ml/minute – now contains
40.6 mg **inulin**/100 ml since plasma is now diluted by the reabsorption of water only.

$$\left(\frac{267.5}{659} \times 100\right) = 40.6$$

CALCULATION
Plasma contained
50 mg **inulin**/100 ml (P)
Urine contained
6250 mg **inulin**/100 ml (U)
Urine excreted at rate of
1 ml/minute (V)
∴ **inulin clearance** or **glomerular filtration**

$$\text{rate} = \frac{6250 \times 1}{50} \quad \text{i.e.} \quad \frac{UV}{P}$$

= 125 ml/minute

This idea of clearance can be applied to other substances naturally present such as **urea**, or artificially introduced, such as **diodone**.

UREA 'CLEARANCE'

Urea, like inulin, is filtered by the renal corpuscle. Unlike inulin some urea is reabsorbed back into the blood stream from the tubules. See substance 'B' on page 186.

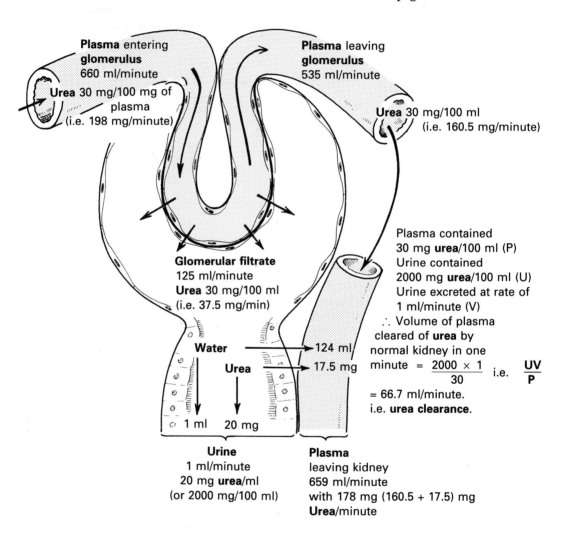

Plasma entering
glomerulus
660 ml/minute
Urea 30 mg/100 mg of
plasma
(i.e. 198 mg/minute)

Plasma leaving
glomerulus
535 ml/minute
Urea 30 mg/100 ml
(i.e. 160.5 mg/minute)

Glomerular filtrate
125 ml/minute
Urea 30 mg/100 ml
(i.e. 37.5 mg/min)

Plasma contained
30 mg **urea**/100 ml (P)
Urine contained
2000 mg **urea**/100 ml (U)
Urine excreted at rate of
1 ml/minute (V)
∴ Volume of plasma
cleared of **urea** by
normal kidney in one
minute $= \dfrac{2000 \times 1}{30}$ i.e. $\dfrac{UV}{P}$
= 66.7 ml/minute.
i.e. **urea clearance**.

Water → 124 ml
Urea → 17.5 mg

1 ml   20 mg

Urine
1 ml/minute
20 mg **urea**/ml
(or 2000 mg/100 ml)

Plasma
leaving kidney
659 ml/minute
with 178 mg (160.5 + 17.5) mg
Urea/minute

Urea clearance is used as a test of renal function.

PAH 'CLEARANCE'

Certain special substances are filtered by the renal corpuscle and the rest that escapes filtration is then secreted totally from the peritubular blood into the tubule. Thus the renal artery contains the substance but the renal vein contains none. **Para-aminohippuric acid (PAH)** and **diodone** are such substances. The 'Plasma Clearance' of these substances measures the **renal plasma flow** rate. Compare this with substance 'C' on page 186.

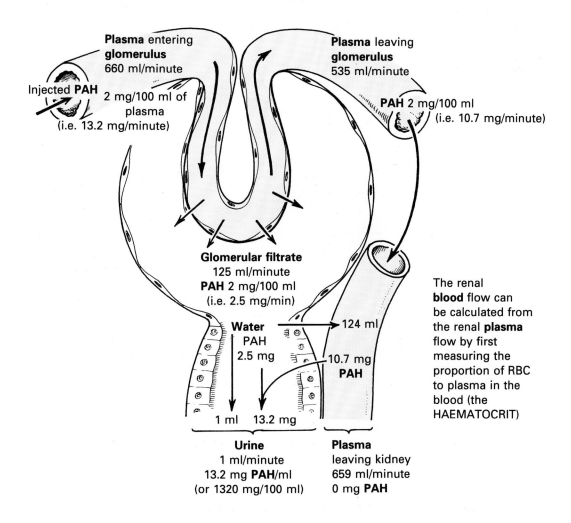

Plasma entering **glomerulus** 660 ml/minute

Injected **PAH** 2 mg/100 ml of plasma (i.e. 13.2 mg/minute)

Plasma leaving **glomerulus** 535 ml/minute

PAH 2 mg/100 ml (i.e. 10.7 mg/minute)

Glomerular filtrate 125 ml/minute **PAH** 2 mg/100 ml (i.e. 2.5 mg/min)

Water PAH 2.5 mg

124 ml

10.7 mg **PAH**

1 ml   13.2 mg

Urine 1 ml/minute 13.2 mg **PAH**/ml (or 1320 mg/100 ml)

Plasma leaving kidney 659 ml/minute 0 mg **PAH**

The renal **blood** flow can be calculated from the renal **plasma** flow by first measuring the proportion of RBC to plasma in the blood (the HAEMATOCRIT)

Complete clearance of **PAH** from plasma in one passage through normal kidney gauges not only glomerular filtrating power but also the efficiency of the tubular epithelium to secrete.

URINARY BLADDER AND URETERS

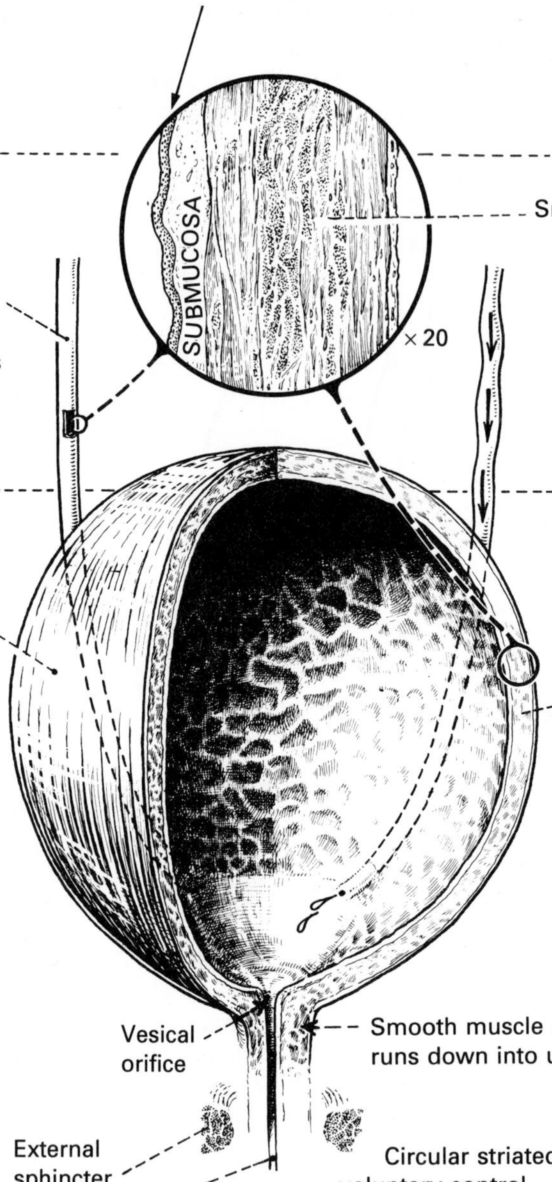

A resistant, distensible **transitional epithelium** lines all urinary passages.

URETERS - - - - - - -
Long, narrow
muscular
tubes
with outer
fibrous tissue
coat and
inner mucous
membrane

SUBMUCOSA

× 20

- - - **convey urine from
kidneys to bladder**.
Smooth muscle coats – slow
waves of contraction
(every 10 seconds) propel
urine along ureter.
1–5 small 'spurts' enter
bladder per minute.

BLADDER - - - - - -
Hollow
muscular
organ

- - - **acts as reservoir for
urine**.
[Size and position vary
with amount of urine stored
(120–320 cc).]

Smooth muscle coats –
distend as urine collects;
contract periodically to
expel urine to urethra.

Vesical
orifice

- - Smooth muscle of bladder wall
runs down into urethra.

External
sphincter

Circular striated muscle (under
voluntary control – central nervous
system)

URETHRA <- -
Membranous tube

**conveys urine to
exterior**.

STORAGE AND EXPULSION OF URINE

Urine is formed continuously by the kidneys. It collects, drop by drop, in the urinary bladder which expands to hold about 300 ml. When the bladder is full the desire to void urine is experienced.

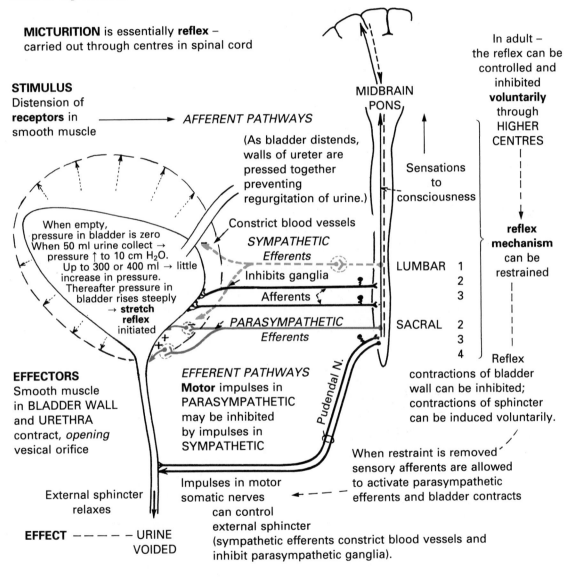

MICTURITION is essentially **reflex** – carried out through centres in spinal cord

In adult –
the reflex can be controlled and inhibited **voluntarily** through HIGHER CENTRES

STIMULUS
Distension of **receptors** in smooth muscle

AFFERENT PATHWAYS

(As bladder distends, walls of ureter are pressed together preventing regurgitation of urine.)

MIDBRAIN PONS

Sensations to consciousness

reflex mechanism can be restrained

When empty, pressure in bladder is zero
When 50 ml urine collect → pressure ↑ to 10 cm H₂O.
Up to 300 or 400 ml → little increase in pressure.
Thereafter pressure in bladder rises steeply → **stretch reflex** initiated

Constrict blood vessels
SYMPATHETIC Efferents
Inhibits ganglia
Afferents
PARASYMPATHETIC Efferents

LUMBAR 1
        2
        3

SACRAL 2
        3
        4

Reflex contractions of bladder wall can be inhibited; contractions of sphincter can be induced voluntarily.

EFFECTORS
Smooth muscle in BLADDER WALL and URETHRA contract, *opening* vesical orifice

EFFERENT PATHWAYS
Motor impulses in PARASYMPATHETIC may be inhibited by impulses in SYMPATHETIC

Pudendal N.

When restraint is removed sensory afferents are allowed to activate parasympathetic efferents and bladder contracts

External sphincter relaxes

EFFECT – – – – URINE VOIDED

Impulses in motor somatic nerves can control external sphincter (sympathetic efferents constrict blood vessels and inhibit parasympathetic ganglia).

When bladder is empty and beginning to fill –
Inhibition of parasympathetic
Activation of sympathetic } Relaxation of bladder wall.

URINE

VOLUME: In **adult**
1000–1500 ml/24 hours

SPECIFIC GRAVITY: 1.010–1.035

} Vary with fluid intake and with fluid output from other routes – skin, lungs, gut.
[Volume reduced during sleep and muscular exercise:
specific gravity greater on protein diet.]

REACTION: Usually slightly acid – (pH 4.5–8)

Varies with diet
[acid on ordinary mixed diet: alkaline on vegetarian diet].

COLOUR:
Yellow due to **urochrome** pigment – probably from destruction of tissue protein.
More concentrated and **darker** in early morning – less water excreted at night but unchanged amounts of urinary solids.

ODOUR:
Aromatic when fresh → **ammoniacal** on standing due to bacterial decomposition of **urea** to **ammonia**.

COMPOSITION

Water --- 1000–1500 ml/24 h

Inorganic substances millimoles excreted in 24 h

Sodium -------- 200
Chloride -------- 200
Calcium ---------- 5
Potassium ------- 50
Phosphates ------ 25
Sulphates -------- 50

[These figures are approximate and vary widely in healthy individuals]

Organic substances

Urea ----------- 400 -- derived from breakdown of protein – therefore varies with protein in diet.
Uric Acid -------- 4 -- comes from purine of food and body tissues.
Creatinine ------- 10 -- from breakdown of body tissues; uninfluenced by amount of dietary protein.
Ammonia -------- 40 -- formed in kidney from glutamine brought to it by blood stream; varies with amounts of acid substances requiring neutralization in the kidney.

[In the **newborn**, volume and specific gravity are low and composition varies.]

ENDOCRINE SYSTEM

ENDOCRINE SYSTEM

The **DUCTLESS GLANDS** produce **hormones** ('chemical messengers') which they pass into the **blood stream** for **general circulation** to excite or inhibit the activity of other organs or tissues.

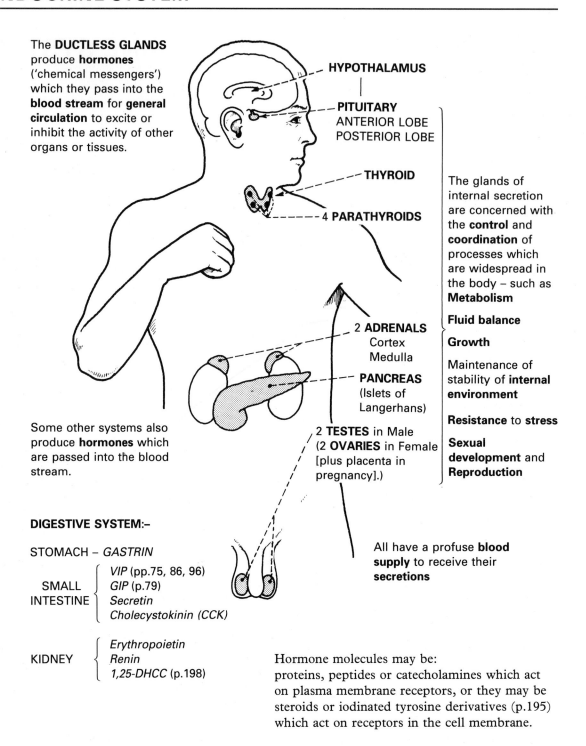

HYPOTHALAMUS

PITUITARY
ANTERIOR LOBE
POSTERIOR LOBE

THYROID

4 **PARATHYROIDS**

The glands of internal secretion are concerned with the **control** and **coordination** of processes which are widespread in the body – such as **Metabolism**

Fluid balance

Growth

Maintenance of stability of **internal environment**

Resistance to **stress**

Sexual development and **Reproduction**

2 **ADRENALS**
Cortex
Medulla

PANCREAS
(Islets of Langerhans)

2 **TESTES** in Male
(2 **OVARIES** in Female
[plus placenta in pregnancy].)

Some other systems also produce **hormones** which are passed into the blood stream.

All have a profuse **blood supply** to receive their **secretions**

DIGESTIVE SYSTEM:–

STOMACH – *GASTRIN*

SMALL
INTESTINE
{ *VIP* (pp.75, 86, 96)
GIP (p.79)
Secretin
Cholecystokinin (CCK)

KIDNEY
{ *Erythropoietin*
Renin
1,25-DHCC (p.198)

Hormone molecules may be: proteins, peptides or catecholamines which act on plasma membrane receptors, or they may be steroids or iodinated tyrosine derivatives (p.195) which act on receptors in the cell membrane.

THYROID

STRUCTURE:

2 LOBES (joined by ISTHMUS) composed of

lie in
front of
TRACHEA

FOLLICLES
lined by
CUBICAL
EPITHELIUM

(NO DUCTS)

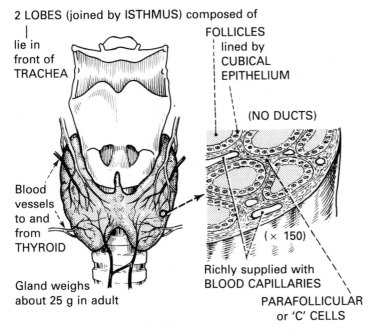

Blood
vessels
to and
from
THYROID

Gland weighs
about 25 g in adult

(× 150)

Richly supplied with
BLOOD CAPILLARIES

PARAFOLLICULAR
or 'C' CELLS

FUNCTION:

Cubical epithelium extracts from the blood stream and concentrates *IODIDE* (**iodide trapping**)

$\downarrow \leftarrow$ oxidised by peroxidase

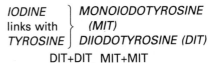

IODINE
links with
TYROSINE

MONOIODOTYROSINE (MIT)
DIIODOTYROSINE (DIT)

DIT+DIT   MIT+MIT

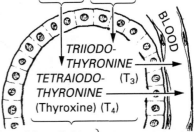

*TRIIODO-
THYRONINE*   (T_3)
*TETRAIODO-
THYRONINE*
(Thyroxine) (T_4)

BLOOD

Stored in colloid
linked with protein
THYROGLOBULIN

*when required
a protein-splitting
enzyme releases*
T_3 and T_4

REGULATION OF SECRETION:

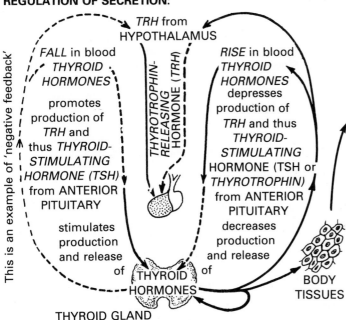

TRH from
HYPOTHALAMUS

FALL in blood
*THYROID
HORMONES*

promotes
production of
TRH and
thus *THYROID-
STIMULATING
HORMONE (TSH)*
from ANTERIOR
PITUITARY

stimulates
production
and release
of

THYROTROPHIN-
RELEASING
HORMONE (TRH)

RISE in blood
*THYROID
HORMONES*
depresses
production of
TRH and thus
*THYROID-
STIMULATING
HORMONE (TSH or
THYROTROPHIN)*
from ANTERIOR
PITUITARY
decreases
production
and release
of

This is an example of 'negative feedback'

THYROID
HORMONES

THYROID GLAND

BODY
TISSUES

T_3 and T_4 are carried by the blood to all body tissues. T_4 is usually converted in the cell cytoplasm to T_3 which binds to receptors in the **nuclei**. This complex binds to DNA and increases specific genes which increase mRNA and ribosomal RNA and hence protein synthesis. **Oxygen consumption, heat production** and **metabolism** are increased. Normal thyroid output is required for normal **growth**.

(**Parafollicular** cells secrete calcitonin – which **lowers blood calcium** by suppressing calcium mobilization from bone and by increasing **calcium excretion** in the urine.)

Increased O_2 consumption is due to an increase in the size and number of mitochondria, in Na^+, K^+-ATPase activity and the rates of glucose and fatty acid oxidation and synthesis.

UNDERACTIVITY OF THYROID

If the thyroid shows atrophy or destruction of its secretory cells or is inadequately stimulated, the syndrome of hypothyroidism develops because of lack of thyrotrophin-releasing hormone from the hypothalamus or thyroid-stimulating hormone from the anterior pituitary.

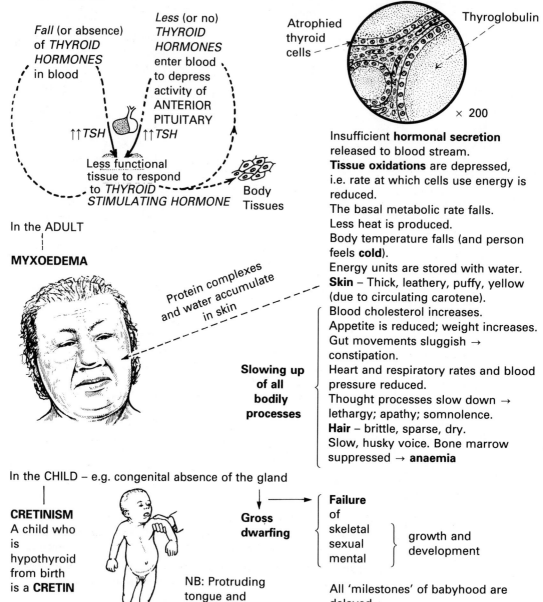

Fall (or absence) of *THYROID HORMONES* in blood

Less (or no) *THYROID HORMONES* enter blood to depress activity of ANTERIOR PITUITARY

↑↑*TSH*   ↑↑*TSH*

Less functional tissue to respond to *THYROID STIMULATING HORMONE*

Body Tissues

Atrophied thyroid cells

Thyroglobulin

× 200

Insufficient **hormonal secretion** released to blood stream.
Tissue oxidations are depressed, i.e. rate at which cells use energy is reduced.
The basal metabolic rate falls.
Less heat is produced.
Body temperature falls (and person feels **cold**).
Energy units are stored with water.
Skin – Thick, leathery, puffy, yellow (due to circulating carotene).
Blood cholesterol increases.
Appetite is reduced; weight increases.
Gut movements sluggish → constipation.
Heart and respiratory rates and blood pressure reduced.
Thought processes slow down → lethargy; apathy; somnolence.
Hair – brittle, sparse, dry.
Slow, husky voice. Bone marrow suppressed → **anaemia**

In the ADULT

MYXOEDEMA

Protein complexes and water accumulate in skin

Slowing up of all bodily processes

In the CHILD – e.g. congenital absence of the gland

CRETINISM
A child who is hypothyroid from birth is a **CRETIN**

NB: Protruding tongue and pot belly.

Gross dwarfing

Failure of skeletal sexual mental } growth and development

All 'milestones' of babyhood are delayed.

THYROXINE (taken by mouth) restores individuals to normal.

OVERACTIVITY OF THYROID

Commonest form is **Graves' disease**. Produces increased thyroid hormone secretion (**thyrotoxicosis**), enlarged thyroid (**goitre**) and protrusion of eyeballs (**exophthalmos**). The disease is caused by production of antibodies against the person's own thyroid cells (i.e. an autoimmune disease). These antibodies, *thyroid-stimulating immunoglobulins (TSI)*, act like *thyroid-stimulating hormone (TSH)* and release thyroid hormones (T_3 and T_4).

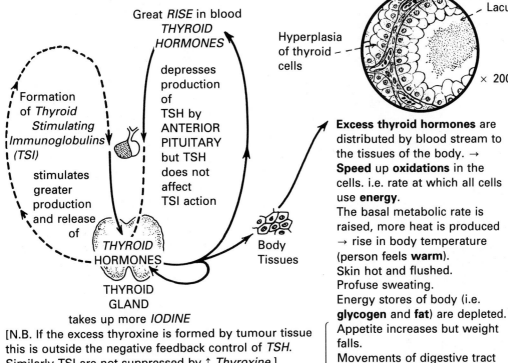

Great *RISE* in blood *THYROID HORMONES*

depresses production of TSH by ANTERIOR PITUITARY but TSH does not affect TSI action

Formation of *Thyroid Stimulating Immunoglobulins (TSI)*

stimulates greater production and release of

THYROID HORMONES

THYROID GLAND
takes up more *IODINE*

Hyperplasia of thyroid cells

Lacunae

× 200

Body Tissues

[N.B. If the excess thyroxine is formed by tumour tissue this is outside the negative feedback control of *TSH*. Similarly TSI are not suppressed by ↑ *Thyroxine*.]

Excess thyroid hormones are distributed by blood stream to the tissues of the body. →
Speed up **oxidations** in the cells. i.e. rate at which all cells use **energy**.
The basal metabolic rate is raised, more heat is produced → rise in body temperature (person feels **warm**).
Skin hot and flushed.
Profuse sweating.
Energy stores of body (i.e. **glycogen** and **fat**) are depleted.
Appetite increases but weight falls.
Movements of digestive tract are increased → diarrhoea.
Heart and respiratory rates rise.
Blood pressure is raised. A fine muscular tremor and nervousness are marked.
Person becomes excitable, irritable and apprehensive.

Speeding up of all bodily processes

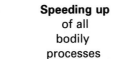

Goitre

CVS symptoms very important. T_3 and T_4 increase cAMP and number of β adrenergic receptors in heart, thus increase heart's sensitivity to *adrenaline*. Blocked by β-receptor blocking agents.

[**Exophthalmos** (protrusion of eyeballs) may be due to an action of an antibody against a protein of the extraocular muscles and the connective tissue behind the eye which causes these tissues to swell. It is not due to an excess of thyroid hormones.]

Surgical removal of part or all of the overactive gland or destruction by radioactive iodine reduces the thyroid activity.

PARATHYROIDS

Four small glands composed of cords of chief cells which secrete a peptide –
parathyroid hormone – **parathormone or PTH**

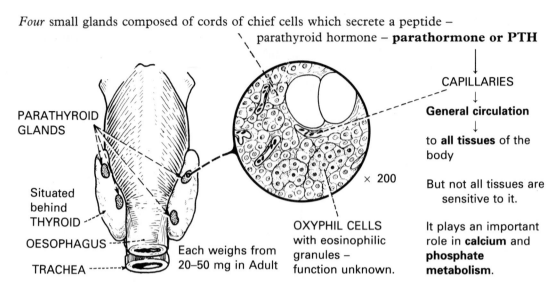

CAPILLARIES

General circulation

to **all tissues** of the body

But not all tissues are sensitive to it.

It plays an important role in **calcium** and **phosphate metabolism**.

PARATHYROID GLANDS

Situated behind THYROID

OESOPHAGUS

TRACHEA

Each weighs from 20–50 mg in Adult

OXYPHIL CELLS with eosinophilic granules – function unknown.

× 200

Three hormones, *parathormone, 1, 25-dihydroxycholecalciferol* (1,25-DHCC) and *calcitonin* act on **kidney** and **gut** to keep blood ionized **calcium** constant (necessary for normal nerve and muscle excitability, blood coagulation and formation of bone and teeth).

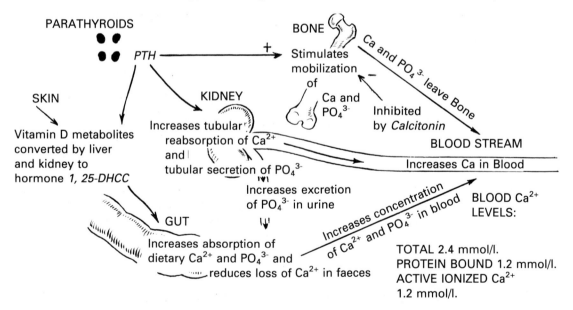

PARATHYROIDS

PTH

BONE

Stimulates mobilization of Ca and PO_4^{3-}

Ca and PO_4^{3-} leave Bone

Inhibited by *Calcitonin*

SKIN

Vitamin D metabolites converted by liver and kidney to hormone *1, 25-DHCC*

KIDNEY

Increases tubular reabsorption of Ca^{2+} and tubular secretion of PO_4^{3-}

Increases excretion of PO_4^{3-} in urine

BLOOD STREAM

Increases Ca in Blood

Increases concentration of Ca^{2+} and PO_4^{3-} in blood

BLOOD Ca^{2+} LEVELS:

GUT

Increases absorption of dietary Ca^{2+} and PO_4^{3-} and reduces loss of Ca^{2+} in faeces

TOTAL 2.4 mmol/l.
PROTEIN BOUND 1.2 mmol/l.
ACTIVE IONIZED Ca^{2+} 1.2 mmol/l.

In bones and kidneys PTH activates adenylate cyclase, thus increasing cAMP. **Osteoblast** cells are responsible for bone formation and differentiate into osteocytes (p.19). PTH inhibits synthesis of new bone by osteoblasts: **osteoclasts** resorb (break down) bone.

Calcium ions in extracellular fluid control parathyroid activity. $\uparrow Ca^{2+}$ depresses PTH secretion. $\downarrow Ca^{2+}$ increases PTH secretion.

UNDERACTIVITY OF PARATHYROIDS

Atrophy or removal of parathyroid tissue causes a fall in **blood calcium** level and increased excitability of neuromuscular tissue. This leads to severe convulsive disorder – **tetany**.

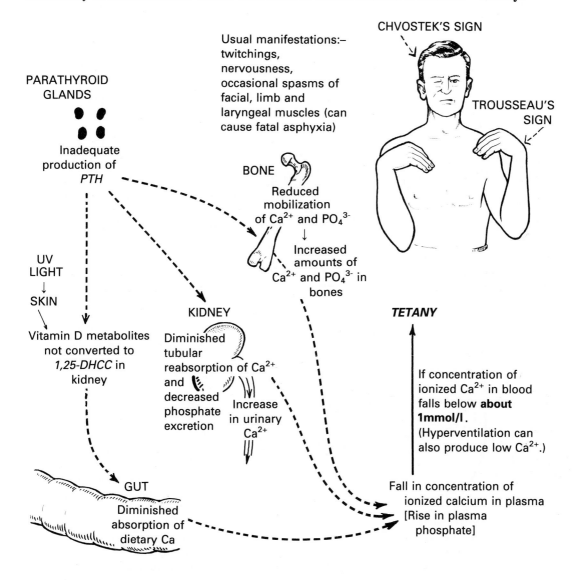

PARATHYROID
GLANDS

Inadequate
production of
PTH

Usual manifestations:–
twitchings,
nervousness,
occasional spasms of
facial, limb and
laryngeal muscles (can
cause fatal asphyxia)

CHVOSTEK'S SIGN

TROUSSEAU'S
SIGN

BONE

Reduced
mobilization
of Ca^{2+} and PO_4^{3-}

Increased
amounts of
Ca^{2+} and PO_4^{3-} in
bones

UV
LIGHT
↓
SKIN
↓
Vitamin D metabolites
not converted to
1,25-DHCC in
kidney

KIDNEY

Diminished
tubular
reabsorption of Ca^{2+}
and
decreased
phosphate
excretion

Increase
in urinary
Ca^{2+}

TETANY

If concentration of
ionized Ca^{2+} in blood
falls below **about
1mmol/l**.
(Hyperventilation can
also produce low Ca^{2+}.)

GUT

Diminished
absorption of
dietary Ca

Fall in concentration of
ionized calcium in plasma
[Rise in plasma
phosphate]

[Note the inverse relationship between plasma calcium and inorganic phosphate]

Symptoms are relieved by injection of large doses of calcium and a Vit.D compound.

OVERACTIVITY OF PARATHYROIDS

Overactivity of the parathyroids (due often to tumour) leads to rise in **blood calcium** level which may produce **renal stones**, kidney damage and perhaps **osteitis fibrosa cystica**.

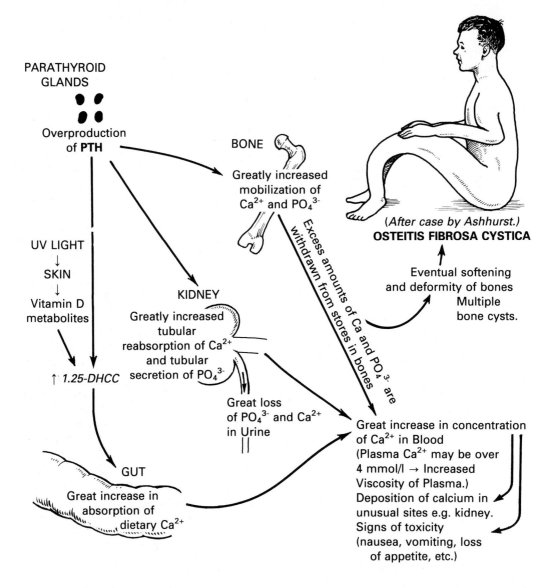

PARATHYROID
GLANDS

Overproduction
of **PTH**

UV LIGHT
↓
SKIN
↓
Vitamin D
metabolites

↑ *1.25-DHCC*

BONE
Greatly increased
mobilization of
Ca^{2+} and PO_4^{3-}

KIDNEY
Greatly increased
tubular
reabsorption of Ca^{2+}
and tubular
secretion of PO_4^{3-}

Great loss
of PO_4^{3-} and Ca^{2+}
in Urine

GUT
Great increase in
absorption of
dietary Ca^{2+}

Excess amounts of Ca and PO_4^{3-} are
withdrawn from stores in bones

(After case by Ashhurst.)
OSTEITIS FIBROSA CYSTICA

Eventual softening
and deformity of bones
Multiple
bone cysts.

Great increase in concentration
of Ca^{2+} in Blood
(Plasma Ca^{2+} may be over
4 mmol/l → Increased
Viscosity of Plasma.)
Deposition of calcium in
unusual sites e.g. kidney.
Signs of toxicity
(nausea, vomiting, loss
of appetite, etc.)

The increased level of blood calcium eventually leads to excessive loss of **calcium** in **urine** (in spite of ↑ reabsorption) and also of **water** since the salts are excreted in solution. **Polyuria, dehydration** and **thirst** result. Most cases are diagnosed before bone disease develops.

Excision of the overactive parathyroid tissue abolishes syndrome.

ADRENAL CORTEX

The adrenal cortex is essential for life. It plays an important role in states of stress.

There are *TWO* adrenal glands.
They lie close to the kidneys.

Each has an outer CORTEX
and an inner

MEDULLA

RIGHT
KIDNEY

LEFT
KIDNEY

CAPSULE
ZONA
GLOMERULOSA

ZONA
FASCICULATA

CORTEX

ZONA
RETICULARIS

MEDULLA

× 80

Secretion from the adrenal cortex is under the control of *adreno-corticotrophic hormone (ACTH, corticotrophin)* from the anterior pituitary (AP).

The adrenal cortex secretes **steroid hormones** derived from **cholesterol**. Their effects are mediated by receptors *inside* cells of all tissues of the body.
There are three classes of adrenal hormone.

1. *MINERALOCORTICOIDS*
Especially *aldosterone* but also *deoxycorticosterone*.
– chief action on **kidney tubules**.

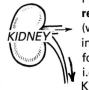
KIDNEY

Promote **retention** of Na^+ (with water) in exchange for K^+ and H^+ i.e. ↑ loss of K^+ and H^+

2. *GLUCOCORTICOIDS*
Especially *cortisol* (hydrocortisone) but also *corticosterone* causes protein catabolism

LIVER

Amino acids so formed are used to make **glucose** in **liver**. Increases **blood sugar**.

They also have anti-insulin, anti-inflammatory and anti-allergic actions; are necessary for noradrenaline and adrenaline actions; reduce circulating eosinophils.

3. *ANDROGENS* (sex hormones)
Especially *dehydroepiandrosterone* but also *androstenedione*
(Oestrogen produced from this in the circulation.)
Promote protein anabolism and growth (anabolic steroids). Have minor effects on reproductive function.

Stress acts via HYPOTHALAMUS

FALL in blood *CORTICOIDS*

corticotrophin-releasing hormone

RISE in blood *CORTICOIDS*

promotes production of *ACTH*

depresses production of *ACTH*

stimulates production and release of

CORTICOIDS

ADRENAL GLAND

Circulates bound to corticosteroid binding globulin CBG

This reciprocal relationship between A.P. and adrenal cortex leads to balanced effects on →

Na^+ balance and extracellular fluid volume

carbohydrate, fat and protein metabolism

Secretion of *aldosterone* from the zona glomerulosa is controlled not only by *ACTH* but also by (a) *Angiotensin II* released by the **renin-angiotensin system** (page 183) following blood or fluid loss and (b) increase in plasma potassium.

UNDERACTIVITY OF ADRENAL CORTEX

Atrophy of the adrenal cortex can be caused by autoimmune disease or destruction by tuberculosis or cancer. Total absence of adrenal hormones is rapidly fatal.

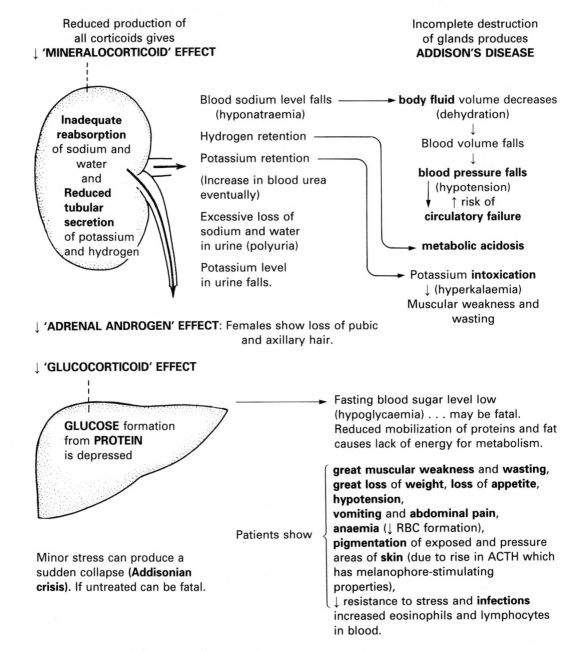

Reduced production of all corticoids gives
↓ 'MINERALOCORTICOID' EFFECT

Incomplete destruction of glands produces
ADDISON'S DISEASE

Inadequate reabsorption of sodium and water and **Reduced tubular secretion** of potassium and hydrogen

Blood sodium level falls (hyponatraemia) ⟶ **body fluid** volume decreases (dehydration)
↓
Blood volume falls
↓
blood pressure falls (hypotension)
↑ risk of **circulatory failure**

Hydrogen retention
Potassium retention
(Increase in blood urea eventually)
Excessive loss of sodium and water in urine (polyuria)
Potassium level in urine falls.

metabolic acidosis

Potassium **intoxication** ↓ (hyperkalaemia) Muscular weakness and wasting

↓ 'ADRENAL ANDROGEN' EFFECT: Females show loss of pubic and axillary hair.

↓ 'GLUCOCORTICOID' EFFECT

GLUCOSE formation from **PROTEIN** is depressed

Fasting blood sugar level low (hypoglycaemia) . . . may be fatal. Reduced mobilization of proteins and fat causes lack of energy for metabolism.

Patients show {
great muscular weakness and **wasting**, **great loss** of **weight**, **loss** of **appetite**, **hypotension**, **vomiting** and **abdominal pain**, **anaemia** (↓ RBC formation), **pigmentation** of exposed and pressure areas of **skin** (due to rise in ACTH which has melanophore-stimulating properties), ↓ resistance to stress and **infections** increased eosinophils and lymphocytes in blood.

Minor stress can produce a sudden collapse (**Addisonian crisis**). If untreated can be fatal.

Administration of *cortisol*, a synthetic mineralocorticoid, and sodium chloride restores individual to normal.

OVERACTIVITY OF ADRENAL CORTEX

Overactivity or tumour of adrenal cortex may give **excess secretion** of any or all of the corticoids:

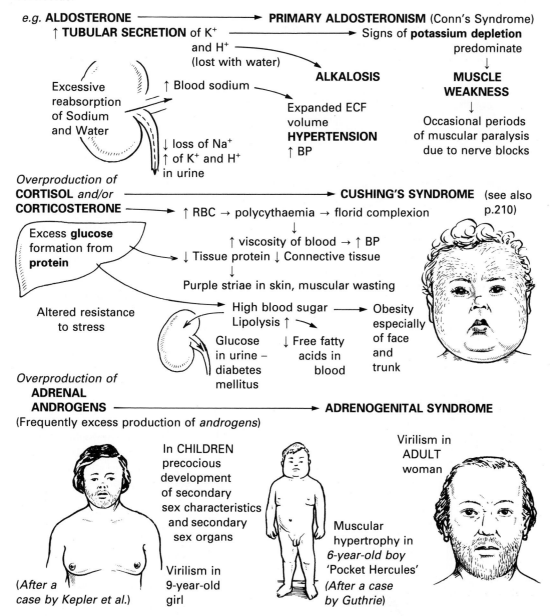

e.g. **ALDOSTERONE** ⟶ **PRIMARY ALDOSTERONISM** (Conn's Syndrome)

↑ **TUBULAR SECRETION** of K^+ ⟶ Signs of **potassium depletion** predominate

and H^+ (lost with water) ⟶ **ALKALOSIS**

↓

MUSCLE WEAKNESS

↓

Occasional periods of muscular paralysis due to nerve blocks

Excessive reabsorption of Sodium and Water

↑ Blood sodium

Expanded ECF volume **HYPERTENSION** ↑ BP

↓ loss of Na^+ ↑ of K^+ and H^+ in urine

Overproduction of **CORTISOL** *and/or* **CORTICOSTERONE** ⟶ **CUSHING'S SYNDROME** (see also p.210)

↑ RBC → polycythaemia → florid complexion

↓

↑ viscosity of blood → ↑ BP

↓ Tissue protein ↓ Connective tissue

↓

Purple striae in skin, muscular wasting

Excess **glucose** formation from **protein**

Altered resistance to stress

High blood sugar

Lipolysis ↑

Glucose in urine – diabetes mellitus

↓ Free fatty acids in blood

Obesity especially of face and trunk

Overproduction of **ADRENAL ANDROGENS** ⟶ **ADRENOGENITAL SYNDROME**

(Frequently excess production of *androgens*)

In CHILDREN precocious development of secondary sex characteristics and secondary sex organs

Virilism in 9-year-old girl

(*After a case by Kepler et al.*)

Muscular hypertrophy in *6-year-old boy* 'Pocket Hercules' (*After a case by Guthrie*)

Virilism in ADULT woman

Administration of *cortisone* depresses pituitary secretion of *ACTH* → inhibits production of the abnormal steroids.

Removal of the over-secreting tissue or tumour restores individual. In **secondary** hyperaldosteronism *excess aldosterone* is the result of *increased* **renin** and **angiotensin II** secretion.

ADRENAL MEDULLA

The adrenal medulla arises from the same primitive tissue as the postganglionic cells of the sympathetic nervous system.

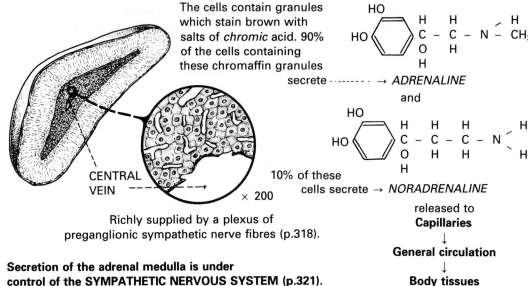

The cells contain granules which stain brown with salts of *chromic* acid. 90% of the cells containing these chromaffin granules

secrete $\cdots\cdots \to$ *ADRENALINE*

and

10% of these cells secrete $\to$ *NORADRENALINE*

released to
Capillaries
↓
General circulation
↓
Body tissues

CENTRAL VEIN

× 200

Richly supplied by a plexus of preganglionic sympathetic nerve fibres (p.318).

Secretion of the adrenal medulla is under control of the SYMPATHETIC NERVOUS SYSTEM (p.321).

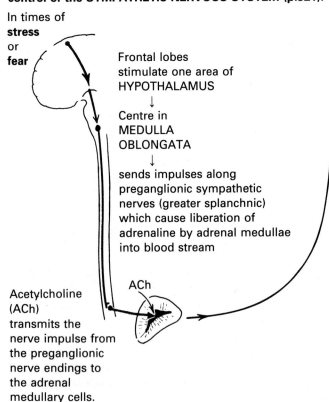

In times of
stress
or
fear

Frontal lobes stimulate one area of HYPOTHALAMUS
↓
Centre in MEDULLA OBLONGATA
↓
sends impulses along preganglionic sympathetic nerves (greater splanchnic) which cause liberation of adrenaline by adrenal medullae into blood stream

ACh

Acetylcholine (ACh) transmits the nerve impulse from the preganglionic nerve endings to the adrenal medullary cells.

Adrenaline reinforces action of sympathetic nervous system in preparing the various **systems** of the **body** to react efficiently in emergencies and stress (p.205).

There is some evidence to suggest that adrenaline and noradrenaline are released separately, e.g. stimulation of another part of the hypothalamus apparently leads to release of noradrenaline into blood stream
↓
general vasoconstriction
↓
rise in blood pressure.

ADRENALINE

Under quiet resting conditions the blood contains very little *adrenaline*. During excitement or circumstances which demand special efforts *adrenaline* is released into the blood stream, and is responsible for the following actions summed up as the **'fight or flight' function** of the adrenal medullae. These actions are produced via α and β adrenergic receptors although adrenaline has a greater affinity for β receptors than α receptors.

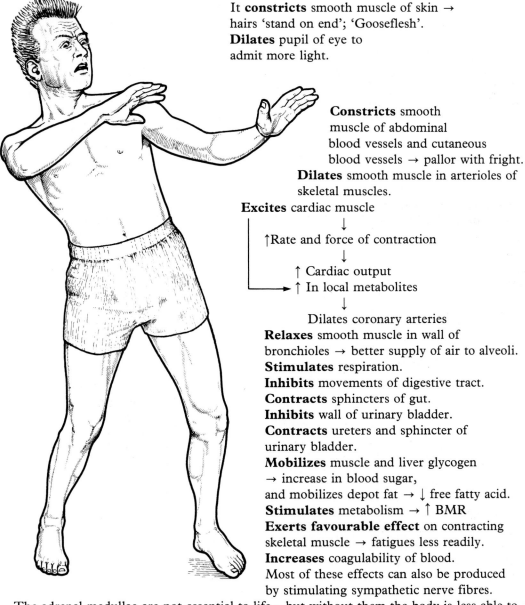

It **constricts** smooth muscle of skin →
hairs 'stand on end'; 'Gooseflesh'.
Dilates pupil of eye to
admit more light.

Constricts smooth
muscle of abdominal
blood vessels and cutaneous
blood vessels → pallor with fright.
Dilates smooth muscle in arterioles of
skeletal muscles.
Excites cardiac muscle
↓
↑Rate and force of contraction
↓
↑ Cardiac output
↑ In local metabolites
↓
Dilates coronary arteries
Relaxes smooth muscle in wall of
bronchioles → better supply of air to alveoli.
Stimulates respiration.
Inhibits movements of digestive tract.
Contracts sphincters of gut.
Inhibits wall of urinary bladder.
Contracts ureters and sphincter of
urinary bladder.
Mobilizes muscle and liver glycogen
→ increase in blood sugar,
and mobilizes depot fat → ↓ free fatty acid.
Stimulates metabolism → ↑ BMR
Exerts favourable effect on contracting
skeletal muscle → fatigues less readily.
Increases coagulability of blood.
Most of these effects can also be produced
by stimulating sympathetic nerve fibres.

The adrenal medullae are not essential to life – but without them the body is less able to face emergencies and conditions of stress.

DEVELOPMENT OF PITUITARY

The pituitary gland consists of **anterior, intermediate** and **posterior** parts which differ in **origin, structure** and **function**.

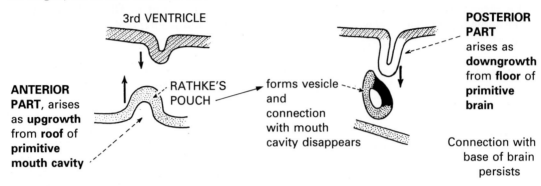

ANTERIOR PART, arises as **upgrowth** from **roof** of **primitive mouth cavity**

3rd VENTRICLE

RATHKE'S POUCH → forms vesicle and connection with mouth cavity disappears

POSTERIOR PART arises as **downgrowth** from **floor** of **primitive brain**

Connection with base of brain persists

The **two parts meet and fuse**

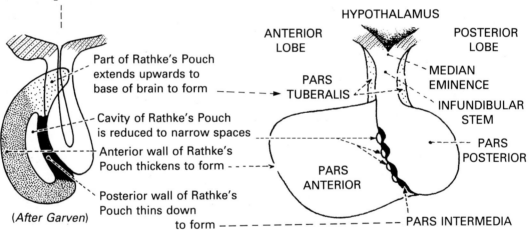

Part of Rathke's Pouch extends upwards to base of brain to form – – – – – ▶ PARS TUBERALIS

Cavity of Rathke's Pouch is reduced to narrow spaces

Anterior wall of Rathke's Pouch thickens to form – – – – ▶ PARS ANTERIOR

Posterior wall of Rathke's Pouch thins down to form – – – – – – – – – – – – PARS INTERMEDIA

(*After Garven*)

HYPOTHALAMUS

ANTERIOR LOBE

POSTERIOR LOBE

MEDIAN EMINENCE

INFUNDIBULAR STEM

PARS POSTERIOR

Pars tuberalis + infundibular stem = **infundibulum** or **pituitary stalk**.
Neurohypophysis = pars posterior (posterior or neural lobe) + infundibular stem + median eminence.
Adenohypophysis = pars anterior (pars distalis or glandularis) + pars tuberalis (pars intermedia is also sometimes included).
The **adult pituitary (hypophysis)** is a small (8 × 12 mm) oval gland which lies in the **Sella Turcica** – a small cavity in the bone at the base of the skull. It weighs only 500 mg but, along with the adjacent hypothalamus, it exerts a major control over endocrine function. Their close interdependence has resulted in the adoption of the term '**hypothalamo-hypophysial system**'.

ANTERIOR PITUITARY

This is the **master gland** of the **endocrine system**. It regulates the activity of other endocrine glands, including the gonads, and influences **all metabolic processes** including **growth**.

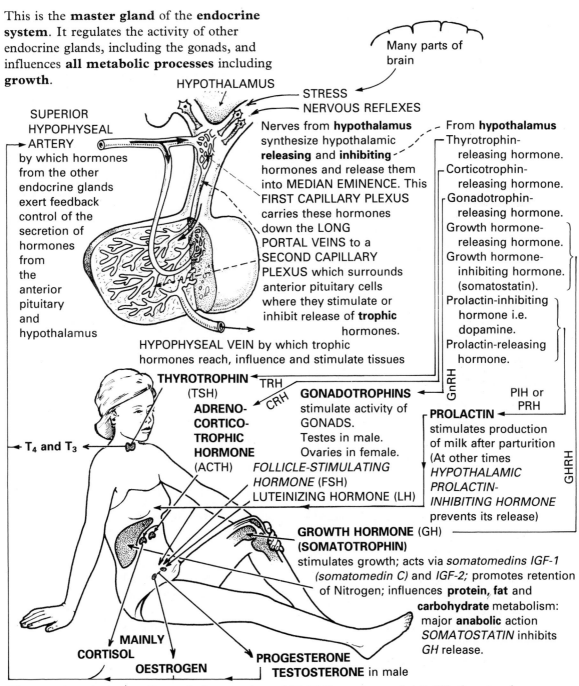

Many parts of brain

HYPOTHALAMUS

STRESS
NERVOUS REFLEXES

SUPERIOR HYPOPHYSEAL ARTERY by which hormones from the other endocrine glands exert feedback control of the secretion of hormones from the anterior pituitary and hypothalamus

Nerves from **hypothalamus** synthesize hypothalamic **releasing** and **inhibiting** hormones and release them into MEDIAN EMINENCE. This FIRST CAPILLARY PLEXUS carries these hormones down the LONG PORTAL VEINS to a SECOND CAPILLARY PLEXUS which surrounds anterior pituitary cells where they stimulate or inhibit release of **trophic** hormones.

From **hypothalamus**
Thyrotrophin-releasing hormone.
Corticotrophin-releasing hormone.
Gonadotrophin-releasing hormone.
Growth hormone-releasing hormone.
Growth hormone-inhibiting hormone. (somatostatin).
Prolactin-inhibiting hormone i.e. dopamine.
Prolactin-releasing hormone.

HYPOPHYSEAL VEIN by which trophic hormones reach, influence and stimulate tissues

THYROTROPHIN (TSH)

TRH
CRH

GnRH

PIH or PRH

ADRENO-CORTICO-TROPHIC HORMONE (ACTH)

GONADOTROPHINS stimulate activity of GONADS. Testes in male. Ovaries in female. *FOLLICLE-STIMULATING HORMONE* (FSH) LUTEINIZING HORMONE (LH)

PROLACTIN stimulates production of milk after parturition (At other times *HYPOTHALAMIC PROLACTIN-INHIBITING HORMONE* prevents its release)

GHRH

T_4 and T_3

GROWTH HORMONE (GH) (SOMATOTROPHIN) stimulates growth; acts via *somatomedins IGF-1 (somatomedin C)* and *IGF-2;* promotes retention of Nitrogen; influences **protein, fat** and **carbohydrate** metabolism: major **anabolic** action *SOMATOSTATIN* inhibits *GH* release.

MAINLY CORTISOL
OESTROGEN
PROGESTERONE
TESTOSTERONE in male

The anterior pituitary cell population consists of 15-20% corticotrophs, 3-5% thyrotrophs, 10-15% gonadotrophs, 40-50% somatotrophs, 10-25% mammotrophs; identified by immunohistochemistry. (*IGF-1 = insulin-like growth factor I*).

207

UNDERACTIVITY OF ANTERIOR PITUITARY

Deficiency or absence
of **somatotroph** cells
↓
Underproduction of *growth
hormone (somatotrophin)*
↓
PITUITARY DWARF
(Lorain Dwarf)
Delayed skeletal
growth and
retarded sexual
development
but alert, intelligent,
well proportioned
child.

Destructive disease of part of anterior
pituitary (usually with damage to
posterior pituitary and/or hypothalamus)
↓
Underproduction of *growth* and other
endocrine-trophic hormones
↓
FRÖHLICH'S DWARF

Stunting of growth,
obesity (large
appetite for sugar);
arrested sexual
development;
lethargic;
somnolent;
mentally
subnormal.

If atrophy of
other
endocrine
glands
↓
Signs of
deficiency
of their
hormones.

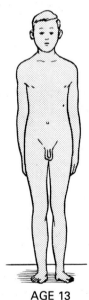

AGE 13

NORMAL CHILD
AGE 13

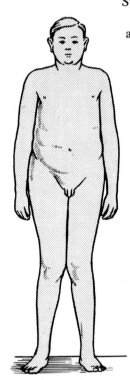

AGE 13

Replacement therapy
restores growth and
development pattern
to normal.

Short stature of Pygmies
is due to a genetic defect
which prevents *IGF-1* being
produced by *growth hormone.*

In the **LARON syndrome** *GH*
levels are normal but *IGF-1*
levels are low.

A similar condition occurs in adults
without dwarfing but with suppression
of sex functions and regression of
secondary sex characterics.

Growth and *gonadotrophic hormones*
aid in restoring patient to normal.

OVERACTIVITY OF PITUITARY SOMATOTROPH CELLS

Functional overactivity (or tumour) chiefly of the **SOMATOTROPH** cells of the anterior pituitary
leads to ⟶ **GIANTISM** in the CHILD: **ACROMEGALY** in the ADULT.

Overproduction of *growth Hormone*

↑ *IGF-1 (somatomedin C)*

Stimulates protein synthesis.
Influences carbohydrate and
fat metabolism and mitosis
of **ALL CELLS** of the body

Overgrowth of all body tissues

Onset before
bony epiphyses have
closed at puberty

Onset after puberty

Bones thicken
especially of
**face, jaw, ⟶
nose, hands**
and **feet**

Long bones
grow in length
(Height 7–8 feet)
Overgrowth of
MUSCLES

Overgrowth of
SOFT TISSUES ⟶
| and
INTERNAL ORGANS
(e.g. Heart,
Spleen,
Stomach,
etc.)

Coarse thick
SKIN

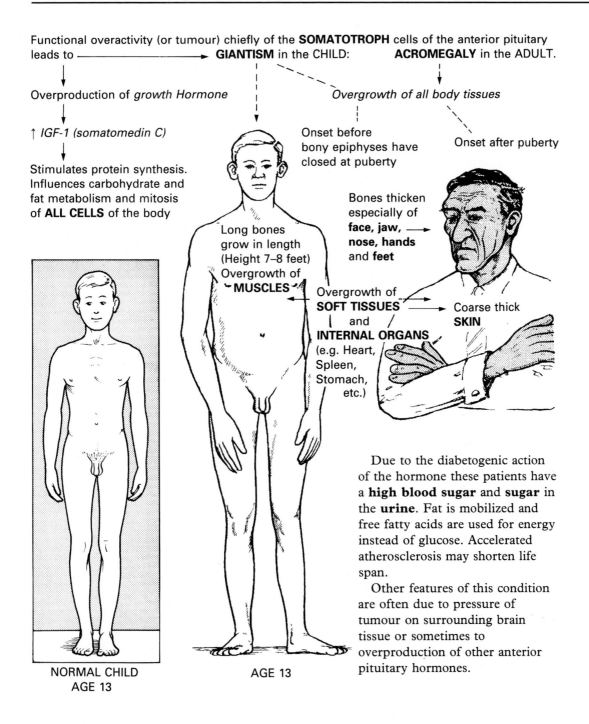

NORMAL CHILD
AGE 13

AGE 13

Due to the diabetogenic action
of the hormone these patients have
a **high blood sugar** and **sugar** in
the **urine**. Fat is mobilized and
free fatty acids are used for energy
instead of glucose. Accelerated
atherosclerosis may shorten life
span.

Other features of this condition
are often due to pressure of
tumour on surrounding brain
tissue or sometimes to
overproduction of other anterior
pituitary hormones.

Destruction of the overactive tissue – usually by surgery or radiation therapy – prevents
progress of the condition.

OVERACTIVITY OF PITUITARY CORTICOTROPH CELLS

Overactivity (often due to tumour) of the **corticotroph** cells of the anterior pituitary gives

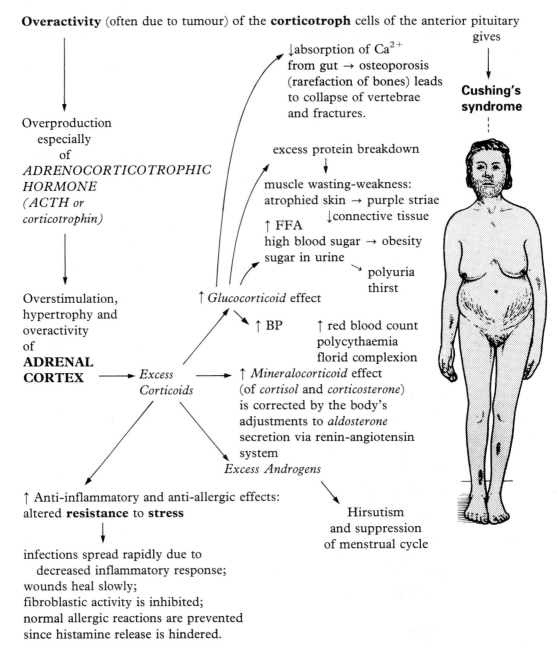

Overproduction
  especially
    of
*ADRENOCORTICOTROPHIC
HORMONE
(ACTH or
corticotrophin)*

↓absorption of Ca^{2+}
from gut → osteoporosis
(rarefaction of bones) leads
to collapse of vertebrae
and fractures.

**Cushing's
syndrome**

excess protein breakdown

muscle wasting-weakness:
atrophied skin → purple striae
  ↓connective tissue
↑ FFA
high blood sugar → obesity
sugar in urine
  ⟶ polyuria
    thirst

Overstimulation,
hypertrophy and
overactivity
of
**ADRENAL
CORTEX** ⟶ *Excess
Corticoids* ⟶

↑ *Glucocorticoid* effect

↑ BP   ↑ red blood count
    polycythaemia
    florid complexion

↑ *Mineralocorticoid* effect
(of *cortisol* and *corticosterone*)
is corrected by the body's
adjustments to *aldosterone*
secretion via renin-angiotensin
system

Excess Androgens

↑ Anti-inflammatory and anti-allergic effects:
altered **resistance** to **stress**

Hirsutism
and suppression
of menstrual cycle

infections spread rapidly due to
  decreased inflammatory response;
wounds heal slowly;
fibroblastic activity is inhibited;
normal allergic reactions are prevented
since histamine release is hindered.

  This condition is usually indistinguishable clinically from that seen in primary
overactivity or tumour of the **adrenal cortex** itself. It can be produced by
administration of large doses of *glucocorticoids*.
  The syndrome is shown here in the adult woman.

Overproduction of thyroid stimulating hormone → Overactivity of thyroid gland.

PANHYPOPITUITARISM

Complete atrophy (or insufficiency) of all secreting cells of anterior pituitary in adult
produces **SIMMOND'S DISEASE**

Appearance of premature senility

Failure to
**produce
any hormones** ⟶ Features usually
associated with
very **old age**

Lack of
growth hormone
Grave upset in
tissue metabolism ⟶ { **Hair** grey, sparse:
loss of body hair.
Skin dry, sallow,
wrinkled.
Body emaciated
(great loss of weight)
Bones frail

Lack of
gonadotrophins ⟶ **Sex organs** atrophy.
Menstruation ceases.
Reproductive cycle stops.
Secondary sex characteristics
gradually regress.

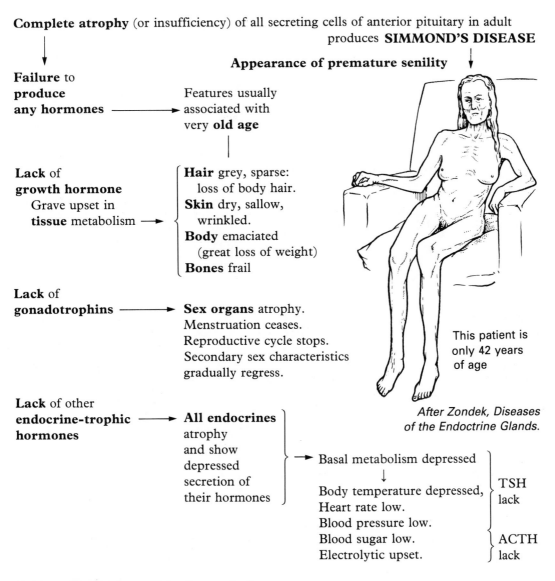

This patient is
only 42 years
of age

*After Zondek, Diseases
of the Endoctrine Glands.*

Lack of other
endocrine-trophic ⟶ **All endocrines**
hormones atrophy
and show
depressed
secretion of
their hormones

⟶ Basal metabolism depressed
↓
Body temperature depressed,   } **TSH**
Heart rate low.   lack
Blood pressure low.
Blood sugar low.   } **ACTH**
Electrolytic upset.   } lack

Subject may die due to lack of control of
metabolism. If less severe, symptoms of lack of only
one or two pituitary hormones may predominate.

Anterior pituitary hormones may relieve the condition but rarely succeed in completely
restoring the patient to normal.

211

POSTERIOR PITUITARY

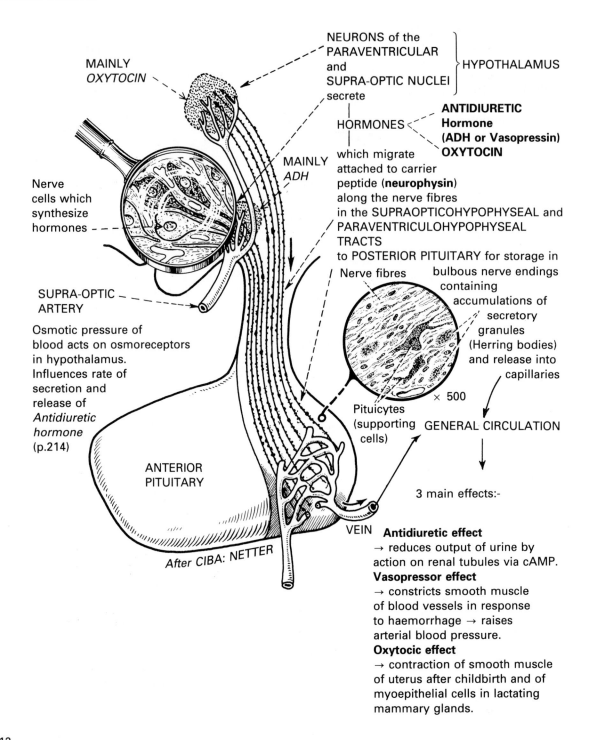

MAINLY
OXYTOCIN

NEURONS of the
PARAVENTRICULAR
and
SUPRA-OPTIC NUCLEI } HYPOTHALAMUS

secrete

HORMONES {
ANTIDIURETIC
Hormone
(ADH or Vasopressin)
OXYTOCIN

MAINLY
ADH

which migrate
attached to carrier
peptide (**neurophysin**)
along the nerve fibres
in the SUPRAOPTICOHYPOPHYSEAL and
PARAVENTRICULOHYPOPHYSEAL
TRACTS
to POSTERIOR PITUITARY for storage in
bulbous nerve endings
containing
accumulations of
secretory
granules
(Herring bodies)
and release into
capillaries

Nerve fibres

Nerve
cells which
synthesize
hormones – – –

SUPRA-OPTIC
ARTERY

Osmotic pressure of
blood acts on osmoreceptors
in hypothalamus.
Influences rate of
secretion and
release of
Antidiuretic
hormone
(p.214)

ANTERIOR
PITUITARY

× 500

Pituicytes
(supporting
cells)

GENERAL CIRCULATION

VEIN

After CIBA: NETTER

3 main effects:-

Antidiuretic effect
→ reduces output of urine by
action on renal tubules via cAMP.
Vasopressor effect
→ constricts smooth muscle
of blood vessels in response
to haemorrhage → raises
arterial blood pressure.
Oxytocic effect
→ contraction of smooth muscle
of uterus after childbirth and of
myoepithelial cells in lactating
mammary glands.

OXYTOCIN

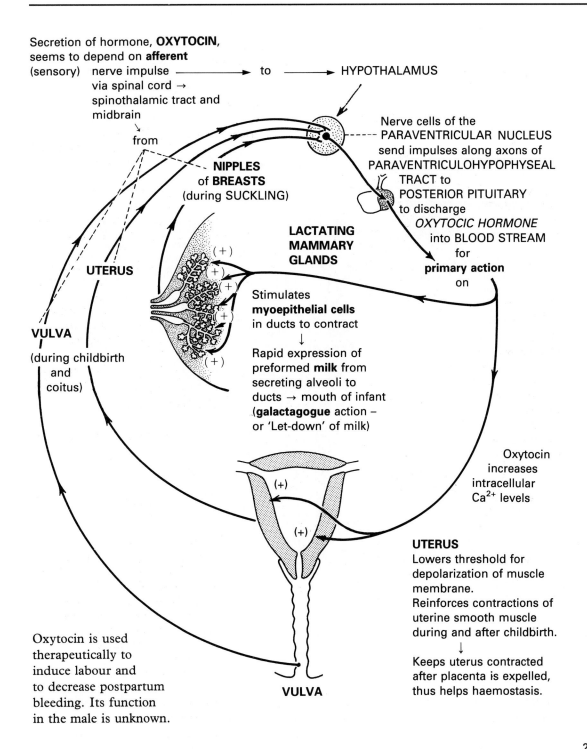

Secretion of hormone, **OXYTOCIN**, seems to depend on **afferent** (sensory) nerve impulse ⟶ to ⟶ HYPOTHALAMUS via spinal cord → spinothalamic tract and midbrain

from

Nerve cells of the PARAVENTRICULAR NUCLEUS send impulses along axons of PARAVENTRICULOHYPOPHYSEAL TRACT to POSTERIOR PITUITARY to discharge *OXYTOCIC HORMONE* into BLOOD STREAM for **primary action** on

NIPPLES of **BREASTS** (during SUCKLING)

LACTATING MAMMARY GLANDS

(+) (+) (+) (+) (+)

Stimulates **myoepithelial cells** in ducts to contract
↓
Rapid expression of preformed **milk** from secreting alveoli to ducts → mouth of infant (**galactagogue** action – or 'Let-down' of milk)

UTERUS

VULVA
(during childbirth and coitus)

(+)

(+)

Oxytocin increases intracellular Ca^{2+} levels

VULVA

UTERUS
Lowers threshold for depolarization of muscle membrane.
Reinforces contractions of uterine smooth muscle during and after childbirth.
↓
Keeps uterus contracted after placenta is expelled, thus helps haemostasis.

Oxytocin is used therapeutically to induce labour and to decrease postpartum bleeding. Its function in the male is unknown.

ANTIDIURETIC HORMONE (ADH)

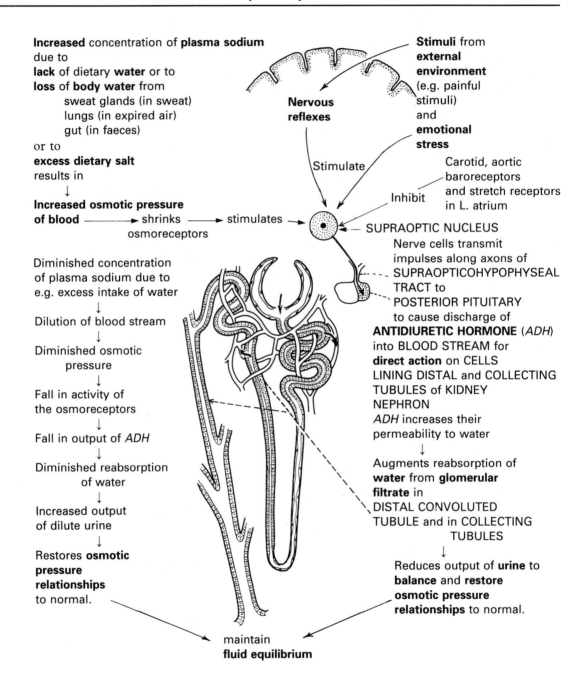

Increased concentration of **plasma sodium**
due to
lack of dietary **water** or to
loss of **body water** from
    sweat glands (in sweat)
    lungs (in expired air)
    gut (in faeces)
or to
excess dietary salt
results in
↓
**Increased osmotic pressure
of blood** ⟶ shrinks ⟶ stimulates ⟶
    osmoreceptors

**Nervous
reflexes**

Stimulate

Stimuli from
**external
environment**
(e.g. painful
stimuli)
and
**emotional
stress**

Carotid, aortic
baroreceptors
and stretch receptors
in L. atrium

Inhibit

— SUPRAOPTIC NUCLEUS
Nerve cells transmit
impulses along axons of
SUPRAOPTICOHYPOPHYSEAL
TRACT to
POSTERIOR PITUITARY
to cause discharge of
ANTIDIURETIC HORMONE (*ADH*)
into BLOOD STREAM for
direct action on CELLS
LINING DISTAL and COLLECTING
TUBULES of KIDNEY
NEPHRON
ADH increases their
permeability to water
↓
Augments reabsorption of
water from **glomerular
filtrate** in
DISTAL CONVOLUTED
TUBULE and in COLLECTING
    TUBULES
↓
Reduces output of **urine** to
balance and **restore
osmotic pressure
relationships** to normal.

Diminished concentration
of plasma sodium due to
e.g. excess intake of water
↓
Dilution of blood stream
↓
Diminished osmotic
    pressure
↓
Fall in activity of
the osmoreceptors
↓
Fall in output of *ADH*
↓
Diminished reabsorption
    of water
↓
Increased output
of dilute urine
↓
Restores **osmotic
pressure
relationships**
to normal.

maintain
fluid equilibrium

ADH binds to V_2 receptors on capillary side of duct cells → activates adenylate cyclase →
increases cyclic AMP → activates a protein kinase on luminal side of cell which results in
the insertion of vesicles containing water channels into the apical membrane of the cell →
provides a rapid mechanism for increasing permeability of cell membrane to water.

UNDERACTIVITY OF POSTERIOR PITUITARY

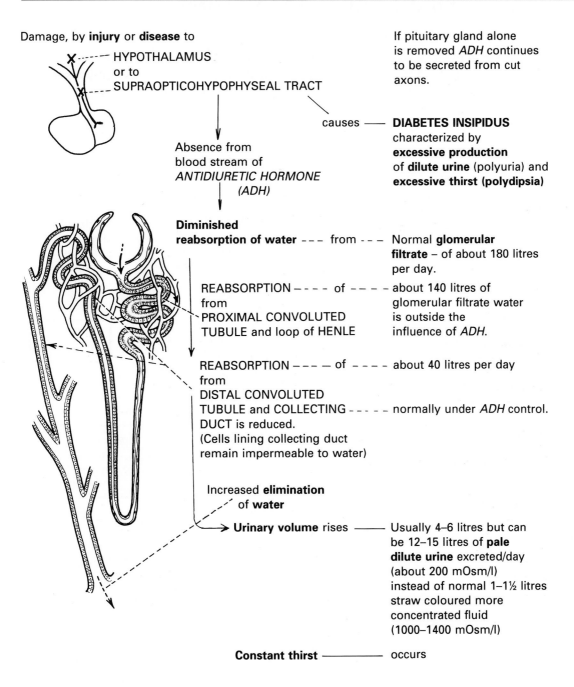

Damage, by **injury** or **disease** to

HYPOTHALAMUS
or to
SUPRAOPTICOHYPOPHYSEAL TRACT

If pituitary gland alone
is removed *ADH* continues
to be secreted from cut
axons.

causes ———— **DIABETES INSIPIDUS**
characterized by
excessive production
of **dilute urine** (polyuria) and
excessive thirst (polydipsia)

Absence from
blood stream of
ANTIDIURETIC HORMONE
(ADH)

**Diminished
reabsorption of water** - - - from - - - Normal **glomerular
filtrate** – of about 180 litres
per day.

REABSORPTION - - - - of - - - - about 140 litres of
from   glomerular filtrate water
PROXIMAL CONVOLUTED   is outside the
TUBULE and loop of HENLE   influence of *ADH*.

REABSORPTION - - - — of - - - - about 40 litres per day
from
DISTAL CONVOLUTED
TUBULE and COLLECTING - - - - - normally under *ADH* control.
DUCT is reduced.
(Cells lining collecting duct
remain impermeable to water)

Increased **elimination**
of **water**

Urinary volume rises ———— Usually 4–6 litres but can
be 12–15 litres of **pale
dilute urine** excreted/day
(about 200 mOsm/l)
instead of normal 1–1½ litres
straw coloured more
concentrated fluid
(1000–1400 mOsm/l)

Constant thirst ———————— occurs

Replacement of *ADH* restores the elimination of water and symptoms of thirst to normal.

ALDOSTERONE AND ANTIDIURETIC HORMONE (ADH) IN THE MAINTENANCE OF BLOOD VOLUME

A reduction in the total volume of **extracellular fluid** (e.g. after haemorrhage or loss of isotonic secretions from the gut in vomiting or diarrhoea) leads to chain of **compensatory** mechanisms in which *aldosterone* plays an important role. See pages 183 and 185.

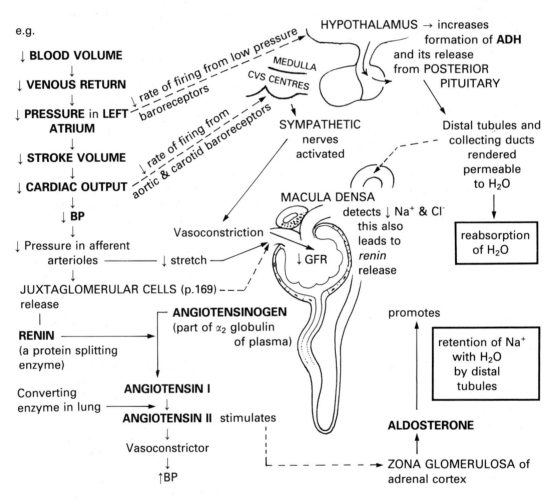

Decreased pressure in atria decreases release of atrial natriuretic peptide from the atria, thus decreasing excretion of Na^+.

These measures serve to maintain **blood volume** till the long term replacement of the lost RBC, plasma proteins and electrolytes can be achieved.

PANCREAS: ISLETS OF LANGERHANS

ISLETS OF LANGERHANS make up 1–2% of pancreatic tissue. Consist of four cell types: A(α) secrete *glucagon*, B(β) secrete *insulin*, D(δ) secrete *somatostatin*, F secrete *pancreatic polypeptide* (regulates release of digestive enzymes of pancreas).

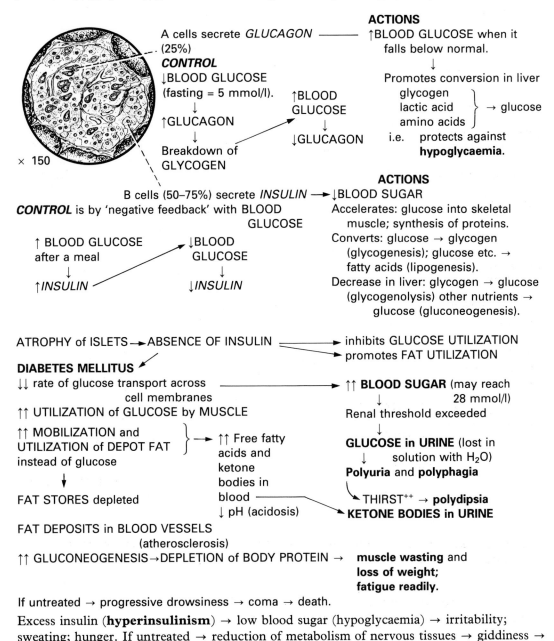

A cells secrete *GLUCAGON*
(25%)

CONTROL
↓BLOOD GLUCOSE
(fasting = 5 mmol/l).
↓
↑GLUCAGON
↓
Breakdown of
GLYCOGEN

↑BLOOD
GLUCOSE
↓
↓GLUCAGON

× 150

ACTIONS
↑BLOOD GLUCOSE when it
falls below normal.
↓
Promotes conversion in liver
glycogen
lactic acid } → glucose
amino acids
i.e. protects against
hypoglycaemia.

B cells (50–75%) secrete *INSULIN* → ↓BLOOD SUGAR

CONTROL is by 'negative feedback' with BLOOD
GLUCOSE

↑ BLOOD GLUCOSE
after a meal
↓
↑*INSULIN*

↓BLOOD
GLUCOSE
↓
↓*INSULIN*

ACTIONS
Accelerates: glucose into skeletal
muscle; synthesis of proteins.
Converts: glucose → glycogen
(glycogenesis); glucose etc. →
fatty acids (lipogenesis).
Decrease in liver: glycogen → glucose
(glycogenolysis) other nutrients →
glucose (gluconeogenesis).

ATROPHY of ISLETS → ABSENCE OF INSULIN → inhibits GLUCOSE UTILIZATION
→ promotes FAT UTILIZATION

DIABETES MELLITUS
↓↓ rate of glucose transport across
cell membranes
↑↑ UTILIZATION of GLUCOSE by MUSCLE

↑↑ MOBILIZATION and
UTILIZATION of DEPOT FAT
instead of glucose
↓
FAT STORES depleted

} → ↑↑ Free fatty
acids and
ketone
bodies in
blood
↓ pH (acidosis)

↑↑ **BLOOD SUGAR** (may reach
↓ 28 mmol/l)
Renal threshold exceeded
↓
GLUCOSE in URINE (lost in
↓ solution with H_2O)
Polyuria and **polyphagia**

THIRST++ → **polydipsia**
KETONE BODIES in URINE

FAT DEPOSITS in BLOOD VESSELS
(atherosclerosis)
↑↑ GLUCONEOGENESIS → DEPLETION of BODY PROTEIN →   **muscle wasting** and
loss of weight;
fatigue readily.

If untreated → progressive drowsiness → coma → death.

Excess insulin (**hyperinsulinism**) → low blood sugar (hypoglycaemia) → irritability; sweating; hunger. If untreated → reduction of metabolism of nervous tissues → giddiness → coma → death. *Somatostatin* prevents excessive levels of nutrients in plasma by reducing rate of food digestion and absorption – Inhibits insulin and glucagon secretion.

CHAPTER 9

REPRODUCTIVE SYSTEM

MALE REPRODUCTIVE SYSTEM

PRIMARY SEX ORGANS → produce the MALE GERM CELLS – **SPERMATOZOA**
TESTES (Two)   and the MALE SEX HORMONE – **TESTOSTERONE**

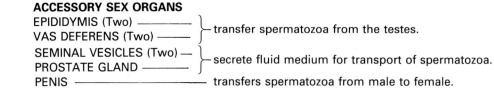

Testosterone $\xrightarrow{\text{5}\alpha\text{–reductase}}$ dihydrotestosterone

These bind to intracellular receptors and the complexes thus formed bind to DNA and are responsible for maturation at puberty of:

ACCESSORY SEX ORGANS
EPIDIDYMIS (Two) ———— ⎫
VAS DEFERENS (Two) ——— ⎬ transfer spermatozoa from the testes.
SEMINAL VESICLES (Two) — ⎫
PROSTATE GLAND ———— ⎬ secrete fluid medium for transport of spermatozoa.
PENIS ———————————— transfers spermatozoa from male to female.

and appearance of
SECONDARY SEX CHARACTERISTICS
Laryngeal changes → deep voice.
Growth of pubic, axillary and facial hair.
Receding hair at temples.
Increase in muscle and
skeletal mass (protein anabolism)
giving growth spurt and
characteristic male shape
of body.
Sex drive.   Aggression.
Increased sebaceous
gland secretion –
oversecretion causes
acne.

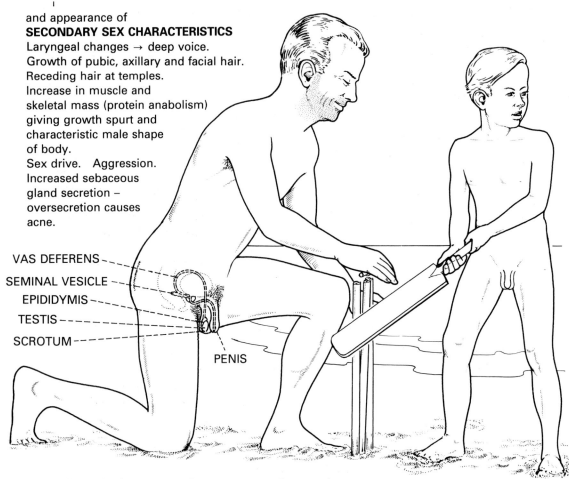

VAS DEFERENS
SEMINAL VESICLE
EPIDIDYMIS
TESTIS
SCROTUM
PENIS

In the male the process of spermatogenesis starts just after puberty and is normally continuous until old age.

TESTIS

There are two TESTES (singular: testis).
These produce the MALE GERM CELLS:-

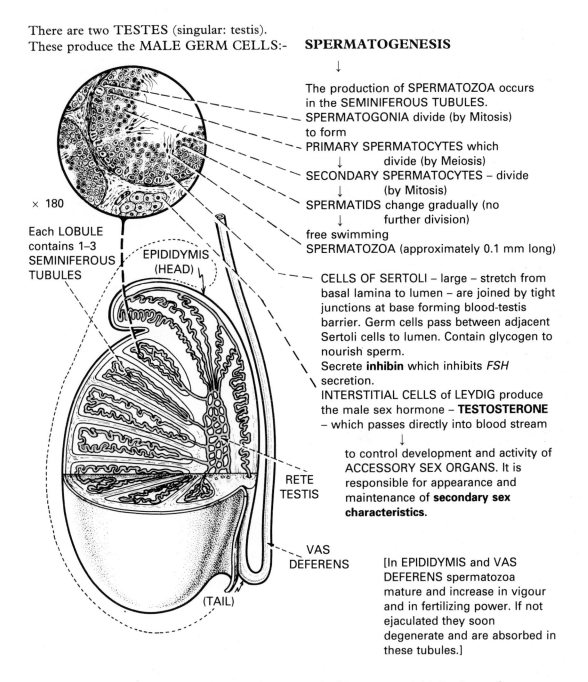

× 180

Each LOBULE
contains 1–3
SEMINIFEROUS
TUBULES

EPIDIDYMIS
(HEAD)

RETE
TESTIS

VAS
DEFERENS

(TAIL)

SPERMATOGENESIS
↓

The production of SPERMATOZOA occurs
in the SEMINIFEROUS TUBULES.
SPERMATOGONIA divide (by Mitosis)
to form
PRIMARY SPERMATOCYTES which
↓   divide (by Meiosis)
SECONDARY SPERMATOCYTES – divide
↓   (by Mitosis)
SPERMATIDS change gradually (no
↓   further division)
free swimming
SPERMATOZOA (approximately 0.1 mm long)

CELLS OF SERTOLI – large – stretch from
basal lamina to lumen – are joined by tight
junctions at base forming blood-testis
barrier. Germ cells pass between adjacent
Sertoli cells to lumen. Contain glycogen to
nourish sperm.
Secrete **inhibin** which inhibits *FSH*
secretion.
INTERSTITIAL CELLS of LEYDIG produce
the male sex hormone – **TESTOSTERONE**
– which passes directly into blood stream
↓
to control development and activity of
ACCESSORY SEX ORGANS. It is
responsible for appearance and
maintenance of **secondary sex
characteristics.**

[In EPIDIDYMIS and VAS
DEFERENS spermatozoa
mature and increase in vigour
and in fertilizing power. If not
ejaculated they soon
degenerate and are absorbed in
these tubules.]

Events occurring in the testes are under **control** of **hormones**, chiefly those of
ANTERIOR PITUITARY and the HYPOTHALAMUS.

MALE ACCESSORY SEX ORGANS

These are the organs adapted for **transfer** of live **spermatozoa** from male to female.

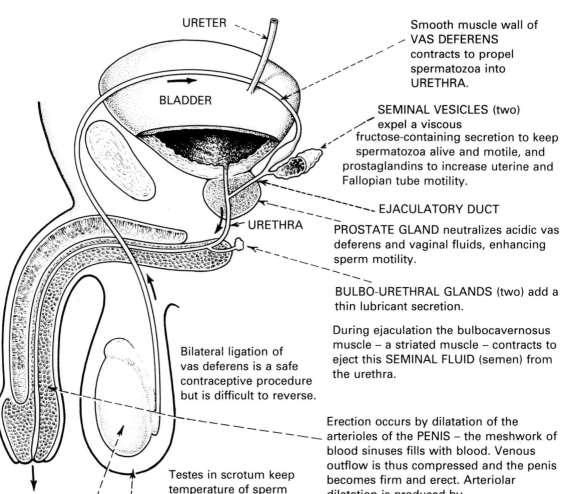

URETER

BLADDER

URETHRA

TESTIS

SCROTUM

Smooth muscle wall of
VAS DEFERENS
contracts to propel
spermatozoa into
URETHRA.

SEMINAL VESICLES (two)
expel a viscous
fructose-containing secretion to keep
spermatozoa alive and motile, and
prostaglandins to increase uterine and
Fallopian tube motility.

EJACULATORY DUCT

PROSTATE GLAND neutralizes acidic vas
deferens and vaginal fluids, enhancing
sperm motility.

BULBO-URETHRAL GLANDS (two) add a
thin lubricant secretion.

During ejaculation the bulbocavernosus
muscle – a striated muscle – contracts to
eject this SEMINAL FLUID (semen) from
the urethra.

Bilateral ligation of
vas deferens is a safe
contraceptive procedure
but is difficult to reverse.

Erection occurs by dilatation of the
arterioles of the PENIS – the meshwork of
blood sinuses fills with blood. Venous
outflow is thus compressed and the penis
becomes firm and erect. Arteriolar
dilatation is produced by
parasympathetic nerves releasing
acetylcholine and VIP and nonadrenergic –
noncholinergic nerves releasing the
powerful vasodilator nitric oxide (EDRF).
2–4 ml of SEMINAL FLUID containing
several hundred million spermatozoa are
deposited in the female vagina.

Testes in scrotum keep
temperature of sperm
2°C below normal body
temperature.
Necessary for fertility.

Sperm must remain in female tract for
several hours to acquire ability to
penetrate ovum – **capacitation**.

222

CONTROL OF EVENTS IN THE TESTIS

Between the ages of 13 and 16 years the hypothalamus begins to secrete *gonadotrophin-releasing hormone (GnRH)* which travels via the portal veins (p.207) and releases from the anterior pituitary 1. *follicle-stimulating hormone (FSH)*, which stimulates sperm production in the testis, and 2. *luteinizing hormone (LH)* – often called, in the male, *interstitial cell stimulating hormone (ICSH)* since it stimulates these cells to secrete *testosterone*.

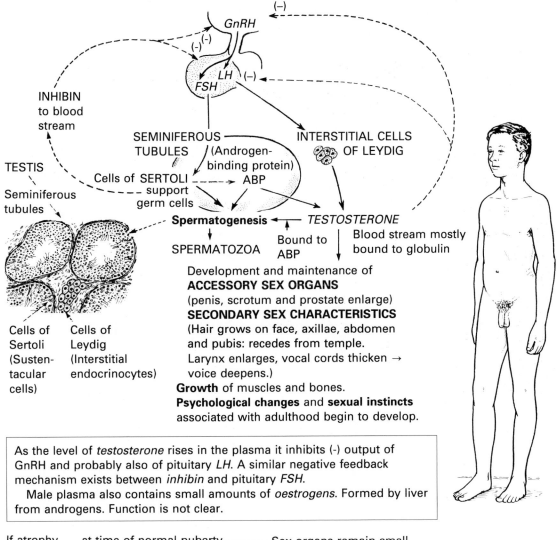

As the level of *testosterone* rises in the plasma it inhibits (-) output of GnRH and probably also of pituitary *LH*. A similar negative feedback mechanism exists between *inhibin* and pituitary *FSH*.

Male plasma also contains small amounts of *oestrogens*. Formed by liver from androgens. Function is not clear.

If atrophy of testes occurs
at time of normal puberty —— Sex organs remain small.
Secondary sex characteristics fail to develop.
after puberty → Spermatogenesis stops → Sterility.
Testosterone production falls → Atrophy of secondary sex organs.

Injections of *Testosterone* in cases of delayed puberty → Changes associated with puberty.
Use of *inhibin* as a male contraceptive hormone is a possibility.

223

FEMALE REPRODUCTIVE SYSTEM

PRIMARY SEX ORGANS ————————————————▶ produce the FEMALE GERM CELLS – **OVA**
OVARIES (two)   and the FEMALE SEX HORMONES. –
                                                                 OESTROGENS and **PROGESTERONE**

At puberty, secretions of *GnRH, LH,*
FSH and oestrogens increase.
Oestrogen is the main factor responsible
for maturation at puberty of:

ACCESSORY SEX ORGANS
FALLOPIAN TUBES (two) – – – – for the transfer of the ova from ovaries.
VAGINA – – – – – – – – – – – for the reception of the male germ cells.
UTERUS – – – – – – – – – – – for the nutrition and development of the
                             fertilized egg cell → developing embryo.
MAMMARY GLANDS (two) – – – – for the nutrition of the new individual after birth.

and
appearance and
maintenance of
SECONDARY SEX
CHARACTERISTICS

Development of
breasts.
Typical feminine
proportions of body,
narrow shoulders,
broad hips.

Androgens from
adrenal cortex
are responsible
for sex drive
and growth of
pubic and axillary
hair.

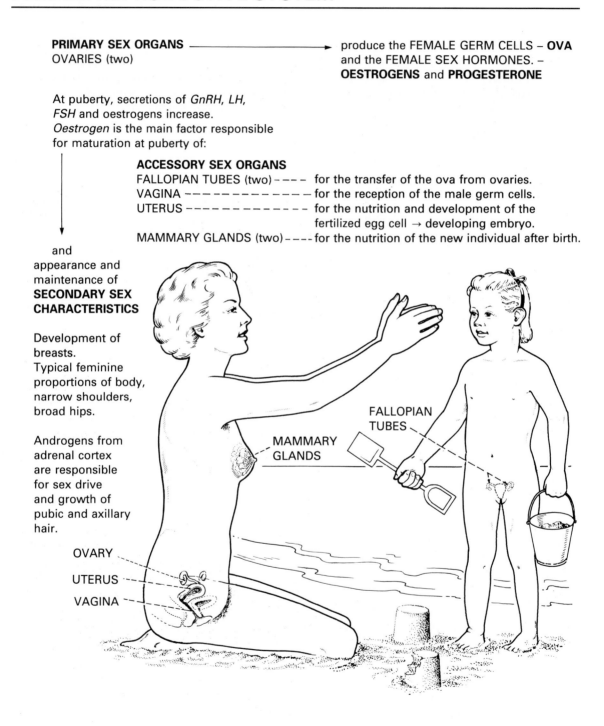

FALLOPIAN
TUBES

MAMMARY
GLANDS

OVARY

UTERUS

VAGINA

In the female the cyclical production of ova starts just after puberty and continues
(unless interrupted by pregnancy or disease) until the menopause.

ADULT PELVIC SEX ORGANS IN ORDINARY FEMALE CYCLE

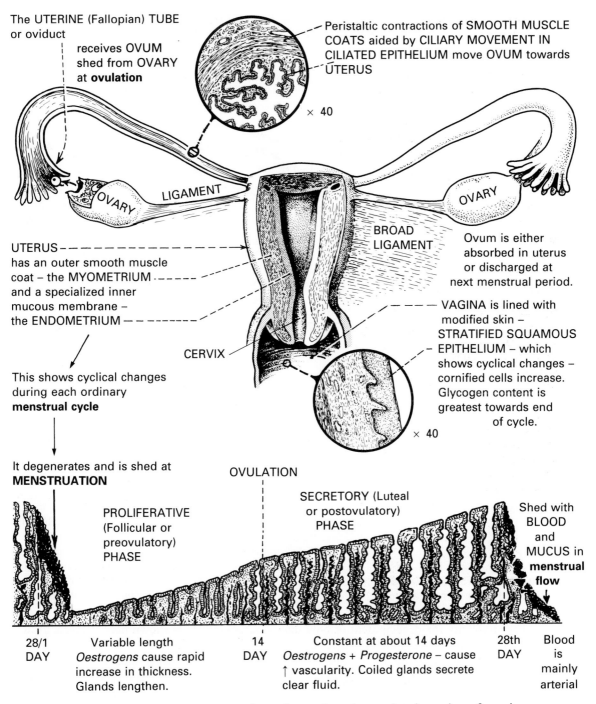

The UTERINE (Fallopian) TUBE or oviduct

receives OVUM shed from OVARY at **ovulation**

Peristaltic contractions of SMOOTH MUSCLE COATS aided by CILIARY MOVEMENT IN CILIATED EPITHELIUM move OVUM towards UTERUS

× 40

LIGAMENT

OVARY

OVARY

BROAD LIGAMENT

Ovum is either absorbed in uterus or discharged at next menstrual period.

UTERUS –
has an outer smooth muscle coat – the MYOMETRIUM – and a specialized inner mucous membrane – the ENDOMETRIUM – –

VAGINA is lined with modified skin – STRATIFIED SQUAMOUS EPITHELIUM – which shows cyclical changes – cornified cells increase. Glycogen content is greatest towards end of cycle.

CERVIX

× 40

This shows cyclical changes during each ordinary **menstrual cycle**

It degenerates and is shed at **MENSTRUATION**

OVULATION

PROLIFERATIVE (Follicular or preovulatory) PHASE

SECRETORY (Luteal or postovulatory) PHASE

Shed with BLOOD and MUCUS in **menstrual flow**

| 28/1 DAY | Variable length *Oestrogens* cause rapid increase in thickness. Glands lengthen. | 14 DAY | Constant at about 14 days *Oestrogens* + *Progesterone* – cause ↑ vascularity. Coiled glands secrete clear fluid. | 28th DAY | Blood is mainly arterial |

Rhythmical changes occur in uterus, uterine tubes and vagina under the action of ovarian hormones.

225

OVARY IN ORDINARY ADULT CYCLE

There are *two* OVARIES. These produce the Female GERM CELLS. The production of OVA is a cyclical process – **OOGENESIS**.

1. FORMATION – PRIMORDIAL GERM CELLS divide to produce oogonia which develop into primary oocytes by age of 6 months.

2. GROWTH
OOCYTE with single layer of cells – the precursors of granulosa cells – is PRIMORDIAL FOLLICLE. GRANULOSA CELLS multiply and first a primary follicle then a SECONDARY FOLLICLE are created. CUMULUS OOPHORUS (attaches OOCYTE to wall of follicle) and GRANULOSA CELLS take androgens produced by the THECA INTERNA and convert them to OESTROGENS – partly stored in FOLLICULAR FLUID in enlarging antrum of developing GRAAFIAN FOLLICLE – partly absorbed into blood vessels of THECA INTERNA.
↓
GENERAL CIRCULATION
↓
Controls changes in ACCESSORY SEX ORGANS in first half of menstrual cycle.

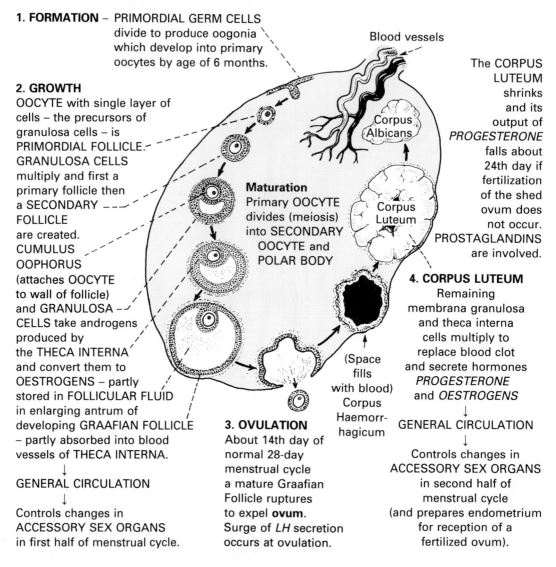

Blood vessels

Corpus Albicans

Maturation
Primary OOCYTE divides (meiosis) into SECONDARY OOCYTE and POLAR BODY

Corpus Luteum

(Space fills with blood)
Corpus Haemorr-hagicum

3. OVULATION
About 14th day of normal 28-day menstrual cycle a mature Graafian Follicle ruptures to expel **ovum**. Surge of *LH* secretion occurs at ovulation.

The CORPUS LUTEUM shrinks and its output of *PROGESTERONE* falls about 24th day if fertilization of the shed ovum does not occur. PROSTAGLANDINS are involved.

4. CORPUS LUTEUM
Remaining membrana granulosa and theca interna cells multiply to replace blood clot and secrete hormones *PROGESTERONE* and *OESTROGENS*
↓
GENERAL CIRCULATION
↓
Controls changes in ACCESSORY SEX ORGANS in second half of menstrual cycle (and prepares endometrium for reception of a fertilized ovum).

For simplicity the development of only one Graafian follicle is shown here. Several grow in each cycle but in the human subject usually only one follicle ruptures: the others atrophy. Strictly speaking, each month it is a secondary oocyte that is shed at ovulation. If fertilized, the secondary oocyte acquires a full complement of chromosomes and is then an **ovum**. However the term 'ovum' is used loosely here as in other texts.

Events in the ovary are under control of anterior pituitary hormones *FSH* and *LH*, and hypothalamic *Gonadotrophin-Releasing Hormone (GnRH)*.

OVARY IN PREGNANCY

When pregnancy occurs the ordinary ovarian cycle is suspended.

After the first 14 days the developing placenta secretes the hormone
HUMAN CHORIONIC GONADOTROPHIN (hCG).

Under its influence
the CORPUS LUTEUM ———— continues to grow and secrete *oestrogens, progesterone* and
relaxin until it may come to occupy 30–50% of the total volume of
the ovary.

hCG can be detected in urine
14 days after conception. Basis
of pregnancy test.

The large amount of
PROGESTERONE

reaches its peak
at about
6 weeks after
conception

helps to maintain the
PREGNANCY in its
early stages and is
essential for
development of the
PLACENTA – the
special structure
through which the
child receives its
nourishment from
the mother. The
placenta also
produces
progesterone which
gradually takes over
from the

falls off
about
2nd
month

Diminishes
in size

CORPUS LUTEUM ———— ceases to
contribute
significantly
after 4th month.

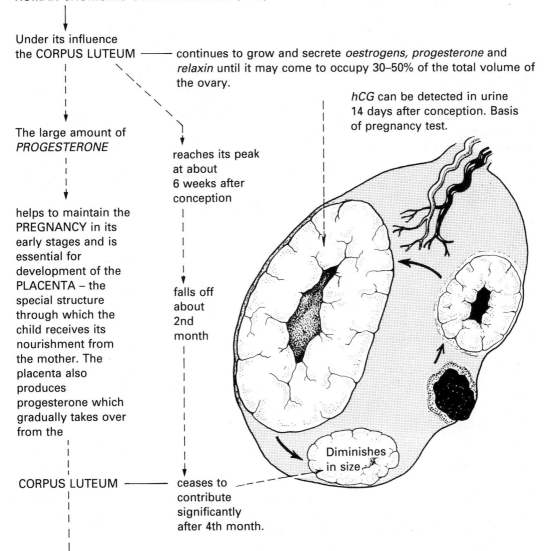

PLACENTAL PROGESTERONE takes over to maintain the pregnancy. Increases resting
membrane potential of uterine muscle; hence decreases its excitability. Also decreases its
sensitivity to *oxytocin* and its number of oestrogen receptors. Helps prepare mammary glands
for lactation.

RELAXIN – secreted by corpus luteum and placenta. Ensures uterine quiescence and prevents
early abortion of the pregnancy. Relaxes pelvic bones and ligaments. Softens cervix.

CONTROL OF EVENTS IN THE OVARY

Between the ages of 10 and 14 years the HYPOTHALAMUS begins to secrete *GONADOTROPHIN-RELEASING HORMONE (GnRH)* in varying periodic surges. The girl enters puberty. Thereafter the cycle is controlled thus:

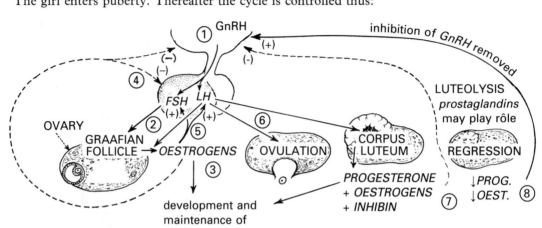

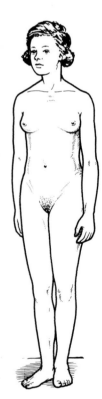

1. The cycle begins with a rise in *GnRH*.
2. This increases *LH* and *FSH* secretion. *LH* acts on the theca interna cells which produce androgens. Androgens are converted to oestrogens by granulosa cells under the influence of *FSH*.
3. The oestrogens enter the circulation.
4. As the level of oestrogen rises it first inhibits (-) output of *GnRH*, *FSH* and *LH*.
5. About the 12th or 13th day the prolonged high level of oestrogen, by enhancing the sensitivity of *LH*-releasing mechanism to *GnRH*, causes a positive feedback (+) effect.
6. A sudden surge of *LH* (and of *FSH*) secretion leads to ovulation nine hours later and the formation of the CORPUS LUTEUM.
7. As the level of progesterone rises (along with oestrogen) it inhibits (-) *GnRH*, *LH* and *FSH*. Secretion of *inhibin* by the granulosa cells increases during the luteal phase and inhibits secretion of *FSH*.
8. A few days before menstruation the corpus luteum involutes. As the levels of progesterone and oestrogen fall, *GnRH* is freed from inhibition. The cycle starts again.

OVARIAN HORMONES

The ovarian cycle is repeated monthly from **puberty** to the **menopause** unless interrupted by **pregnancy** or **disease**.

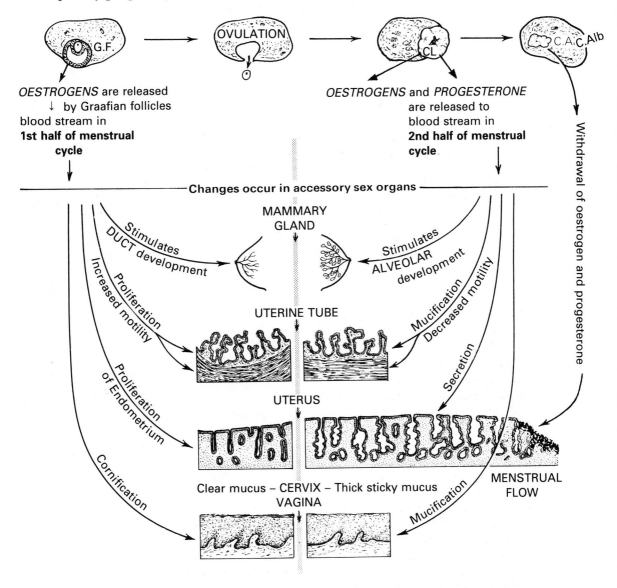

OESTROGENS are released
↓ by Graafian follicles
blood stream in
**1st half of menstrual
cycle**

OESTROGENS and *PROGESTERONE*
are released to
blood stream in
**2nd half of menstrual
cycle**.

Withdrawal of oestrogen and progesterone

——— Changes occur in accessory sex organs ———

MAMMARY
GLAND

Stimulates
DUCT development

Stimulates
ALVEOLAR
development

Proliferation
Increased motility

Mucification
Decreased motility

UTERINE TUBE

Proliferation
of Endometrium

Secretion

UTERUS

MENSTRUAL
FLOW

Cornification

Clear mucus – CERVIX – Thick sticky mucus
VAGINA

Mucification

Ovarian hormones are therefore directly responsible for regular cycle of events in accessory sex organs.

There are three natural oestrogens: *oestradiol* is the major and most potent. It is formed from androgen precursors, as is a second called *oestrone*. Oestrone is metabolized to *oestriol* mainly in the liver.

DEVELOPMENT OF UTERUS AND UTERINE TUBES

The **uterus** (or womb) is the organ which bears the developing child till birth.

IN CHILDHOOD –
it is a small undeveloped organ
situated deep in the pelvis.

Outer walls of
smooth muscle –
the MYOMETRIUM

Inner lining or
Mucous membrane –
the ENDOMETRIUM

AT PUBERTY
(Adolescence)

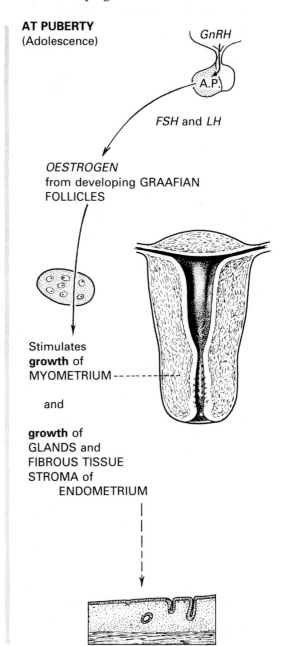

GnRH

A.P.

FSH and LH

OESTROGEN
from developing GRAAFIAN
FOLLICLES

Stimulates
growth of
MYOMETRIUM

and

growth of
GLANDS and
FIBROUS TISSUE
STROMA of
ENDOMETRIUM

MATURE UTERUS AND UTERINE TUBES

IN MATURITY

[From puberty to menopause
(unless interrupted by
pregnancy or disease) –
when ovarian cycle is
fully established]

GnRH

AP

FSH

LH

Fimbriated
end of tube
receives OVUM
at OVULATION

Released to
abdominal
cavity

OESTROGEN and *PROGESTERONE*

stimulate
further
growth of
MYOMETRIUM

stimulates
regeneration
of glands and
fibrous tissue
in ENDOMETRIUM
in first half of
menstrual cycle

stimulates
secretion
of
glands of
ENDOMETRIUM
in second half of
of menstrual cycle

MENSTRUATION

If fertilization does not take place
the OVUM, which is about 100 μm in
diameter (*cf* RBC = 7μm), is either
absorbed in uterus or discharged
at next menstrual period.

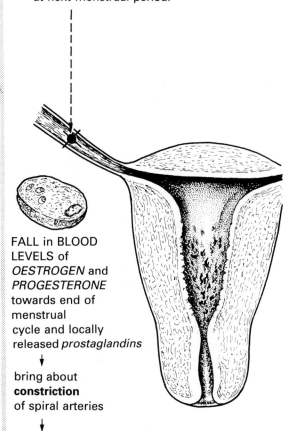

FALL in BLOOD
LEVELS of
OESTROGEN and
PROGESTERONE
towards end of
menstrual
cycle and locally
released *prostaglandins*

↓

bring about
constriction
of spiral arteries

↓

Degeneration and
breakdown of glands and other
tissues of ENDOMETRIUM to give
Menstrual flow.

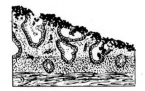

231

UTERINE TUBES IN CYCLE ENDING IN PREGNANCY

The fimbriated end of the **uterine tube** receives the **ovum** at **ovulation. Peristaltic** contractions of the muscular tube aided by ciliary movements of its lining cells transfer the **ovum** towards the **uterus**. The uterine tube also transmits **spermatazoa** towards the **ovum**.

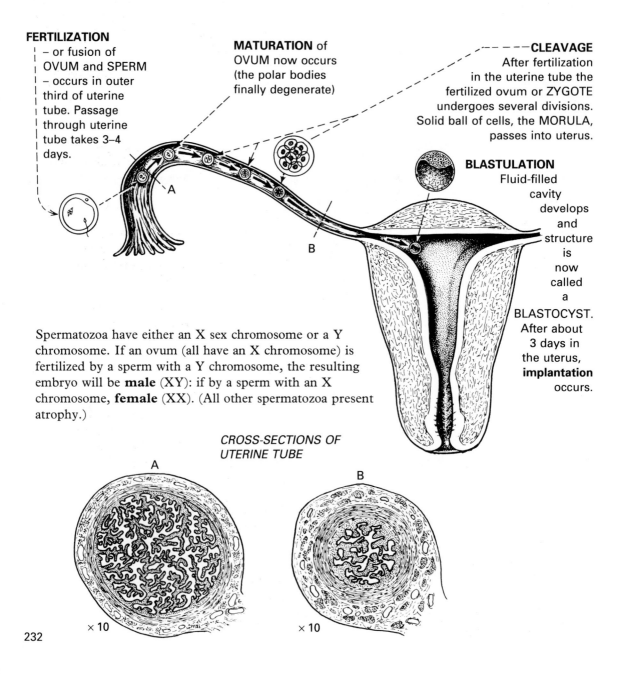

FERTILIZATION
– or fusion of OVUM and SPERM – occurs in outer third of uterine tube. Passage through uterine tube takes 3–4 days.

MATURATION of OVUM now occurs (the polar bodies finally degenerate)

CLEAVAGE
After fertilization in the uterine tube the fertilized ovum or ZYGOTE undergoes several divisions. Solid ball of cells, the MORULA, passes into uterus.

BLASTULATION
Fluid-filled cavity develops and structure is now called a BLASTOCYST. After about 3 days in the uterus, **implantation** occurs.

Spermatozoa have either an X sex chromosome or a Y chromosome. If an ovum (all have an X chromosome) is fertilized by a sperm with a Y chromosome, the resulting embryo will be **male** (XY): if by a sperm with an X chromosome, **female** (XX). (All other spermatozoa present atrophy.)

CROSS-SECTIONS OF UTERINE TUBE

A

B

× 10

× 10

UTERUS AFTER FERTILIZATION – 1

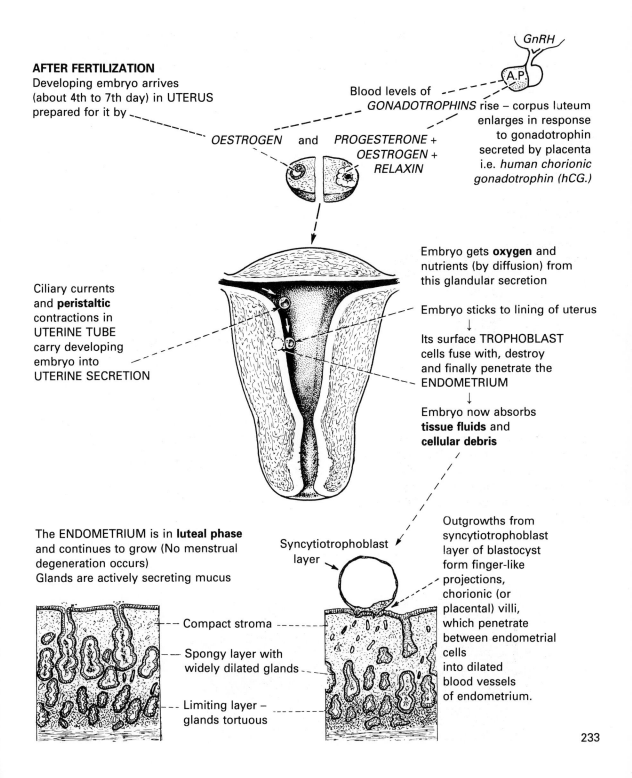

GnRH

A.P.

AFTER FERTILIZATION
Developing embryo arrives
(about 4th to 7th day) in UTERUS
prepared for it by

Blood levels of
GONADOTROPHINS rise – corpus luteum
enlarges in response
to gonadotrophin
secreted by placenta
i.e. *human chorionic
gonadotrophin (hCG.)*

OESTROGEN and *PROGESTERONE +
OESTROGEN +
RELAXIN*

Embryo gets **oxygen** and
nutrients (by diffusion) from
this glandular secretion

Ciliary currents
and **peristaltic**
contractions in
UTERINE TUBE
carry developing
embryo into
UTERINE SECRETION

Embryo sticks to lining of uterus
↓
Its surface TROPHOBLAST
cells fuse with, destroy
and finally penetrate the
ENDOMETRIUM
↓
Embryo now absorbs
tissue fluids and
cellular debris

The ENDOMETRIUM is in **luteal phase**
and continues to grow (No menstrual
degeneration occurs)
Glands are actively secreting mucus

Syncytiotrophoblast
layer

Outgrowths from
syncytiotrophoblast
layer of blastocyst
form finger-like
projections,
chorionic (or
placental) villi,
which penetrate
between endometrial
cells
into dilated
blood vessels
of endometrium.

- - - Compact stroma - - - -

- Spongy layer with
widely dilated glands - -

- Limiting layer –
glands tortuous

233

UTERUS AFTER FERTILIZATION – 2

IMPLANTATION
Embryo invades
ENDOMETRIUM (which
is now called the
DECIDUA).
Prostaglandins released
by endometrial cells
facilitate this process.

GnRH

A.P.

Blood levels of
GONADOTROPHINS
continue to rise

PLACENTATION
PROGESTERONE is necessary
for the development of the
PLACENTA – the special organ
through which the developing
child receives nourishment
from the mother

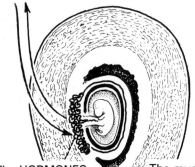

OESTROGEN, PROGESTERONE and *RELAXIN*

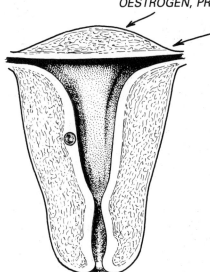

The HORMONES
of the PLACENTA
help to maintain
the
PREGNANCY

The myometrial
smooth muscle
cells increase
in number and size

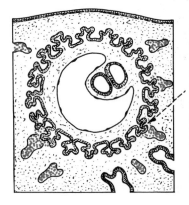

CHORIONIC VILLI –
Finger-like
projections from
the embryo have
invaded
mother's
endometrial
blood vessels.
Proteolytic
enzymes aid
this process.

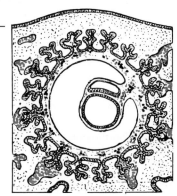

Blood vessels
develop in the
CHORIONIC VILLI
which are now
interlocked with
mother's tissues
and surrounded
by mother's
blood.
STRUCTURE
formed
in this way is
the **placenta**.

234   After 2 months the developing embryo is called a **fetus**.

PLACENTA

The **placenta** functions for the **fetus** as alimentary tract, kidneys and lungs.
It increases in weight throughout pregnancy.

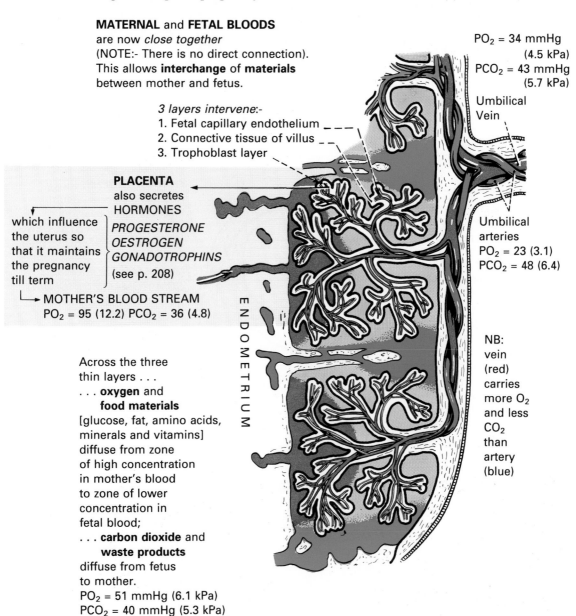

MATERNAL and **FETAL BLOODS**
are now *close together*
(NOTE:- There is no direct connection).
This allows **interchange** of **materials**
between mother and fetus.

3 layers intervene:-
1. Fetal capillary endothelium
2. Connective tissue of villus
3. Trophoblast layer

PLACENTA
also secretes
HORMONES
PROGESTERONE
OESTROGEN
GONADOTROPHINS
(see p. 208)

which influence
the uterus so
that it maintains
the pregnancy
till term

MOTHER'S BLOOD STREAM
PO_2 = 95 (12.2) PCO_2 = 36 (4.8)

PO_2 = 34 mmHg
(4.5 kPa)
PCO_2 = 43 mmHg
(5.7 kPa)

Umbilical
Vein

Umbilical
arteries
PO_2 = 23 (3.1)
PCO_2 = 48 (6.4)

ENDOMETRIUM

NB:
vein
(red)
carries
more O_2
and less
CO_2
than
artery
(blue)

Across the three
thin layers . . .
. . . **oxygen** and
   food materials
[glucose, fat, amino acids,
minerals and vitamins]
diffuse from zone
of high concentration
in mother's blood
to zone of lower
concentration in
fetal blood;
. . . **carbon dioxide** and
   waste products
diffuse from fetus
to mother.
PO_2 = 51 mmHg (6.1 kPa)
PCO_2 = 40 mmHg (5.3 kPa)

Substances of small molecular weight usually pass in either direction by diffusion.
Larger molecules are probably transported by special carrier systems.

UTERUS IN ADVANCED PREGNANCY

AS PREGNANCY ADVANCES

Fetus grows larger and comes to fill UTERINE CAVITY

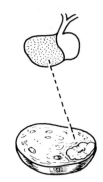

CORPUS LUTEUM remains, but after the 4th month its contribution to *oestrogen and progesterone* supply is dwarfed by that of the placenta.

PLACENTAL HORMONES
(1) *HUMAN CHORIONIC GONADOTROPHIN (hCG)* maintains corpus luteum. Placenta takes over main secretion of (2) *OESTROGENS* and (3) *PROGESTERONE* after the sixth week.
(4) *HUMAN CHORIONIC SOMATOMAMMOTROPHIN (hCS)* or *human placental lactogen (hPL)* 'maternal growth hormone of pregnancy' has anabolic and lactogenic activity.
Retains nitrogen, potassium and calcium and saves glucose for use by fetus.
(5) *RELAXIN* decreases uterine activity – later relaxes pelvic joints, softens and dilates cervix.

Fetus is attached by UMBILICAL CORD to PLACENTA

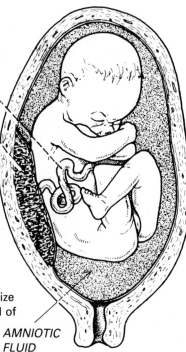

AMNIOTIC FLUID

Fetus is bathed in AMNIOTIC FLUID which is derived from amniotic epithelium, fetal urine and lung fluid and contained within amniotic and chorionic membranes. Maintains fetus in shock-proof, constant temperature environment.

Growth of MYOMETRIUM – increase in number and size of smooth muscle cells and of the blood vessels

Stretching of MYOMETRIUM

Major *oestrogen* of pregnancy is *oestriol*. Synthesized by the placenta from precursors synthesized in the adrenal gland of the fetus.

Amniotic fluid can be sampled – **amniocentesis** – to detect fetal abnormalities.

FETAL CIRCULATION

For the fetus the **placenta** acts as the organ of transfer for oxygen, nutritives and waste products. Only a small volume of blood passes through the fetal lungs.

BLOOD RETURNING TO HEART

... To RIGHT ATRIUM
Small amount from heart, head, neck and arms → S.V.C.
LARGE AMOUNT via UMBILICAL VEINS through LIVER – short circuits to I.V.C. via DUCTUS VENOSUS. Some of this passes to right atrium.
Small amount from abdominal cavity and legs.

... To LEFT ATRIUM
Small amount from 2 lungs
LARGE AMOUNT from INFERIOR VENA CAVA through

FORAMEN OVALE.
(thus by-passing pulmonary circulation)

BLOOD LEAVING HEART

... From RIGHT VENTRICLE
Small amount to 2 lungs
LARGE AMOUNT to AORTA through
↓
DUCTUS ARTERIOSUS
(thus by-passing pulmonary circulation) joins *OUTPUT* from LEFT VENTRICLE
↓
Small amount to heart, head, neck and arms.
LARGE AMOUNT to PLACENTA through UMBILICAL ARTERIES
Small amount to abdominal cavity and legs.

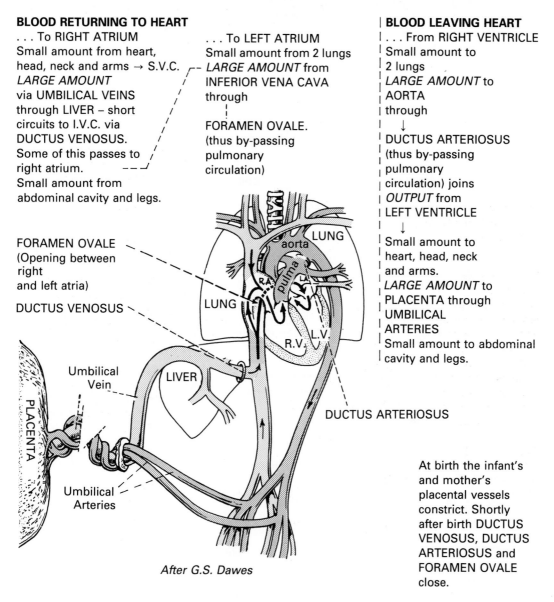

FORAMEN OVALE
(Opening between right and left atria)

DUCTUS VENOSUS

DUCTUS ARTERIOSUS

Umbilical Vein

LIVER

Umbilical Arteries

After G.S. Dawes

At birth the infant's and mother's placental vessels constrict. Shortly after birth DUCTUS VENOSUS, DUCTUS ARTERIOSUS and FORAMEN OVALE close.

Head of fetus receives better oxygenated blood than trunk and lower body. **Oxygenated blood** → umbilical vein → ductus venosus → IVC → R. atrium → foramen ovale → L. atrium → L. ventricle → aorta → **head**.

UTERUS DURING LABOUR

PARTURITION

About 40 weeks after conception the process of **childbirth** begins. When uterine contractions are strong, coordinated and occur at 10–15 min intervals, **labour** has started.

1st stage usually lasts up to 14 hours with a first birth.

MYOMETRIUM
  Uterine muscle is now very greatly
      stretched.
        ↓
Rhythmic contractions which begin to
increase in strength and frequency
        ↓
  Press on amniotic fluid

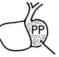

After the 32nd week of pregnancy *relaxin* and *oestrogens* increase *OXYTOCIN* receptors on uterus × 100 and also uterine *PROSTAGLANDIN* synthesis. Both factors increase uterine contractions.

2nd stage LABOUR usually lasts
up to 2 hours with a first birth.

Uterine contractions increase in strength and frequency (aided by voluntary contractions of abdominal muscles).
        ↓
Child is slowly forced through CERVIX and is
delivered from VAGINA.

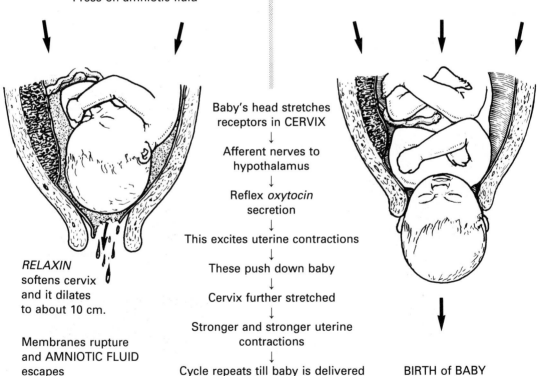

RELAXIN
softens cervix
and it dilates
to about 10 cm.

Membranes rupture
and AMNIOTIC FLUID
escapes

Baby's head stretches
receptors in CERVIX
        ↓
Afferent nerves to
hypothalamus
        ↓
Reflex *oxytocin*
secretion
        ↓
This excites uterine contractions
        ↓
These push down baby
        ↓
Cervix further stretched
        ↓
Stronger and stronger uterine
contractions
        ↓
Cycle repeats till baby is delivered

BIRTH of BABY

UTERUS AFTER PARTURITION

AFTER PARTURITION

3rd stage labour
5–15 minutes
after birth of child

IN PUERPERIUM   (Immediately
following childbirth.)

HYPOTHALAMUS

.... Afferents from
breasts in suckling
and from the
uterus and birth
canal during
parturition

P.P.

Fall in
blood levels
of
OESTROGEN,
PROGESTERONE
and
OTHER PLACENTAL
HORMONES
after loss of
placenta

OXYTOCIN
released to blood stream
stimulates **contractions** of
UTERINE MUSCLE

↓

Detach and **deliver** PLACENTA
and the membranes as the
AFTERBIRTH.

OXYTOCIN
released to
blood stream

MYOMETRIUM
Uterine muscle contracts down
to close off blood vessels torn
and bleeding after separation of
placenta

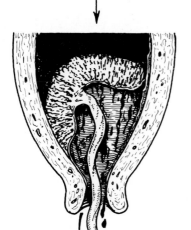

A large part of the endometrium
of pregnancy – i.e. the decidua
– is shed with the placenta.
Only the limiting layer is left.

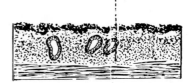

UTERUS – RECOVERY AND MENOPAUSE

INVOLUTION

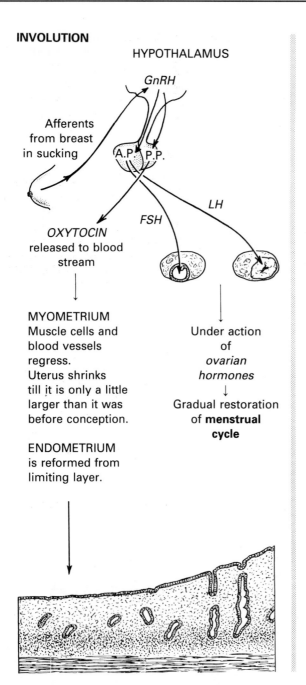

HYPOTHALAMUS

GnRH

Afferents
from breast
in sucking

A.P. P.P.

LH

FSH

OXYTOCIN
released to blood
stream

MYOMETRIUM
Muscle cells and
blood vessels
regress.
Uterus shrinks
till it is only a little
larger than it was
before conception.

ENDOMETRIUM
is reformed from
limiting layer.

Under action
of
*ovarian
hormones*
↓
Gradual restoration
of **menstrual
cycle**

AFTER MENOPAUSE

Ovarian tissue ceases to be
responsive to *anterior pituitary
gonadotrophins*
↓
Fall in production of
oestrogen and *progesterone*
(accompanied by rise in *LH* and
FSH due to absence of feedback
inhibition of these hormones)
↓
Shrinkage of
MYOMETRIUM

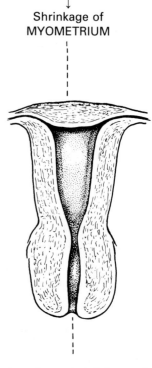

Atrophy and shrinkage of
glands and stroma of
ENDOMETRIUM
↓
Cessation of
menstrual cycle

MAMMARY GLANDS

There are two mammary glands which are modified sweat glands that produce milk.

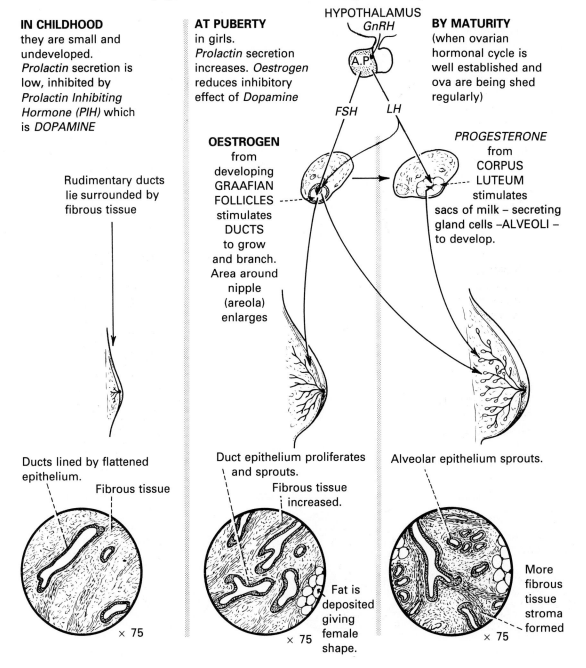

IN CHILDHOOD
they are small and
undeveloped.
Prolactin secretion is
low, inhibited by
*Prolactin Inhibiting
Hormone (PIH)* which
is *DOPAMINE*

Rudimentary ducts
lie surrounded by
fibrous tissue

AT PUBERTY
in girls.
Prolactin secretion
increases. *Oestrogen*
reduces inhibitory
effect of *Dopamine*

HYPOTHALAMUS
GnRH

A.P

FSH   *LH*

OESTROGEN
from
developing
GRAAFIAN
FOLLICLES
stimulates
DUCTS
to grow
and branch.
Area around
nipple
(areola)
enlarges

BY MATURITY
(when ovarian
hormonal cycle is
well established and
ova are being shed
regularly)

PROGESTERONE
from
CORPUS
LUTEUM
stimulates
sacs of milk – secreting
gland cells –ALVEOLI –
to develop.

Ducts lined by flattened
epithelium.

Fibrous tissue

× 75

Duct epithelium proliferates
and sprouts.

Fibrous tissue
increased.

Fat is
deposited
giving
female
shape.

× 75

Alveolar epithelium sprouts.

More
fibrous
tissue
stroma
formed

× 75

241

MAMMARY GLANDS

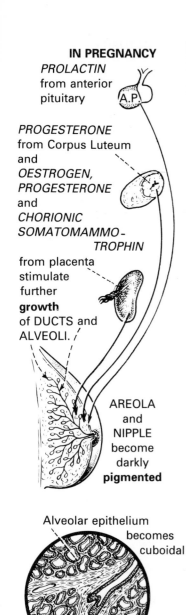

IN PREGNANCY

PROLACTIN from anterior pituitary

PROGESTERONE from Corpus Luteum and *OESTROGEN, PROGESTERONE* and *CHORIONIC SOMATOMAMMO-TROPHIN*

from placenta stimulate further **growth** of DUCTS and ALVEOLI.

AREOLA and NIPPLE become darkly **pigmented**

Alveolar epithelium becomes cuboidal

× 75

Oestrogens and *Progesterone* block milk production by *Prolactin* at this stage.

HYPOTHALAMUS

AFTER CHILDBIRTH

Fall in *OESTROGEN* and *PROGESTERONE* (after loss of placenta) removes their inhibitory influence on *Prolactin*.

A steady increase in *Prolactin* release by anterior pituitary occurs throughout pregnancy and now stimulates prepared

↓

GLAND ALVEOLI to secrete **milk**

Constituents of **MILK** are derived from blood flowing through gland.

Alveolar cells – milk proteins in vesicles released by exocytosis

× 75

Alveolar cells – milk proteins in vesicles released by exocytosis

Hypo-thalamus

PRH

PROLACTIN

OXYTOCIN

Emotional factors influence **LACTATION** – Milk secretion starts 3-4 days after childbirth and is maintained by *Prolactin* surges, set up by suckling. AFFERENT nerve impulses by child **suckling** give rise to reflex EFFERENT nerve impulses to posterior pituitary for the release of *OXYTOCIN* – carried by blood stream to stimulate the 'let-down' of milk which is then more readily available to the suckling child. (see p. 213)

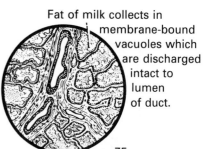

Fat of milk collects in membrane-bound vacuoles which are discharged intact to lumen of duct.

× 75

Afferent impulses cause hypothalamic neurons to release *Prolactin Releasing Hormone (PRH)*

MAMMARY GLANDS

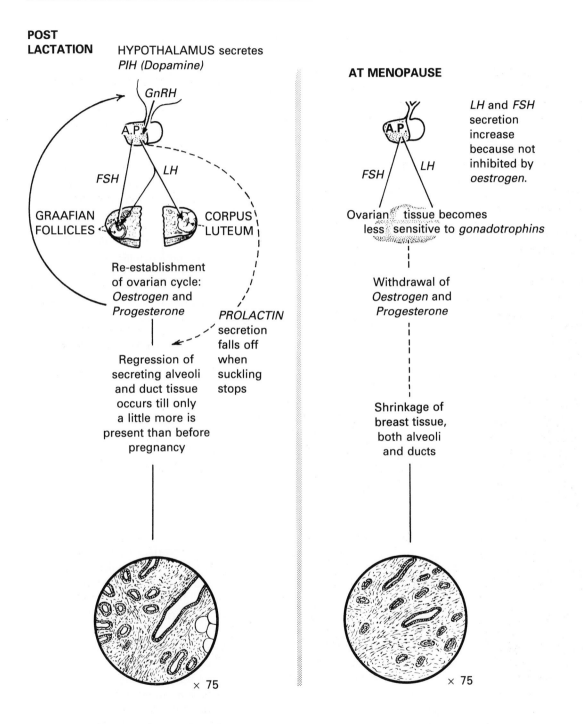

POST LACTATION

HYPOTHALAMUS secretes *PIH (Dopamine)*

GnRH

A.P.

FSH   *LH*

GRAAFIAN FOLLICLES   CORPUS LUTEUM

Re-establishment of ovarian cycle: *Oestrogen* and *Progesterone*

PROLACTIN secretion falls off when suckling stops

Regression of secreting alveoli and duct tissue occurs till only a little more is present than before pregnancy

× 75

AT MENOPAUSE

A.P.

LH and *FSH* secretion increase because not inhibited by *oestrogen*.

FSH   *LH*

Ovarian tissue becomes less sensitive to *gonadotrophins*

Withdrawal of *Oestrogen* and *Progesterone*

Shrinkage of breast tissue, both alveoli and ducts

× 75

MENOPAUSE

Between the ages of 45 and 55 years **ovarian** tissue gradually ceases to respond to stimulation by *anterior pituitary gonadotrophic hormones*.

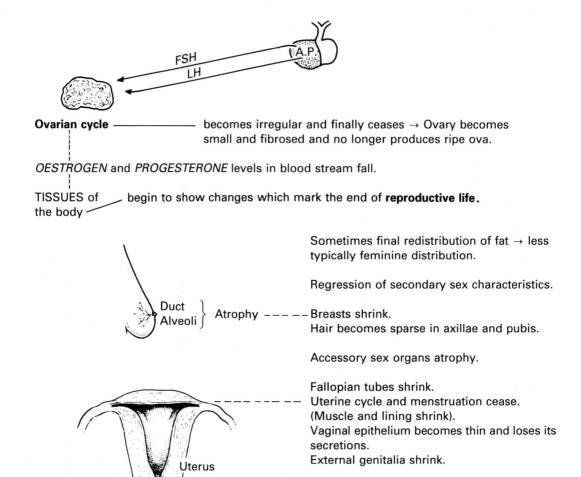

Ovarian cycle —————————— becomes irregular and finally ceases → Ovary becomes small and fibrosed and no longer produces ripe ova.

OESTROGEN and *PROGESTERONE* levels in blood stream fall.

TISSUES of the body — begin to show changes which mark the end of **reproductive life**.

Sometimes final redistribution of fat → less typically feminine distribution.

Regression of secondary sex characteristics.

Duct Alveoli } Atrophy ————Breasts shrink.
Hair becomes sparse in axillae and pubis.

Accessory sex organs atrophy.

Fallopian tubes shrink.
Uterine cycle and menstruation cease. (Muscle and lining shrink).
Vaginal epithelium becomes thin and loses its secretions.
External genitalia shrink.

Uterus

Vagina

Psychological and personality changes
Sexual drive is frequently not diminished – may be increased. Irritability and anxiety attacks may occur accompanied by 'hot flushes' (vasodilatation of arterioles), feeling of warmth and excessive sweating.

Incidence of high blood pressure and atherosclerosis rises to that of men. Marked bone demineralization (**osteoporosis**) occurs, because of oestrogen deficiency. Oestrogen **supplements** reduce many of the symptoms of the menopause but they may occasionally facilitate breast or cervical cancer. Some oestrogen secretion continues. Androgen precursors from ovarian stromal and adrenal cells are converted to *oestrone* by liver and adipose tissue. This diminishes menopausal symptoms. Obese women may therefore suffer less from oestrogen deprivation.

PITUITARY, OVARIAN AND ENDOMETRIAL CYCLES

HYPOTHALAMUS secretes *gonadotrophin-releasing hormone* into hypothalamic-hypophyseal portal circulation (p. 207).

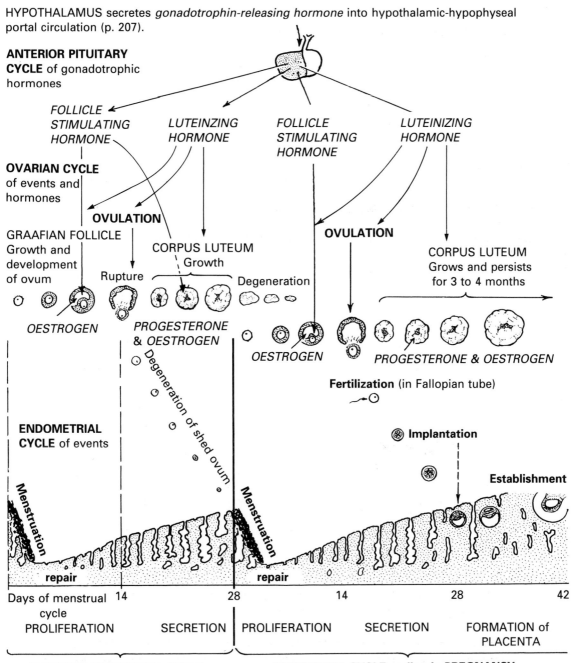

ANTERIOR PITUITARY CYCLE of gonadotrophic hormones

FOLLICLE STIMULATING HORMONE

LUTEINZING HORMONE

FOLLICLE STIMULATING HORMONE

LUTEINZING HORMONE

OVARIAN CYCLE of events and hormones

OVULATION

OVULATION

GRAAFIAN FOLLICLE Growth and development of ovum

CORPUS LUTEUM Growth

CORPUS LUTEUM Grows and persists for 3 to 4 months

Rupture

Degeneration

OESTROGEN

PROGESTERONE & OESTROGEN

OESTROGEN

PROGESTERONE & OESTROGEN

Degeneration of shed ovum

Fertilization (in Fallopian tube)

ENDOMETRIAL CYCLE of events

Implantation

Establishment

Menstruation

Menstruation

repair

repair

Days of menstrual cycle

14   28   14   28   42

PROLIFERATION   SECRETION   PROLIFERATION   SECRETION   FORMATION of PLACENTA

ORDINARY MENSTRUAL CYCLE   **MENSTRUAL CYCLE ending in PREGNANCY**

Secretion of GnRH, and thus LH and FSH, is powerfully inhibited by progesterone and oestrogens. Since these hormones are present in high concentration throughout pregnancy, follicle development, ovulation and menstrual cycles stop for the duration of pregnancy.

245

CHAPTER 10

CENTRAL NERVOUS SYSTEM — LOCOMOTOR SYSTEM

NERVOUS SYSTEM

Most functions of the body are controlled by either the **nervous** or **endocrine** systems. Usually rapid activities, e.g. muscular contraction, are controlled by the nervous system and slower activities, e.g. metabolic functions, are controlled by the endocrine system.

The **NERVOUS** system is specialized in:
(a) **Irritability** – the ability to receive and respond to stimuli from the external and internal environments.
(b) **Conduction** – the ability to transmit signals to and from **central integrating** centres.
(c) **Integration** – the ability to analyse information from the environment in order to generate **behaviour** appropriate to that information.

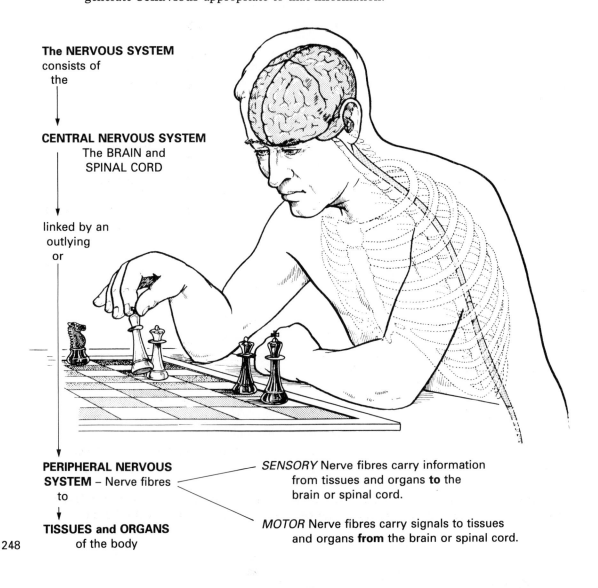

The NERVOUS SYSTEM
consists of
the
↓

CENTRAL NERVOUS SYSTEM
The BRAIN and
SPINAL CORD
↓

linked by an
outlying
or
↓

PERIPHERAL NERVOUS SYSTEM – Nerve fibres
to
↓

TISSUES and ORGANS
of the body

SENSORY Nerve fibres carry information from tissues and organs **to** the brain or spinal cord.

MOTOR Nerve fibres carry signals to tissues and organs **from** the brain or spinal cord.

DEVELOPMENT OF THE NERVOUS SYSTEM

The nervous system develops in the embryo from a simple tube of **ectoderm** – the **primitive neural tube**.

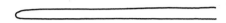

The **cells** forming the wall become the nervous tissue of the **brain** and **spinal cord**. The **canal** becomes distended to form the **ventricles** of the **brain** and the **central canal** of the **spinal cord**:

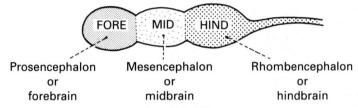

Prosencephalon or forebrain	Mesencephalon or midbrain	Rhombencephalon or hindbrain

Each of these swellings expand mainly by cell division and become more and more complicated:

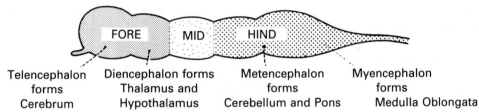

Telencephalon forms Cerebrum	Diencephalon forms Thalamus and Hypothalamus	Metencephalon forms Cerebellum and Pons	Myencephalon forms Medulla Oblongata

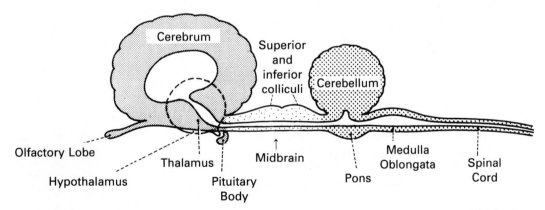

Brainstem = Midbrain + Hindbrain
(see p.253)

There are now many layers of cells forming the brain and spinal cord. The ventricles of the brain and the central canal of the spinal cord are filled with **cerebrospinal fluid**.

CEREBRUM

The largest part of the human brain is the **cerebrum** – made up of **two cerebral hemispheres**. Each of these is divided into **lobes**.

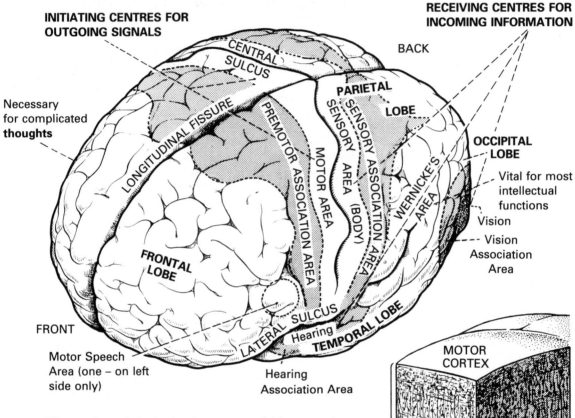

INITIATING CENTRES FOR OUTGOING SIGNALS

RECEIVING CENTRES FOR INCOMING INFORMATION

BACK

Necessary for complicated **thoughts**

CENTRAL SULCUS

PARIETAL LOBE

PREMOTOR ASSOCIATION AREA

LONGITUDINAL FISSURE

MOTOR AREA

SENSORY AREA

SENSORY ASSOCIATION AREA (BODY)

WERNICKE'S AREA

OCCIPITAL LOBE

Vital for most intellectual functions

Vision

Vision Association Area

FRONTAL LOBE

FRONT

Motor Speech Area (one – on left side only)

LATERAL SULCUS

Hearing

TEMPORAL LOBE

Hearing Association Area

MOTOR CORTEX

GREY MATTER

WHITE MATTER

90% of all nerve cells in the body are in the cerebral cortex.

GIANT PYRAMIDAL CELL (BETZ CELL)

The surface of the brain shows many folds or **convolutions**. The raised portions are called **gyri,** the furrows **sulci** or – if particularly deep – **fissures**. The folding has the effect of increasing the amount of **grey matter** present. The grey matter forms the outer layer or **cortex** which has six layers. The cell bodies of its **neurons** are arranged in **modules**, each containing compactly grouped vertical **columns** of pyramidal cells and their axons. Each module is connected to many other modules producing a great **divergence** of input and output. Ascribing specific functions to specific areas of the cortex, although useful, is an oversimplification of the way in which the cortex functions.

Sensory **association** areas provide **analysis** and **interpretation** of sensory experiences.

HORIZONTAL SECTION THROUGH BRAIN

This view shows surface **grey matter** which contains nerve cells and inner **white matter** made up of nerve fibres.

Deep in the substance of the cerebral hemispheres there are **additional** masses of **grey matter**: –

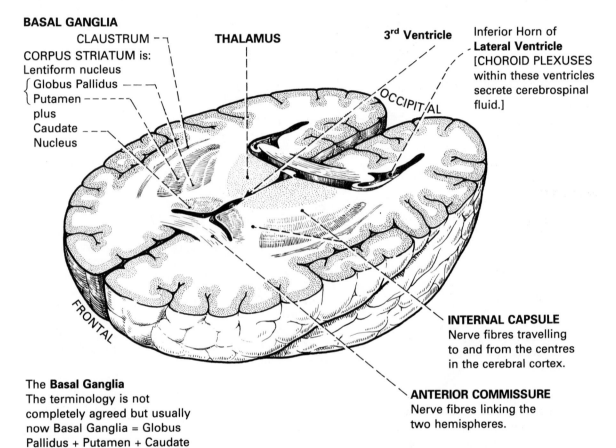

BASAL GANGLIA

CLAUSTRUM

CORPUS STRIATUM is:
Lentiform nucleus
{ Globus Pallidus
{ Putamen
plus
Caudate
Nucleus

THALAMUS

3rd **Ventricle**

Inferior Horn of
Lateral Ventricle
[CHOROID PLEXUSES
within these ventricles
secrete cerebrospinal
fluid.]

OCCIPITAL

FRONTAL

INTERNAL CAPSULE
Nerve fibres travelling
to and from the centres
in the cerebral cortex.

ANTERIOR COMMISSURE
Nerve fibres linking the
two hemispheres.

The **Basal Ganglia**
The terminology is not
completely agreed but usually
now Basal Ganglia = Globus
Pallidus + Putamen + Caudate
nucleus.
Claustrum is often excluded.
Structures associated with
basal ganglia functionally are
subthalamic nucleus and
substantia nigra. This complex
is concerned with **planning**
and **programming voluntary
muscle movement**.

The **Thalamus** is an important relay centre
mainly for sensory fibres but also motor
fibres from the basal ganglia and cerebellum
on their way to the cerebral cortex. Crude
appreciation of touch, pain and temperature
may occur here. It also relays part of the
reticular activating system which controls
the level and state of consciousness. (See
page 253.)

VERTICAL SECTION THROUGH BRAIN

This is a vertical section through the **longitudinal fissure** which separates the two cerebral hemispheres. At the bottom of the cleft are tracts of nerve fibres which link the two hemispheres – the **corpus callosum**.

The **grey matter** in the brainstem is formed by groups of nerve cell bodies called nuclei. These are distributed irregularly through the white matter.

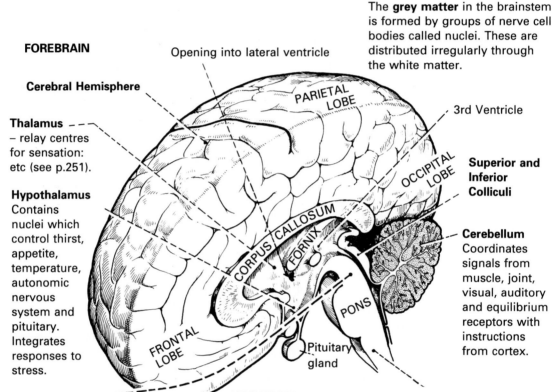

FOREBRAIN

Opening into lateral ventricle

Cerebral Hemisphere

PARIETAL LOBE

3rd Ventricle

Thalamus – – –
– relay centres for sensation: etc (see p.251).

OCCIPITAL LOBE

Superior and Inferior Colliculi

Hypothalamus Contains nuclei which control thirst, appetite, temperature, autonomic nervous system and pituitary. Integrates responses to stress.

CORPUS CALLOSUM

FORNIX

Cerebellum Coordinates signals from muscle, joint, visual, auditory and equilibrium receptors with instructions from cortex.

PONS

FRONTAL LOBE

Pituitary gland

MIDBRAIN
Superior and inferior colliculi are centres for visual and auditory reflexes. Contains nuclei of III, IV cranial nerves, also the red nucleus and substantia nigra which help to control skilled muscular movements. The **white matter** carries nerve fibres linking red nucleus with cerebral cortex, thalamus, cerebellum, corpus striatum and spinal cord. It also carries ascending sensory fibres in lateral and medial lemnisci and descending motor fibres on their way to pons and spinal cord.

HINDBRAIN:
[PONS, CEREBELLUM, MEDULLA OBLONGATA]

Pons: Groups of neurons form sensory nucleus of V and also nuclei of VI and VII cranial nerves. Other nerve cells here relay impulses along their axons to cerebellum and cerebrum. Rubrospinal tract, lateral and medial lemnisci pass through pons as do nerve fibres linking cerebral cortex with medulla oblongata and spinal cord.

Medulla Oblongata
Contains centres controlling heart rate, blood vessels, respiration and nuclei of VIII, IX, X, XI, XII cranial nerves, gracile and cuneate nuclei – second sensory neurons in cutaneous pathways. Tracts of sensory fibres decussate and ascend to other side of cerebral cortex. Some fibres remain uncrossed. The larger part of each motor corticospinal tract crosses and descends in other side of spinal cord.

CORONAL SECTION THROUGH BRAIN

This is a section through the central (transverse) sulcus. It shows the major parts of the brain from another perspective.

LIMBIC SYSTEM Consists of the rim of inner cortex surrounding the corpus callosum and associated deeper structures, the amygdala, the hippocampus, portions of the basal ganglia and thalamus. It is concerned with **emotions**, feeding and sexual behaviour, rage, fear, motivation and learning. The hypothalamus is closely associated with it.

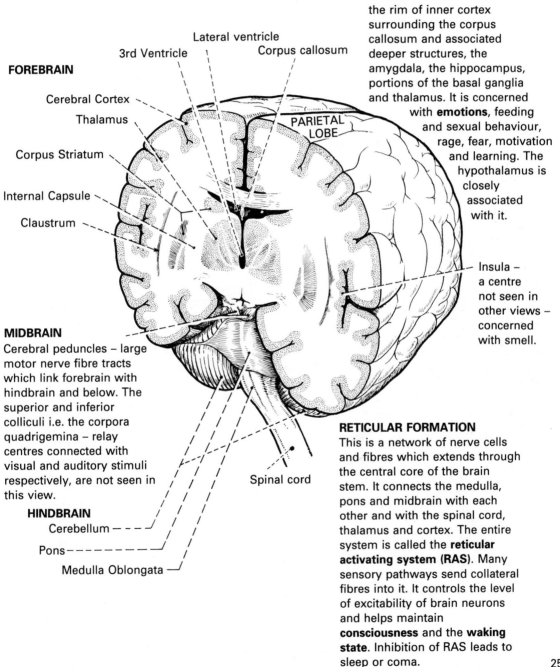

FOREBRAIN

Cerebral Cortex

Thalamus

Corpus Striatum

Internal Capsule

Claustrum

3rd Ventricle

Lateral ventricle

Corpus callosum

PARIETAL LOBE

Insula – a centre not seen in other views – concerned with smell.

MIDBRAIN
Cerebral peduncles – large motor nerve fibre tracts which link forebrain with hindbrain and below. The superior and inferior colliculi i.e. the corpora quadrigemina – relay centres connected with visual and auditory stimuli respectively, are not seen in this view.

HINDBRAIN

Cerebellum

Pons

Medulla Oblongata

Spinal cord

RETICULAR FORMATION
This is a network of nerve cells and fibres which extends through the central core of the brain stem. It connects the medulla, pons and midbrain with each other and with the spinal cord, thalamus and cortex. The entire system is called the **reticular activating system (RAS)**. Many sensory pathways send collateral fibres into it. It controls the level of excitability of brain neurons and helps maintain **consciousness** and the **waking state**. Inhibition of RAS leads to sleep or coma.

CRANIAL NERVES

Twelve pairs of nerves arise directly from the undersurface of the brain to supply head and neck and most of the viscera.

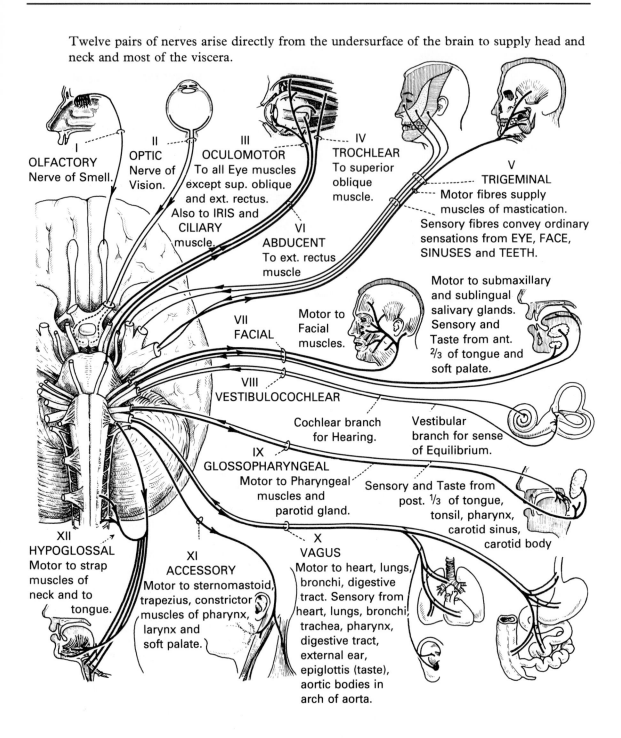

I
OLFACTORY
Nerve of Smell.

II
OPTIC
Nerve of Vision.

III
OCULOMOTOR
To all Eye muscles except sup. oblique and ext. rectus. Also to IRIS and CILIARY muscle.

IV
TROCHLEAR
To superior oblique muscle.

VI
ABDUCENT
To ext. rectus muscle

V
TRIGEMINAL
Motor fibres supply muscles of mastication. Sensory fibres convey ordinary sensations from EYE, FACE, SINUSES and TEETH.

Motor to submaxillary and sublingual salivary glands. Sensory and Taste from ant. 2/3 of tongue and soft palate.

VII
FACIAL

Motor to Facial muscles.

VIII
VESTIBULOCOCHLEAR

Cochlear branch for Hearing.

Vestibular branch for sense of Equilibrium.

IX
GLOSSOPHARYNGEAL
Motor to Pharyngeal muscles and parotid gland.

Sensory and Taste from post. 1/3 of tongue, tonsil, pharynx, carotid sinus, carotid body

XII
HYPOGLOSSAL
Motor to strap muscles of neck and to tongue.

XI
ACCESSORY
Motor to sternomastoid, trapezius, constrictor muscles of pharynx, larynx and soft palate.

X
VAGUS
Motor to heart, lungs, bronchi, digestive tract. Sensory from heart, lungs, bronchi, trachea, pharynx, digestive tract, external ear, epiglottis (taste), aortic bodies in arch of aorta.

SPINAL CORD

The **spinal cord** lies within the vertebral canal. It is continuous above with the medulla oblongata.

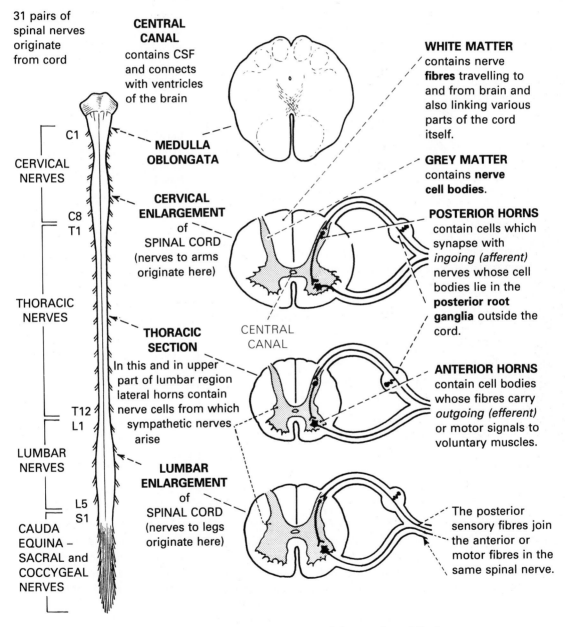

31 pairs of spinal nerves originate from cord

CERVICAL NERVES

C1

C8
T1

THORACIC NERVES

T12
L1

LUMBAR NERVES

L5
S1

CAUDA EQUINA – SACRAL and COCCYGEAL NERVES

CENTRAL CANAL contains CSF and connects with ventricles of the brain

MEDULLA OBLONGATA

CERVICAL ENLARGEMENT of SPINAL CORD (nerves to arms originate here)

THORACIC SECTION
In this and in upper part of lumbar region lateral horns contain nerve cells from which sympathetic nerves arise

LUMBAR ENLARGEMENT of SPINAL CORD (nerves to legs originate here)

CENTRAL CANAL

WHITE MATTER contains nerve **fibres** travelling to and from brain and also linking various parts of the cord itself.

GREY MATTER contains **nerve cell bodies**.

POSTERIOR HORNS contain cells which synapse with *ingoing (afferent)* nerves whose cell bodies lie in the **posterior root ganglia** outside the cord.

ANTERIOR HORNS contain cell bodies whose fibres carry *outgoing (efferent)* or motor signals to voluntary muscles.

The posterior sensory fibres join the anterior or motor fibres in the same spinal nerve.

The spinal nerves travel to all parts of the trunk and limbs.

255

SYNAPSE

The structural unit of the nervous system is the **neuron** or nerve cell. See page 17. Neurons are linked together in the nervous system . . .

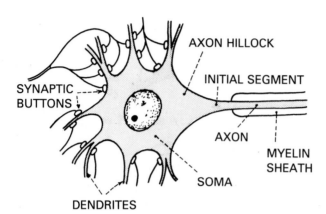

AXON HILLOCK

INITIAL SEGMENT

SYNAPTIC
BUTTONS

AXON

MYELIN
SHEATH

SOMA

DENDRITES

The AXON of a neuron ends in small swellings – SYNAPTIC BUTTONS or END FEET. These terminate very close to the DENDRITES, SOMA or AXON of the next cell. In most cases there is no direct protoplasmic union between neurons at the **synapse** though connection of neurons by **gap junctions** (page 24) sometimes occurs.

One neuron usually connects with a great many others, often widely scattered in different parts of the brain and spinal cord. In this way intricate chains of nerve cells forming complex pathways for *incoming* and *outgoing* information can be built up within the central nervous system.

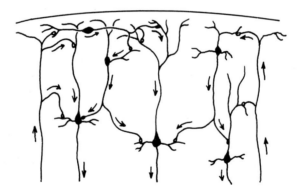

When the **nerve impulse** – a small brief change in membrane potential – reaches a synapse it causes the release from the nerve endings of a **chemical** substance, a chemical transmitter or neurotransmitter, which diffuses across the gap and alters the membrane potential of the next neuron. This alteration of potential spreads across the **soma** of the next neuron and, if large enough, generates more nerve impulses at its **axon hillock-initial segment**. These impulses then travel along the next axon.

A synapse permits transmission of the impulse in one direction only.

REFLEX ACTION

The **neuron** is the **anatomical** or **structural unit** of the nervous system: the **nervous reflex** is the **physiological** or **functional unit**.

A nervous reflex is an involuntary action caused by the stimulation of a **receptor** at the end of an *afferent (sensory)* nerve axon.

The structural basis of reflex action is the reflex arc. In its simplest form this consists of: –

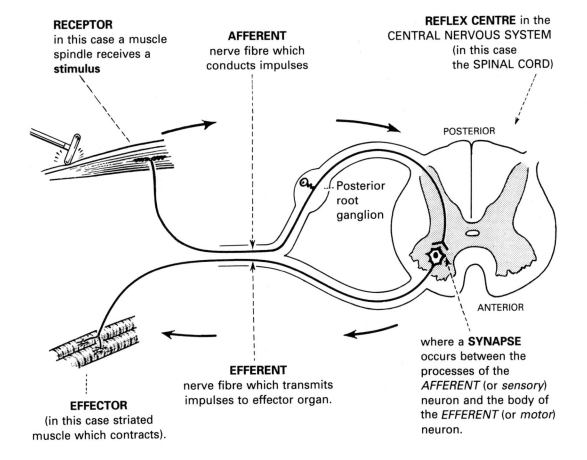

RECEPTOR
in this case a muscle spindle receives a **stimulus**

AFFERENT
nerve fibre which conducts impulses

REFLEX CENTRE in the CENTRAL NERVOUS SYSTEM (in this case the SPINAL CORD)

POSTERIOR

Posterior root ganglion

ANTERIOR

where a **SYNAPSE** occurs between the processes of the *AFFERENT* (or *sensory*) neuron and the body of the *EFFERENT* (or *motor*) neuron.

EFFERENT
nerve fibre which transmits impulses to effector organ.

EFFECTOR
(in this case striated muscle which contracts).

Reflexes form the basis of all central nervous system (CNS) activity. They occur at all levels of the brain and spinal cord. Important bodily functions such as movements of respiration, digestion, etc., are all controlled through reflexes. We are made aware of some reflex acts; others occur without our being conscious of them.

STRETCH REFLEXES

In man a very few **reflex arcs** involve *two neurons only*. Two examples elicited by doctors when testing the nervous system are: –

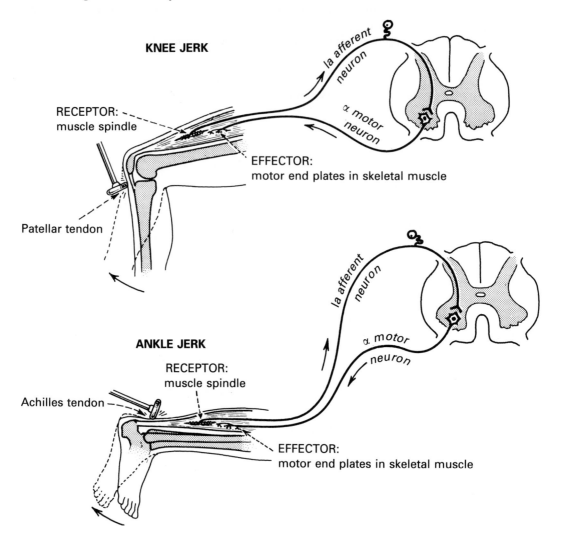

KNEE JERK

RECEPTOR:
muscle spindle

Ia afferent neuron

α motor neuron

EFFECTOR:
motor end plates in skeletal muscle

Patellar tendon

ANKLE JERK

RECEPTOR:
muscle spindle

Achilles tendon

Ia afferent neuron

α motor neuron

EFFECTOR:
motor end plates in skeletal muscle

When the tendon is sharply tapped the **muscle** is **stretched** (NB: the **stimulus** is by **stretch** of the **muscle spindle**.) Nerve impulses pass into the spinal cord – and out to the muscle which then contracts. This is a **monosynaptic** reflex since there is only one synapse in the reflex pathway.

SPINAL REFLEXES

In most **reflex arcs** in man *afferent* and *efferent neurons* are linked by at least one **interneuron**.

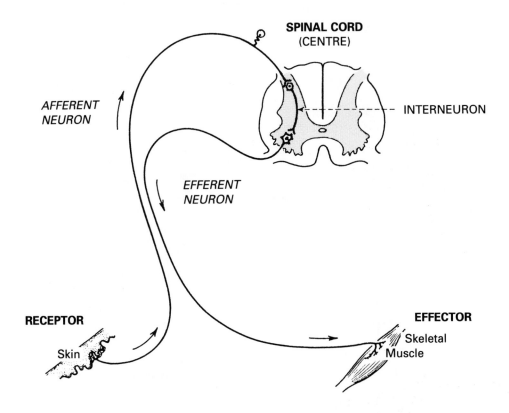

A chain of **many** interneurons is frequently found.

'EDIFICE' OF THE CNS *(After R.C. Garry)*

In the majority of reflex arcs in man a chain of many connector neurons is found. There may be link-ups with various levels of the brain and spinal cord.

This diagram gives a highly simplified concept of the type of **link-up** which can occur between different levels of the central nervous system.

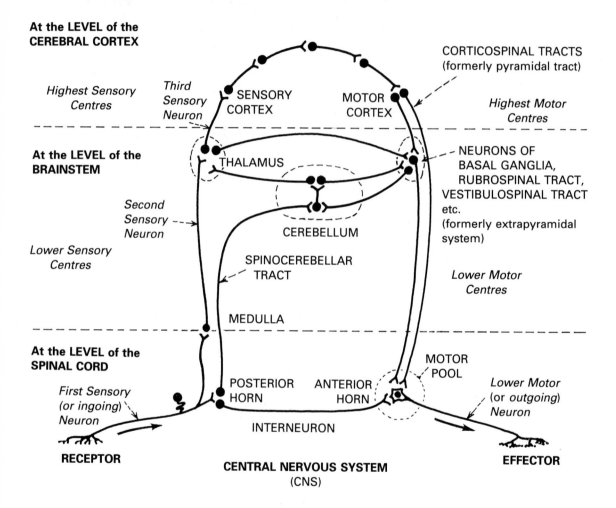

At the LEVEL of the CEREBRAL CORTEX

Highest Sensory Centres

Third Sensory Neuron

SENSORY CORTEX

MOTOR CORTEX

CORTICOSPINAL TRACTS (formerly pyramidal tract)

Highest Motor Centres

At the LEVEL of the BRAINSTEM

THALAMUS

NEURONS OF BASAL GANGLIA, RUBROSPINAL TRACT, VESTIBULOSPINAL TRACT etc. (formerly extrapyramidal system)

Second Sensory Neuron

CEREBELLUM

Lower Sensory Centres

SPINOCEREBELLAR TRACT

Lower Motor Centres

MEDULLA

At the LEVEL of the SPINAL CORD

MOTOR POOL

First Sensory (or ingoing) Neuron

POSTERIOR HORN

ANTERIOR HORN

Lower Motor (or outgoing) Neuron

INTERNEURON

RECEPTOR

CENTRAL NERVOUS SYSTEM (CNS)

EFFECTOR

Every receptor neuron is thus potentially linked in the CNS with a large number of effector organs all over the body, and every effector neuron is similarly in communication with receptors all over the body.

Centres in the brain and brain stem can thus modify reflex acts which occur through the spinal cord. These centres can send 'suppressing' or 'facilitating' impulses along their pathways to the cells in the spinal cord.

REFLEX ACTION

Most **reflex actions** in man involve several **reflex arcs**.

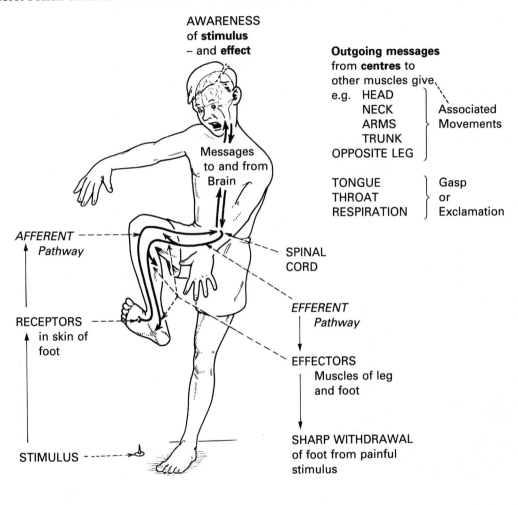

AWARENESS
of **stimulus**
– and **effect**

Outgoing messages
from **centres** to
other muscles give,
e.g. HEAD
NECK
ARMS   } Associated
TRUNK   Movements
OPPOSITE LEG

TONGUE   } Gasp
THROAT   } or
RESPIRATION } Exclamation

Messages
to and from
Brain

AFFERENT
Pathway

SPINAL
CORD

EFFERENT
Pathway

RECEPTORS
in skin of
foot

EFFECTORS
Muscles of leg
and foot

STIMULUS

SHARP WITHDRAWAL
of foot from painful
stimulus

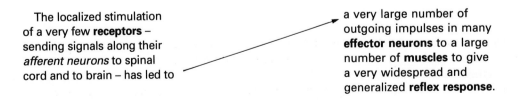

The localized stimulation of a very few **receptors** – sending signals along their *afferent neurons* to spinal cord and to brain – has led to a very large number of outgoing impulses in many **effector neurons** to a large number of **muscles** to give a very widespread and generalized **reflex response**.

This is possible because each receptor neuron is potentially connected within the central nervous system to many effector neurons.

ARRANGEMENT OF NEURONS

Some of the ways in which neurons can be linked are indicated here: –

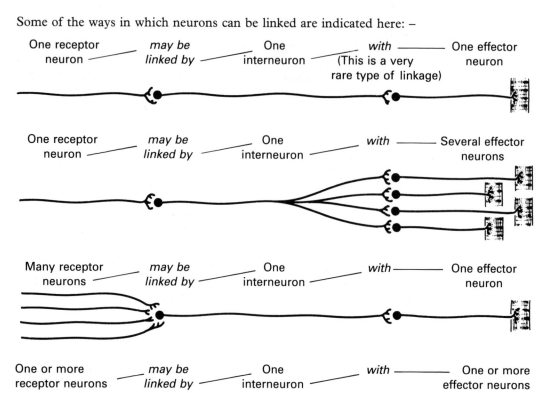

| One receptor neuron | may be linked by | One interneuron | with (This is a very rare type of linkage) | One effector neuron |

| One receptor neuron | may be linked by | One interneuron | with | Several effector neurons |

| Many receptor neurons | may be linked by | One interneuron | with | One effector neuron |

| One or more receptor neurons | may be linked by | One interneuron | with | One or more effector neurons |

Other neurons synapsing with the effector neuron(s) may give a complex link-up with centres at higher and lower levels of the brain and spinal cord.

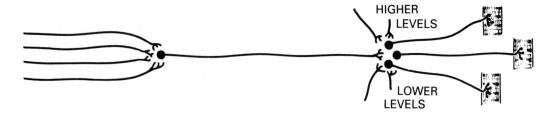

HIGHER LEVELS

LOWER LEVELS

Through such 'functional' link-ups, neurons in different parts of the central nervous system, when active, can influence each other. This makes it possible for **'conditioned' reflexes** to become established (for simple example see p. 75).

Such reflexes probably form the basis of all training so that it becomes difficult to say where **reflex** (or **involuntary**) behaviour ends and purely **voluntary** behaviour begins.

RECEPTOR OR GENERATOR POTENTIALS AND ADAPTATION

The term **receptor** can refer to a membrane protein to which a ligand attaches (p.69). It can also refer to a **sensory** nerve ending which has ion channels opened by an environmental stimulus e.g. light, taste, pressure etc., causing a change in its membrane potential. This change can generate action potentials in the afferent nerve fibres. There are two structurally different types of sensory receptor. Some, e.g. vision, hearing and taste, have separate receptor cells with invaginations in which sensory axons synapse.

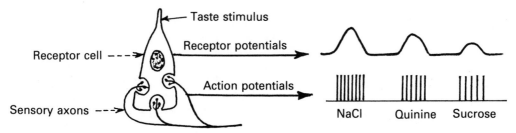

Cell stimulation produces a **receptor** or **generator potential** which is graded (i.e. its size depends on the amount of stimulation) and spreads electrotonically (p.65) over the cell. Neurotransmitter released at the synapses produces a graded depolarization of the neurons. If this is large enough to bring the membrane at the first node of Ranvier (p.67) to threshold, action potentials are initiated.

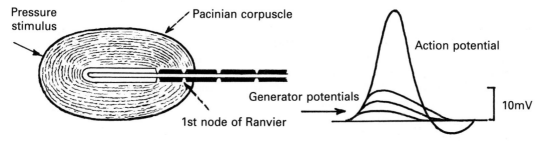

The second type consists of a specialized expansion at the end of a sensory nerve axon e.g. a Pacinian corpuscle (a pressure receptor). When a small amount of pressure is applied to the receptor, electrotonic spread of a generator potential occurs. Increased pressure increases the potential.

If the generator potential reaches 10mV at the first node of Ranvier, an action potential is generated. Further increase in pressure produces a larger generator potential and the nerve fires repetitively and will continue to fire as long as the generator potential remains at or above 10mV.

If a constant stimulus is applied for some time to a receptor, the frequency of the action potentials in the afferent neuron decreases with time. This is called **adaptation.**

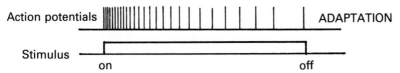

Some receptors are **rapidly** adapting while others are **slowly** adapting.

SENSE ORGANS

Man's awareness of the **world** is limited to those forms of energy, physical or chemical, to which he has receptors designed to respond. (Many 'events' in the Universe go undetected by man because he has no sense organs which can respond to them.)

Each sense organ is designed to respond to one type of stimulation.

EXTEROCEPTORS are stimulated by events in the **external environment**.

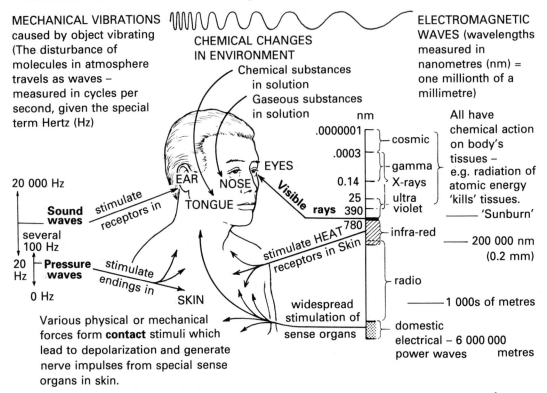

MECHANICAL VIBRATIONS caused by object vibrating (The disturbance of molecules in atmosphere travels as waves – measured in cycles per second, given the special term Hertz (Hz)

CHEMICAL CHANGES IN ENVIRONMENT
- Chemical substances in solution
- Gaseous substances in solution

ELECTROMAGNETIC WAVES (wavelengths measured in nanometres (nm) = one millionth of a millimetre)

20 000 Hz

Sound waves stimulate receptors in

EAR   NOSE   EYES
TONGUE

several 100 Hz

20 Hz   **Pressure waves** stimulate endings in

0 Hz   SKIN

Visible rays   stimulate HEAT receptors in Skin

nm
.0000001   cosmic
.0003   gamma
0.14   X-rays
25   ultra violet
390
780   infra-red

radio

widespread stimulation of sense organs

domestic electrical – 6 000 000 power waves   metres

All have chemical action on body's tissues – e.g. radiation of atomic energy 'kills' tissues.
———— 'Sunburn'

———— 200 000 nm (0.2 mm)

————1 000s of metres

Various physical or mechanical forces form **contact** stimuli which lead to depolarization and generate nerve impulses from special sense organs in skin.

Exteroceptors may convey information to **consciousness** with **awareness** or **sensation** and lead to suitable responses planned **in cerebral cortex** or they may serve as *afferent* pathways for **reflex** (or **involuntary**) **action** with or without rising to consciousness.

PROPRIOCEPTORS are stimulated by changes in **locomotor system** of body

Labyrinth . . . movements and position of head	Sense of **equilibrium** or
Muscles . . . stretch	**balance** and **awareness**
Tendons . . . tension and stretch	of **position** and **movement**
Joints . . . stretch and pressure	of body in space.

INTEROCEPTORS in **viscera** are stimulated by changes in **internal environment** (e.g. by distension in hollow organs).

Much of the proprio- and interoceptor information never rises to consciousness.
Overstimulation of some receptors can give rise to sensation of pain. Some receptors show **adaptation** – if continuously stimulated they send reduced numbers of impulses to the brain

(see p. 263).

SMELL

Smell is a **chemical sense** i.e. the receptors respond to **chemical stimuli** and are thus called chemoreceptors. To arouse the sensation a substance must first be in a **gaseous** state then go into **solution**.

The ORGAN OF SMELL is the NOSE – Also serves as the main air passage to respiratory system.

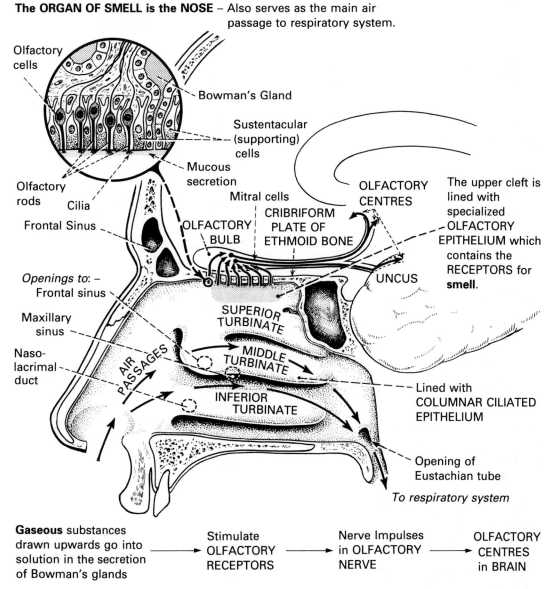

Olfactory cells

Bowman's Gland

Sustentacular (supporting) cells

Mucous secretion

Mitral cells

OLFACTORY CENTRES

The upper cleft is lined with specialized OLFACTORY EPITHELIUM which contains the RECEPTORS for **smell**.

Olfactory rods Cilia

OLFACTORY BULB

CRIBRIFORM PLATE OF ETHMOID BONE

Frontal Sinus

UNCUS

Openings to: – Frontal sinus

SUPERIOR TURBINATE

Maxillary sinus

Naso-lacrimal duct

AIR PASSAGES

MIDDLE TURBINATE

INFERIOR TURBINATE

Lined with COLUMNAR CILIATED EPITHELIUM

Opening of Eustachian tube

To respiratory system

Gaseous substances drawn upwards go into solution in the secretion of Bowman's glands ⟶ Stimulate OLFACTORY RECEPTORS ⟶ Nerve Impulses in OLFACTORY NERVE ⟶ OLFACTORY CENTRES in BRAIN

Axons of receptors enter **olfactory bulb**. Terminations are gathered in clusters called **glomeruli** where they meet dendrites of **mitral** cells whose axons run back in olfactory nerve to terminate in **primary olfactory area** (uncus and adjacent parts of amygdaloid nucleus). These areas are linked to olfactory association areas, hypothalamus, autonomic nuclei and limbic system.

TASTE

Taste is a **chemical** sense, i.e. receptors respond to **chemical stimuli**. To arouse the sensation a substance must be in **solution**.

The essential ORGAN OF TASTE is the TONGUE ———— The **voluntary** muscular organ concerned also in **mastication, swallowing** and **speech**.

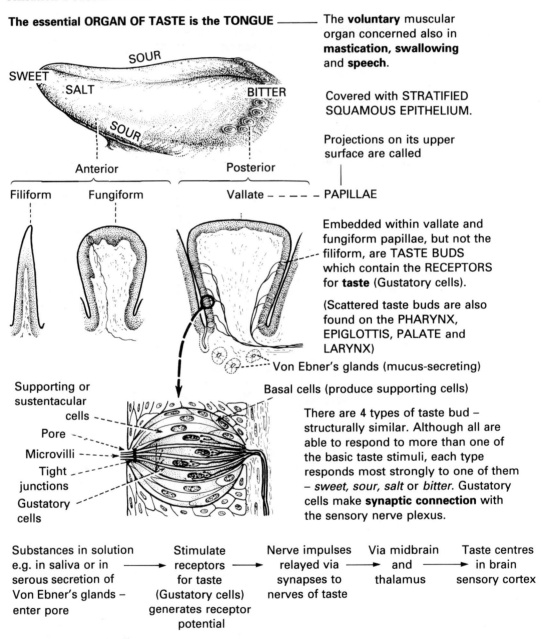

Covered with STRATIFIED SQUAMOUS EPITHELIUM.

Projections on its upper surface are called

PAPILLAE

Embedded within vallate and fungiform papillae, but not the filiform, are TASTE BUDS which contain the RECEPTORS for **taste** (Gustatory cells).

(Scattered taste buds are also found on the PHARYNX, EPIGLOTTIS, PALATE and LARYNX)

Von Ebner's glands (mucus-secreting)

Basal cells (produce supporting cells)

There are 4 types of taste bud – structurally similar. Although all are able to respond to more than one of the basic taste stimuli, each type responds most strongly to one of them – *sweet, sour, salt* or *bitter*. Gustatory cells make **synaptic connection** with the sensory nerve plexus.

Substances in solution e.g. in saliva or in serous secretion of Von Ebner's glands – enter pore ⟶ Stimulate receptors for taste (Gustatory cells) generates receptor potential ⟶ Nerve impulses relayed via synapses to nerves of taste ⟶ Via midbrain and thalamus ⟶ Taste centres in brain sensory cortex

Tastes other than sweet, sour or bitter are probably due to combinations of these with smell or with ordinary skin sensations. Flavours are in large part a combination of taste and smell.

PATHWAYS AND CENTRES FOR TASTE

The **receptors** for **taste** are linked by a chain of three neurons with the **receiving centres** for **taste** in the **cerebral cortex**.

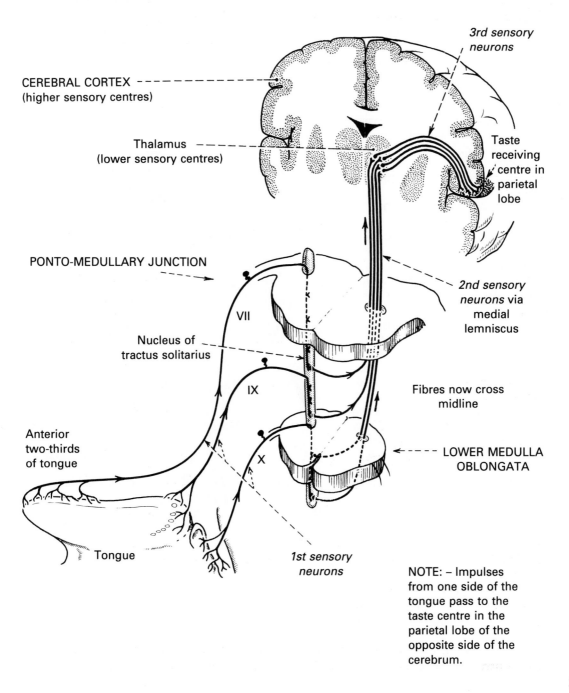

3rd sensory neurons

CEREBRAL CORTEX
(higher sensory centres)

Taste receiving centre in parietal lobe

Thalamus
(lower sensory centres)

PONTO-MEDULLARY JUNCTION

2nd sensory neurons via medial lemniscus

VII

Nucleus of tractus solitarius

IX

Fibres now cross midline

Anterior two-thirds of tongue

X

LOWER MEDULLA OBLONGATA

Tongue

1st sensory neurons

NOTE: – Impulses from one side of the tongue pass to the taste centre in the parietal lobe of the opposite side of the cerebrum.

267

EYE

STRUCTURE
The eyeball has three coats: –

FUNCTION OF PARTS

**1. OUTER COAT –
    SCLERA**
Tough fibrous tissue – – – –
of 'white of eye',
modified
anteriorly
to form the
transparent CORNEA – – – –

[Extrinsic muscles are – – – –
attached to sclera.

**PROTECTIVE
LAYER**
Preserves shape of eyeball and
protects delicate inner layers.

Allows passage of
light rays
Permit and limit movements
of eyeball
within ORBIT.]

**2. MIDDLE COAT –
    CHOROID**
Contains rich blood
supply and melanin.
Circular opening at
front – PUPIL.
Coloured muscular
ring – IRIS – surrounds
pupil.
CILIARY BODY.
CILIARY MUSCLE.
SUSPENSORY
LIGAMENT
suspends

CRYSTALLINE LENS.

CHOROID – Posterior
5/6 of vascular
coat.

**LAYER OF
SUPPLY**
Controls size of
pupil: depth
of focus;
amount of light
entering eye.

Produces
AQUEOUS
HUMOUR.
Circular – has
sphincter-like
action.
Relaxes to allow
curvature of lens
to alter for
accommodation
for **near vision**.
Brings light rays
to focus on
light-sensitive RETINA

**3. INNER COAT –
    the RETINA**
Lines back of eye.
Contains
RECEPTORS for
vision – – – – –

**LIGHT-SENSITIVE
LAYER**
Highly specialized to
respond to stimulation by
light. Convert light energy
into nerve impulses. ——

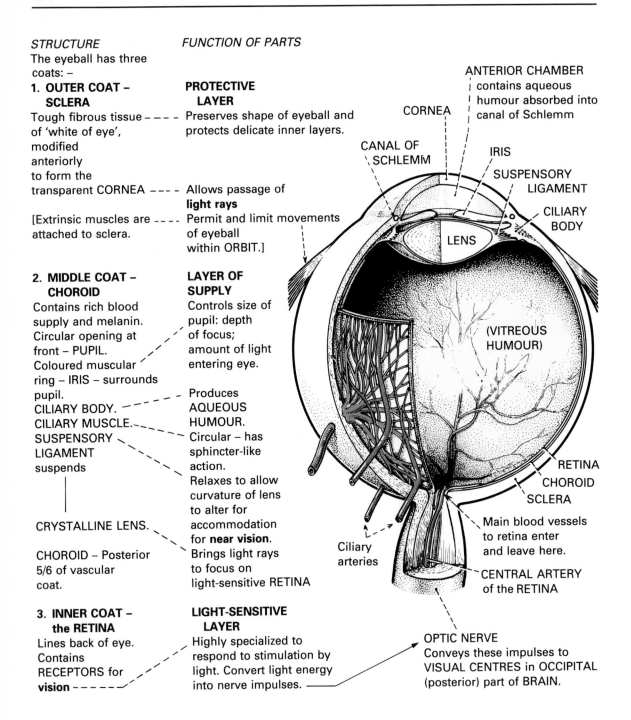

ANTERIOR CHAMBER
contains aqueous
humour absorbed into
canal of Schlemm

CORNEA

CANAL OF
SCHLEMM

IRIS

SUSPENSORY
LIGAMENT

CILIARY
BODY

LENS

(VITREOUS
HUMOUR)

Ciliary
arteries

RETINA
CHOROID
SCLERA

Main blood vessels
to retina enter
and leave here.

CENTRAL ARTERY
of the RETINA

OPTIC NERVE
Conveys these impulses to
VISUAL CENTRES in OCCIPITAL
(posterior) part of BRAIN.

Glaucoma – increased intraocular pressure due to blockage of reabsorption
of aqueous humour into the canal of Schlemm.

PROTECTION OF THE EYE

The hidden posterior 4/5 of the eyeball is encased in a bony socket – the **orbital cavity**. A thick layer of areolar and adipose tissue forms a cushion between bone and eyeball. The exposed anterior 1/5 of the eyeball is protected from injury by: –

The EYELIDS – – – – – – – – – – – – close reflexly to protect eye from dust
    Fringed with EYELASHES   and other foreign particles.

CONJUNCTIVA – – – – – – – – – – – –smooth surfaces which glide over each
    A delicate membrane lining eyelids   other when lids open and close.
and covering exposed surface of eye.

LACRIMAL GLANDS – – – – – – – – – continuously secrete TEARS. These
                                     flow over, wash and lubricate surface
                                     of eye. They contain an **enzyme** –
                                     lysozyme – which destroys bacteria.
                                     Secretion is controlled by parasympathetic
                                     fibres of the facial (VII Cranial) nerve.

TARSAL (or Meibomian) GLANDS - – – – – – – – – – – – – secrete a fluid to prevent lids
(These are embedded in tarsal   from sticking together
plates – connective tissue
giving shape and support
to the eyelids.)

LACRIMAL CANALICULI
  drain tears
  from surface
  of eye

LACRIMAL SAC

NASO-LACRIMAL
  DUCT

Back of NOSE

CONJUNCTIVA

LACRIMAL
GLANDS

LACRIMAL DUCTS

OPENINGS OF
TARSAL GLANDS

ORBICULARIS OCULI
MUSCLE

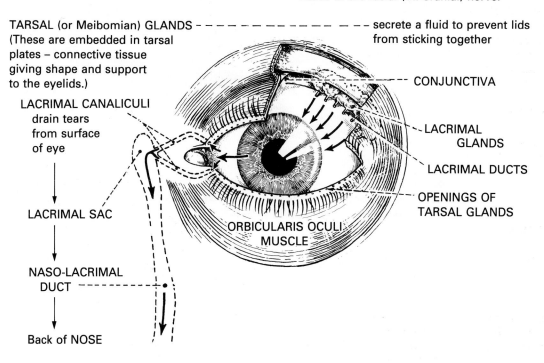

Infection of the tarsal glands produces a cyst on the eyelid called a **chalazion** or **Meibomian cyst**.

The eyelashes have sebacious glands at their base. Infection of these is called a **stye**.

MUSCLES OF EYE

The **eyeballs** are moved by **small muscles** which link the **sclerotic coat** to the **bony socket**.

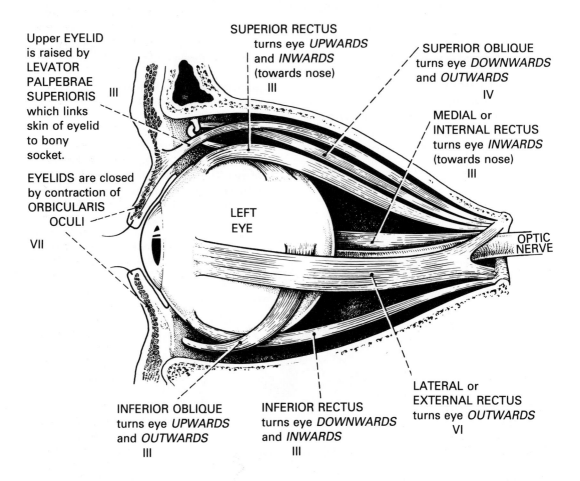

Upper EYELID
is raised by
LEVATOR
PALPEBRAE
SUPERIORIS III
which links
skin of eyelid
to bony
socket.

EYELIDS are closed
by contraction of
ORBICULARIS
OCULI

VII

SUPERIOR RECTUS
turns eye *UPWARDS*
and *INWARDS*
(towards nose)
III

SUPERIOR OBLIQUE
turns eye *DOWNWARDS*
and *OUTWARDS*
IV

MEDIAL or
INTERNAL RECTUS
turns eye *INWARDS*
(towards nose)
III

LEFT
EYE

OPTIC
NERVE

INFERIOR OBLIQUE
turns eye *UPWARDS*
and *OUTWARDS*
III

INFERIOR RECTUS
turns eye *DOWNWARDS*
and *INWARDS*
III

LATERAL or
EXTERNAL RECTUS
turns eye *OUTWARDS*
VI

Acting together, the extrinsic muscles of the eyeballs can bring about **rotatory** movements of the eyes.

The extrinsic muscles are supplied by motor fibres from cranial nerves III, IV and VI.

Because these muscles have to perform very fine and precise movements, the size of their **motor units** is small (see page 304).

CONTROL OF EYE MOVEMENTS

Both eyes must move in a synchronized fashion in order that visual images fall at all times on exactly corresponding points of both retinae.

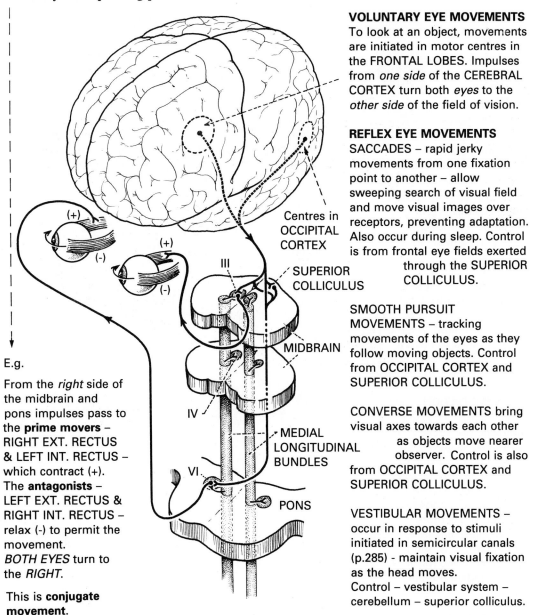

VOLUNTARY EYE MOVEMENTS
To look at an object, movements are initiated in motor centres in the FRONTAL LOBES. Impulses from *one side* of the CEREBRAL CORTEX turn both *eyes* to the *other side* of the field of vision.

REFLEX EYE MOVEMENTS
SACCADES – rapid jerky movements from one fixation point to another – allow sweeping search of visual field and move visual images over receptors, preventing adaptation. Also occur during sleep. Control is from frontal eye fields exerted through the SUPERIOR COLLICULUS.

SMOOTH PURSUIT MOVEMENTS – tracking movements of the eyes as they follow moving objects. Control from OCCIPITAL CORTEX and SUPERIOR COLLICULUS.

CONVERSE MOVEMENTS bring visual axes towards each other as objects move nearer observer. Control is also from OCCIPITAL CORTEX and SUPERIOR COLLICULUS.

VESTIBULAR MOVEMENTS – occur in response to stimuli initiated in semicircular canals (p.285) - maintain visual fixation as the head moves.
Control – vestibular system – cerebellum – superior colliculus.

Centres in
OCCIPITAL
CORTEX

SUPERIOR
COLLICULUS

III

MIDBRAIN

IV

MEDIAL
LONGITUDINAL
BUNDLES

VI

PONS

E.g.

From the *right* side of the midbrain and pons impulses pass to the **prime movers** – RIGHT EXT. RECTUS & LEFT INT. RECTUS – which contract (+).
The **antagonists** – LEFT EXT. RECTUS & RIGHT INT. RECTUS – relax (-) to permit the movement.
BOTH EYES turn to the *RIGHT*.

This is **conjugate movement**.

Centres in midbrain and pons give rise to cranial nerves III, IV and VI, the **final** control paths for all eye muscle movements.

IRIS, LENS AND CILIARY BODY

The **IRIS** is a muscular diaphragm with a central opening – the PUPIL.

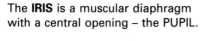
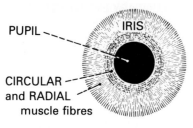

PUPIL

IRIS

CIRCULAR and RADIAL muscle fibres

IRIS controls amount of **light** entering the EYE

CIRCULAR smooth muscle fibres – SPHINCTER PUPILLAE – contract to make pupil smaller in bright light.

RADIAL fibres – DILATOR PUPILLAE – contract to make pupil larger with change from **light** to **dark**: and from **near** to **distant** vision. (also with **fear** and **pain**).

ACCOMMODATION
When CILIARY MUSCLE contracts, SUSPENSORY LIGAMENT is slackened. Tension on CAPSULE of LENS is relaxed. Because lens is elastic, *ANTERIOR* surface springs forwards → LENS becomes more convex especially in its central part. This brings near objects into focus (accommodation reflex).

The **LENS** is a transparent biconvex crystalline disc.

Outer elastic CAPSULE blends with SUSPENSORY LIGAMENT which suspends LENS behind IRIS

The LENS and IRIS are attached to **CILIARY BODY** which contains fibres of SMOOTH MUSCLE

Interior view of ciliary body and lens

LENS

LENS brings **light rays** to a **focus** upside down on the RETINA. To do this under all conditions it must be able to alter its curvature.

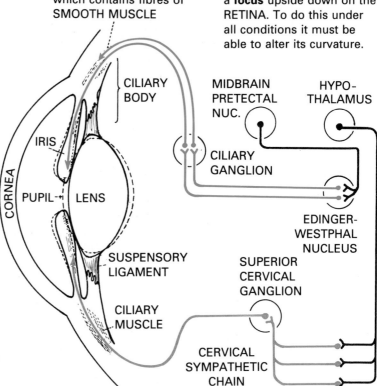

CILIARY BODY

IRIS

CORNEA

PUPIL

LENS

SUSPENSORY LIGAMENT

CILIARY MUSCLE

MIDBRAIN PRETECTAL NUC.

CILIARY GANGLION

SUPERIOR CERVICAL GANGLION

CERVICAL SYMPATHETIC CHAIN

HYPO-THALAMUS

EDINGER-WESTPHAL NUCLEUS

NEAR RESPONSE When subject looks at near objects, in addition to accommodation, visual axes converge and pupils constrict. The latter increases depth of focus.

These changes are brought about reflexly. The *ingoing* impulses travel in the optic nerves. The *outgoing* motor impulses travel in parasympathetic to ciliary body and sphincter pupillae and in sympathetic to dilator pupillae.

ACTION OF LENS

The normal lens brings light rays to a sharp focus upside down on the retina. It can do this whether we are looking at an object far away or one close at hand. The curvature increases reflexly to accommodate for near vision.

The conscious mind learns to interpret the image and project it to its true position in space.

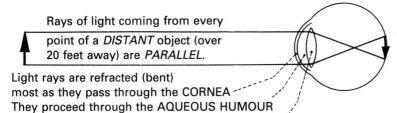

Rays of light coming from every point of a *DISTANT* object (over 20 feet away) are *PARALLEL*.

Light rays are refracted (bent) most as they pass through the CORNEA
They proceed through the AQUEOUS HUMOUR

The LENS refracts them to a sharp focus – upside down and reversed from side to side – on the retina.

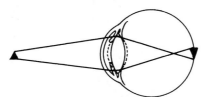

Rays of light coming from a *NEAR* object (less than 20 feet away) *DIVERGE* as they pass to the eye.

A more convex lens is required to bring these rays to a sharp focus on the retina.

If the EYEBALL is *too short*, rays from a distant object are brought into focus *BEHIND* the retina when the ciliary muscle is relaxed.

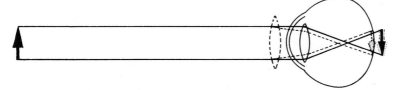

This is longsightedness or **hypermetropia**.

The longsighted eye has to accommodate even for distant vision: i.e. ciliary muscles contract to give a more convex lens and distant objects are then seen clearly. This limits amount of accommodating power left for near objects and the nearest point for sharp vision is then further away. It can be corrected by fitting spectacles with **convex** lenses.

If the EYEBALL is *too long*, rays from a distant object are brought into focus *IN FRONT* of the retina.

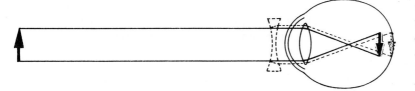

This is shortsightedness or **myopia** – only objects near the eye can be seen clearly. It can be corrected with **concave** lenses.

Total refraction of the optical system = 60 dioptres. The lens contributes 9–10 dioptres – the cornea most of the remainder.

FUNDUS OCULI

Part of the **retina** can be seen by means of an instrument – the **ophthalmoscope** – which shines a beam of light through the **pupil** of the eye on to the retina.

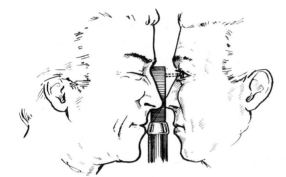

The part of the retina seen in this way is called the **fundus oculi**.

N.B. Observer uses his left eye to look into the patient's left eye and holds the ophthalmoscope in his left hand. Observer uses his right eye to look into patient's right eye and holds the ophthalmoscope in his right hand.

OPTIC DISC The nerve fibres from all parts of the retina converge on this area to leave the eyeball as the OPTIC NERVE. No RODS or CONES overlie the disc so it is not itself sensitive to light, hence it forms a 'BLIND SPOT' on the retina.

RETINAL BLOOD VESSELS enter or leave the eyeball here.

MACULA
The Macula Lutea or 'YELLOW SPOT' marks the location of the FOVEA CENTRALIS – area of acute vision – contains CONES only (the receptors stimulated in bright and coloured light). Few cells and no blood vessels overlie the fovea. When we look at an object the eyes are directed so that the image will fall on the fovea of each eye.

LEFT FUNDUS

EXTRAFOVEAL part of retina – area of less acute vision – CONES become fewer – RODS (the receptors stimulated in **dim light** with no discrimination between **colours**) predominate towards the peripheral part of the retina.

274

RETINA

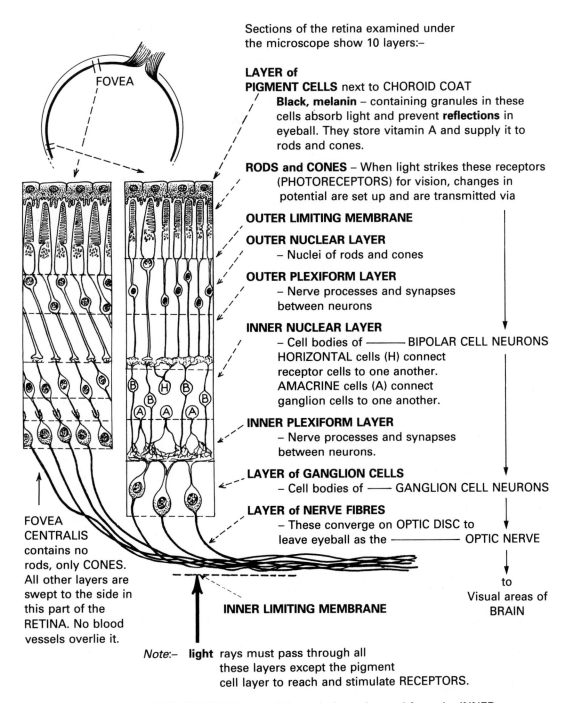

FOVEA

Sections of the retina examined under the microscope show 10 layers:–

LAYER of
PIGMENT CELLS next to CHOROID COAT

Black, melanin – containing granules in these cells absorb light and prevent **reflections** in eyeball. They store vitamin A and supply it to rods and cones.

RODS and CONES – When light strikes these receptors (PHOTORECEPTORS) for vision, changes in potential are set up and are transmitted via

OUTER LIMITING MEMBRANE

OUTER NUCLEAR LAYER
– Nuclei of rods and cones

OUTER PLEXIFORM LAYER
– Nerve processes and synapses between neurons

INNER NUCLEAR LAYER
– Cell bodies of ———— BIPOLAR CELL NEURONS
HORIZONTAL cells (H) connect receptor cells to one another. AMACRINE cells (A) connect ganglion cells to one another.

INNER PLEXIFORM LAYER
– Nerve processes and synapses between neurons.

LAYER of GANGLION CELLS
– Cell bodies of ——— GANGLION CELL NEURONS

LAYER of NERVE FIBRES
– These converge on OPTIC DISC to leave eyeball as the ———— OPTIC NERVE

to
Visual areas of
BRAIN

FOVEA CENTRALIS contains no rods, only CONES. All other layers are swept to the side in this part of the RETINA. No blood vessels overlie it.

INNER LIMITING MEMBRANE

Note:– **light** rays must pass through all these layers except the pigment cell layer to reach and stimulate RECEPTORS.

Supporting cells called MULLER CELLS extend through the retina and form the INNER LIMITING MEMBRANE on the inner surface of the retina and the OUTER LIMITING MEMBRANE in the receptor layer.

275

MECHANISM OF VISION

White light is really due to the fusion of **coloured lights**. These coloured lights are separated by shining a beam of white light through a glass prism. This is called the **visible spectrum**.

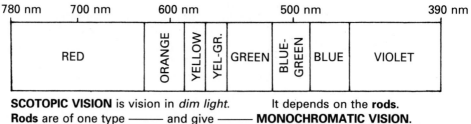

SCOTOPIC VISION is vision in *dim light*.   It depends on the **rods**.
Rods are of one type ——— and give ——— MONOCHROMATIC VISION.

The outer discs of rods and cones contain **photopigments**; these have two parts, a glycoprotein **opsin** and a derivative of vitamin A called **retinal**. In darkness, retinal has a bent shape and is called 11-*cis*-retinal which fits against opsin. When it absorbs light, *cis*-retinal straightens and forms all-*trans*-retinal. This *cis* to *trans* conversion (**isomerization**) is the first step in converting light to an electrical signal in the retina. In darkness, an enzyme reverses the process and re-forms a functional photopigment. The rod photopigment is called **rhodopsin**. Potential changes in the cells of the retina occur as follows:

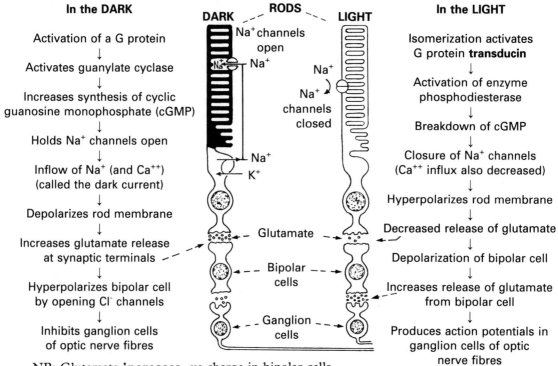

In the DARK

Activation of a G protein
↓
Activates guanylate cyclase
↓
Increases synthesis of cyclic guanosine monophosphate (cGMP)
↓
Holds Na⁺ channels open
↓
Inflow of Na⁺ (and Ca⁺⁺) (called the dark current)
↓
Depolarizes rod membrane
↓
Increases glutamate release at synaptic terminals
↓
Hyperpolarizes bipolar cell by opening Cl⁻ channels
↓
Inhibits ganglion cells of optic nerve fibres

In the LIGHT

Isomerization activates G protein **transducin**
↓
Activation of enzyme phosphodiesterase
↓
Breakdown of cGMP
↓
Closure of Na⁺ channels (Ca⁺⁺ influx also decreased)
↓
Hyperpolarizes rod membrane
↓
Decreased release of glutamate
↓
Depolarization of bipolar cell
↓
Increases release of glutamate from bipolar cell
↓
Produces action potentials in ganglion cells of optic nerve fibres

NB: Glutamate **increases** -ve charge in bipolar cells (hyperpolarization) but **decreases** -ve charge in ganglion cells (depolarization). See page 65. Receptor potentials of the rods and bipolar cells are local, graded potentials. It is only in the ganglion cells that propagated action potentials are generated.

MECHANISM OF VISION

Photopic vision is vision in bright light. It depends on the **cones**.
Cones are of 3 types ———————————— and give **TRICHROMATIC VISION**.

Each type with   Each contains RETINAL, the aldehyde of
  a different   vitamin A, plus one of 3 opsins which filter the
photosensitive   light before it reaches the retinal.
  VISUAL
  PIGMENT— which absorbs light most effectively at a different part of the visible
                  spectrum thus changing its structure.

'*RED*'   responds maximally to *YELLOW-ORANGE* light (558 nm)
'*GREEN*' responds maximally to *GREEN* light (531nm)
'*BLUE*' responds maximally to *BLUE* light (420nm)

Although each type of cone responds **maximally** to one particular wavelength, it does respond to other wavelengths as well. Thus, for any given wavelength, the 3 cone types are excited to different degrees. Hence the sensation of colour is determined by the **pattern** of the frequency of the impulses generated by the **3** cone systems.

All 3 types of CONE are stimulated in roughly equal proportions when WHITE light falls on the retina.

The various types of colour blindness can be explained in terms of the absence or deficiency of one or more of these special receptors.

For any colour there is a **complementary** colour. When these are mixed properly a sensation of white is produced. Black is the sensation produced by the absence of light. However it is a positive sensation since a blind eye does not 'see black' it 'sees nothing'. Compare the blind spot in the normal eye.

A colour sensation has 3 qualities:
(1) **Hue** ———— depends largely on wavelength.
(2) **Saturation** – purity –
                    A 'saturated' colour has no white light mixed with it.
                    An 'unsaturated' colour has some white light mixed with it.
(3) **Intensity** —— brightness – depends largely on 'strength' of the light.

As the intensity of light is reduced the cones cease to respond and the rods take over.

When a person passes from darkness to bright light he is dazzled, but after a short time he sees well again. This adjustment or decrease in sensitivity on exposure to bright light is called **light adaptation** but is, strictly speaking, the disappearance of dark adaptation.

VISUAL PATHWAYS TO THE BRAIN

The **receptors** for **vision** are linked by a chain of neurons with **receiving** and **integrating centres** in the **occipital lobes** of the **cerebral cortex**.

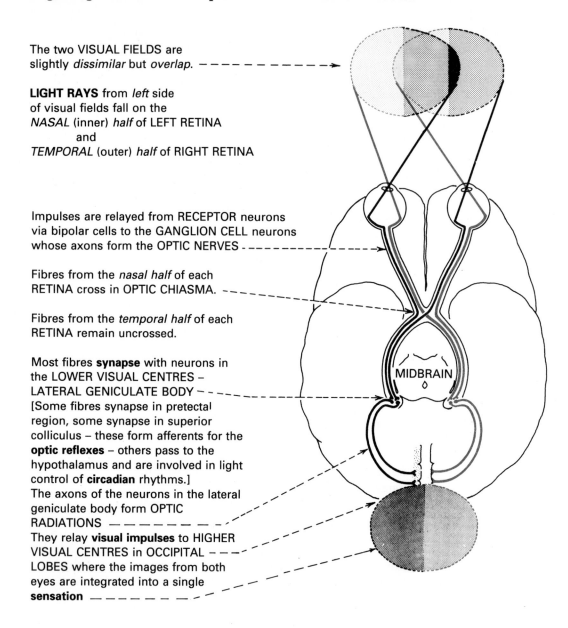

The two VISUAL FIELDS are slightly *dissimilar* but *overlap*. — — — — — — — — — →

LIGHT RAYS from *left* side of visual fields fall on the
NASAL (inner) *half* of LEFT RETINA
            and
TEMPORAL (outer) *half* of RIGHT RETINA

Impulses are relayed from RECEPTOR neurons via bipolar cells to the GANGLION CELL neurons whose axons form the OPTIC NERVES - — — — — — — — — →

Fibres from the *nasal half* of each RETINA cross in OPTIC CHIASMA. — — —

Fibres from the *temporal half* of each RETINA remain uncrossed.

Most fibres **synapse** with neurons in the LOWER VISUAL CENTRES – LATERAL GENICULATE BODY — — — — —
[Some fibres synapse in pretectal region, some synapse in superior colliculus – these form afferents for the **optic reflexes** – others pass to the hypothalamus and are involved in light control of **circadian** rhythms.]
The axons of the neurons in the lateral geniculate body form OPTIC RADIATIONS — — — — — — —
They relay **visual impulses** to HIGHER VISUAL CENTRES in OCCIPITAL — — —
LOBES where the images from both eyes are integrated into a single **sensation** — — — — — —

MIDBRAIN

Note:– One side of the **occipital cortex** receives impressions from the **field of vision** on the opposite side.

STEREOSCOPIC VISION

When we look at some object or scene, the view seen by the **right eye** is slightly different from the view seen by the **left eye**.

These two **dissimilar retinal images** are fused in the visual centres of the brain to give a 3-dimensional picture – an appreciation of *depth* as well as of *height* and *width*.

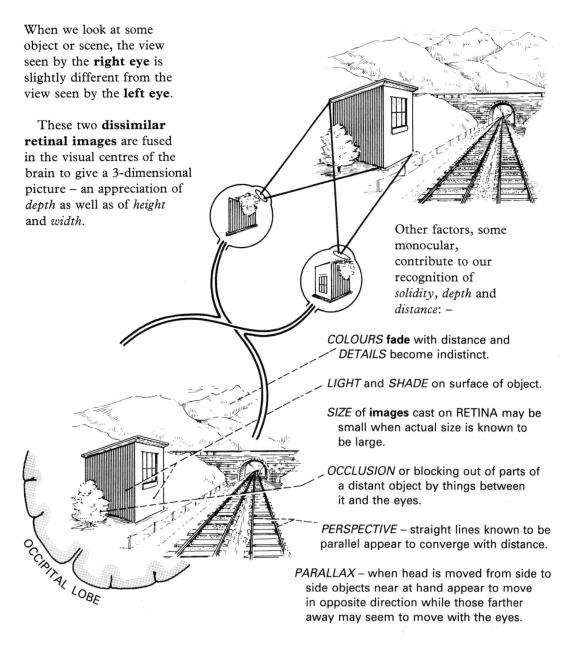

Other factors, some monocular, contribute to our recognition of *solidity, depth* and *distance*: –

COLOURS **fade** with distance and *DETAILS* become indistinct.

LIGHT and *SHADE* on surface of object.

SIZE of **images** cast on RETINA may be small when actual size is known to be large.

OCCLUSION or blocking out of parts of a distant object by things between it and the eyes.

PERSPECTIVE – straight lines known to be parallel appear to converge with distance.

PARALLAX – when head is moved from side to side objects near at hand appear to move in opposite direction while those farther away may seem to move with the eyes.

By complex mental processes these points are interpreted in terms of distance and depth.

LIGHT REFLEX

When **light** falls on the **retina** the **pupils** constrict.

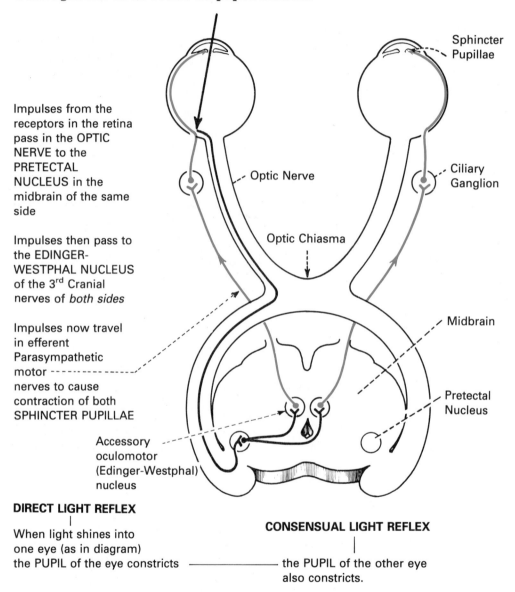

Impulses from the receptors in the retina pass in the OPTIC NERVE to the PRETECTAL NUCLEUS in the midbrain of the same side

Impulses then pass to the EDINGER-WESTPHAL NUCLEUS of the 3rd Cranial nerves of *both sides*

Impulses now travel in efferent Parasympathetic motor nerves to cause contraction of both SPHINCTER PUPILLAE

Sphincter Pupillae

Optic Nerve

Ciliary Ganglion

Optic Chiasma

Midbrain

Pretectal Nucleus

Accessory oculomotor (Edinger-Westphal) nucleus

DIRECT LIGHT REFLEX

When light shines into one eye (as in diagram) the PUPIL of the eye constricts ———————

CONSENSUAL LIGHT REFLEX

the PUPIL of the other eye also constricts.

This cuts down the amount of light entering the eyes and protects the retinae from excessive stimulation. It also increases depth of focus and improves the sharpness of the retinal images.

The **Argyll-Robertson pupil** is one of the signs of cerebral syphilis. In this condition the pupil does *not* constrict in response to light but *does* constrict as part of the **near response** (p. 272). This indicates that the pathways for these two constrictor responses are different.

EAR

The ear has 3 separate parts, each with different roles in the mechanism of **hearing**:–

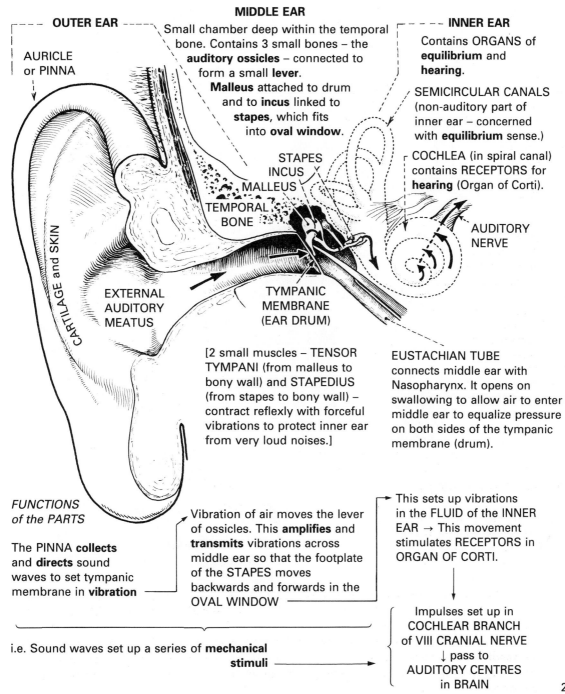

OUTER EAR

AURICLE or PINNA

CARTILAGE and SKIN

EXTERNAL AUDITORY MEATUS

MIDDLE EAR
Small chamber deep within the temporal bone. Contains 3 small bones – the **auditory ossicles** – connected to form a small **lever**. **Malleus** attached to drum and to **incus** linked to **stapes**, which fits into **oval window**.

STAPES
INCUS
MALLEUS
TEMPORAL BONE

TYMPANIC MEMBRANE (EAR DRUM)

INNER EAR
Contains ORGANS of **equilibrium** and **hearing**.

SEMICIRCULAR CANALS (non-auditory part of inner ear – concerned with **equilibrium** sense.)

COCHLEA (in spiral canal) contains RECEPTORS for **hearing** (Organ of Corti).

AUDITORY NERVE

[2 small muscles – TENSOR TYMPANI (from malleus to bony wall) and STAPEDIUS (from stapes to bony wall) – contract reflexly with forceful vibrations to protect inner ear from very loud noises.]

EUSTACHIAN TUBE connects middle ear with Nasopharynx. It opens on swallowing to allow air to enter middle ear to equalize pressure on both sides of the tympanic membrane (drum).

FUNCTIONS of the PARTS

The PINNA **collects** and **directs** sound waves to set tympanic membrane in **vibration**

Vibration of air moves the lever of ossicles. This **amplifies** and **transmits** vibrations across middle ear so that the footplate of the STAPES moves backwards and forwards in the OVAL WINDOW

This sets up vibrations in the FLUID of the INNER EAR → This movement stimulates RECEPTORS in ORGAN OF CORTI.

Impulses set up in COCHLEAR BRANCH of VIII CRANIAL NERVE ↓ pass to AUDITORY CENTRES in BRAIN

i.e. Sound waves set up a series of **mechanical stimuli**

281

COCHLEA

The cochlea is the essential organ of **hearing**.

It consists of:

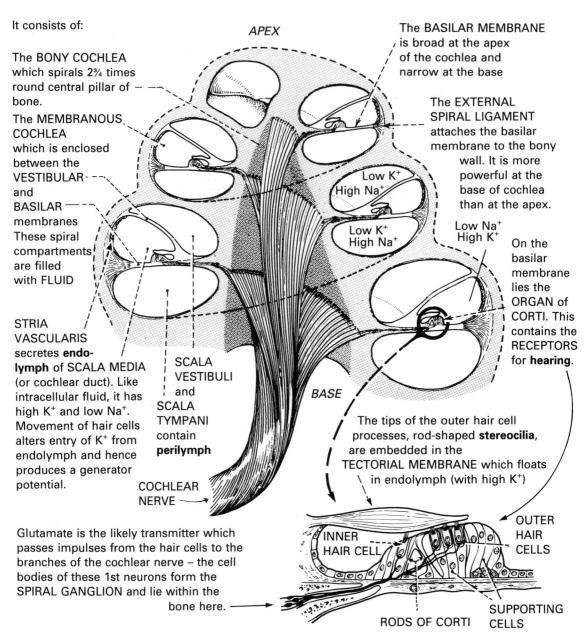

APEX

The BONY COCHLEA which spirals 2¾ times round central pillar of — — bone.

The MEMBRANOUS COCHLEA which is enclosed between the VESTIBULAR- - - - and BASILAR — — membranes These spiral compartments are filled with FLUID

STRIA VASCULARIS secretes **endolymph** of SCALA MEDIA (or cochlear duct). Like intracellular fluid, it has high K^+ and low Na^+. Movement of hair cells alters entry of K^+ from endolymph and hence produces a generator potential.

SCALA VESTIBULI and SCALA TYMPANI contain **perilymph**

COCHLEAR NERVE →

The BASILAR MEMBRANE is broad at the apex of the cochlea and narrow at the base

The EXTERNAL SPIRAL LIGAMENT attaches the basilar membrane to the bony wall. It is more powerful at the base of cochlea than at the apex.

Low K^+ High Na^+

Low K^+ High Na^+

Low Na^+ High K^+

On the basilar membrane lies the ORGAN of CORTI. This contains the RECEPTORS for **hearing**.

BASE

The tips of the outer hair cell processes, rod-shaped **stereocilia**, are embedded in the TECTORIAL MEMBRANE which floats in endolymph (with high K^+)

Glutamate is the likely transmitter which passes impulses from the hair cells to the branches of the cochlear nerve – the cell bodies of these 1st neurons form the SPIRAL GANGLION and lie within the bone here. →

INNER HAIR CELL

OUTER HAIR CELLS

RODS OF CORTI

SUPPORTING CELLS

Inner hair cells are probably the primary sensory cells which generate action potentials. **Outer** hair cells and the afferent fibres from inner hair cells are innervated by cholinergic efferent nerves which may influence basilar membrane vibration pattern to improve hearing.

MECHANISM OF HEARING

This is most readily understood if the **cochlea** is imagined as straightened out:-

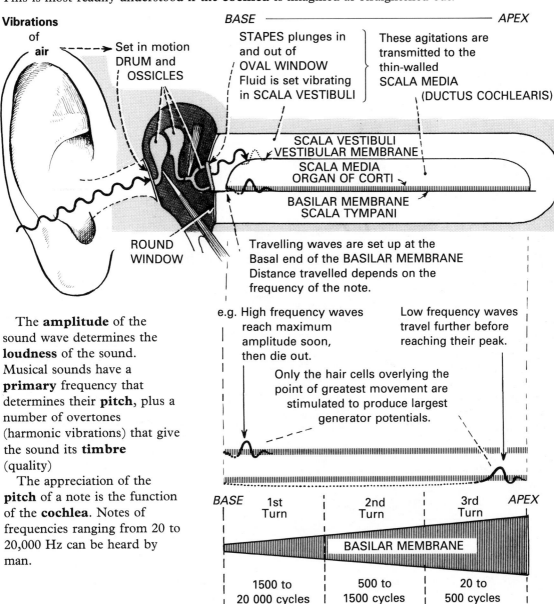

BASE ——————————————————————— *APEX*

STAPES plunges in and out of OVAL WINDOW Fluid is set vibrating in SCALA VESTIBULI

These agitations are transmitted to the thin-walled SCALA MEDIA (DUCTUS COCHLEARIS)

Vibrations of air ---→ Set in motion DRUM and OSSICLES

SCALA VESTIBULI
VESTIBULAR MEMBRANE
SCALA MEDIA
ORGAN OF CORTI
BASILAR MEMBRANE
SCALA TYMPANI

ROUND WINDOW

Travelling waves are set up at the Basal end of the BASILAR MEMBRANE Distance travelled depends on the frequency of the note.

The **amplitude** of the sound wave determines the **loudness** of the sound. Musical sounds have a **primary** frequency that determines their **pitch**, plus a number of overtones (harmonic vibrations) that give the sound its **timbre** (quality)

The appreciation of the **pitch** of a note is the function of the **cochlea**. Notes of frequencies ranging from 20 to 20,000 Hz can be heard by man.

e.g. High frequency waves reach maximum amplitude soon, then die out.

Low frequency waves travel further before reaching their peak.

Only the hair cells overlying the point of greatest movement are stimulated to produce largest generator potentials.

BASE   1st Turn   2nd Turn   3rd Turn   *APEX*

BASILAR MEMBRANE

| 1500 to 20 000 cycles per second (Hz) | 500 to 1500 cycles per second (Hz) | 20 to 500 cycles per second (Hz) |

Bending of stereocilia alters entry of K^+ to the hair cell from the endolymph. When the stereocilia are moved towards the longest stereocilium, **depolarization** is produced. Deflection away from longest stereocilium produces **hyperpolarization**.

AUDITORY PATHWAYS TO BRAIN

The **receptors** for hearing are linked by a chain of **neurons** with the **receiving centres** for hearing in the **temporal lobes** of the **cerebral cortex**.

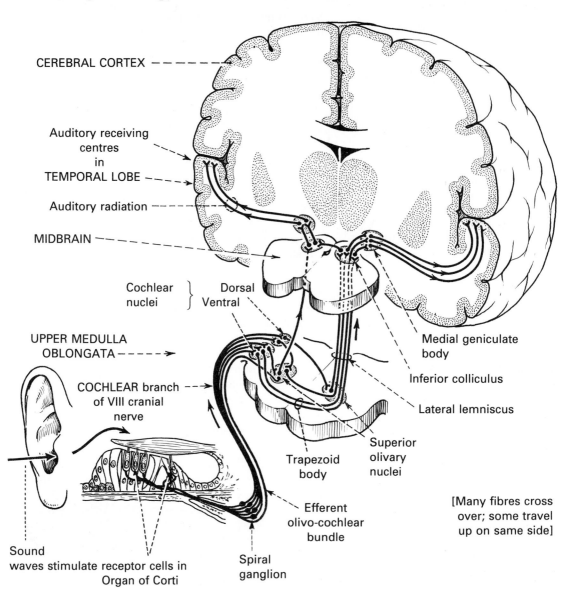

CEREBRAL CORTEX

Auditory receiving
centres
in
TEMPORAL LOBE

Auditory radiation

MIDBRAIN

Cochlear } Dorsal
nuclei { Ventral

UPPER MEDULLA
OBLONGATA

COCHLEAR branch
of VIII cranial
nerve

Medial geniculate
body

Inferior colliculus

Lateral lemniscus

Superior
olivary
nuclei

Trapezoid
body

Efferent
olivo-cochlear
bundle

[Many fibres cross
over; some travel
up on same side]

Sound
waves stimulate receptor cells in
Organ of Corti

Spiral
ganglion

Impulses travel in vestibulo-cochlear nerve (Cranial nerve VIII) and are relayed as shown. Some are sent into the **reticular activating system**.

Efferent fibres arise from the superior olivary nuclei and run in the cochlear nerve to end on the afferent neurons and hair cells of the organ of Corti. They may alter the sensitivity of the hair cells to sound.

VESTIBULAR SYSTEM

The vestibular apparatus is found in the non-auditory part of the inner ear – the labyrinth. It is stimulated by movement or change of position of the head in space enabling balance (equilibrium) to be maintained. It consists of 3 semicircular canals plus an utricle and a saccule.

Three **SEMICIRCULAR CANALS** – in each inner ear – one in each of three planes of space – contain receptors in the form of hair cells.

Membranous tubes continuous with scala media of cochlea containing endolymph embedded in bone surrounded by perilymph.

These receptors, situated in the ampulla of each canal, are stimulated mechanically by the *starting or stopping* of **rotatory** movements of the head in space.

One end of each canal has a swelling – the AMPULLA

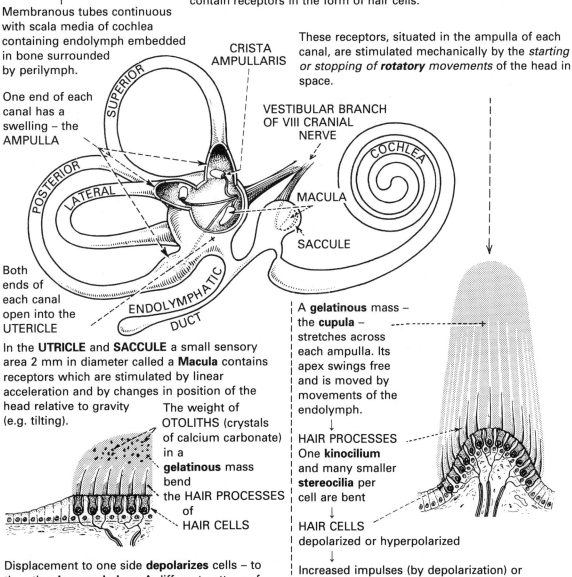

CRISTA AMPULLARIS

VESTIBULAR BRANCH OF VIII CRANIAL NERVE

COCHLEA

MACULA

SACCULE

Both ends of each canal open into the UTERICLE

ENDOLYMPHATIC DUCT

In the **UTRICLE** and **SACCULE** a small sensory area 2 mm in diameter called a **Macula** contains receptors which are stimulated by linear acceleration and by changes in position of the head relative to gravity (e.g. tilting).

The weight of OTOLITHS (crystals of calcium carbonate) in a **gelatinous** mass bend the HAIR PROCESSES of HAIR CELLS

A **gelatinous** mass – the **cupula** – stretches across each ampulla. Its apex swings free and is moved by movements of the endolymph.
↓
HAIR PROCESSES
One **kinocilium** and many smaller **stereocilia** per cell are bent
↓
HAIR CELLS
depolarized or hyperpolarized
↓
Increased impulses (by depolarization) or decreased impulses (by hyperpolarization) conveyed by fibres of the vestibular branch of VIII cranial nerve to centres in the brain.

Displacement to one side **depolarizes** cells – to the other **hyperpolarizes**. A different pattern of excitation occurs for each position of the head. Conveyed by fibres of vestibular branch of VIII cranial nerve to brain.

ORGAN OF EQUILIBRIUM: MECHANISM OF ACTION

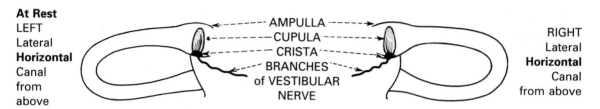

At Rest
LEFT
Lateral
Horizontal
Canal
from
above

AMPULLA
CUPULA
CRISTA
BRANCHES
of VESTIBULAR
NERVE

RIGHT
Lateral
Horizontal
Canal
from above

When head starts to rotate (e.g. to the left) the endolymph in the semicircular canals which lie at right angles to the axis of rotation tends to lag behind the movement of the head – and the CUPULA is displaced, HAIR CELLS are stimulated and *ingoing* impulses form afferent pathways for reflexes leading to alterations in tone of muscles in neck, trunk and limbs to avoid body losing balance.

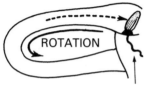

ROTATION

Increased firing

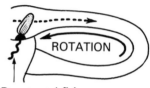

ROTATION

Decreased firing

After the initial inertia is overcome the endolymph no longer lags behind the movement of the head – and the CUPULA is no longer displaced. HAIR CELLS are no longer bent and stimulated.
Nerve fibres no longer send signals to medulla and cerebellum.

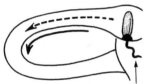

Resting discharge

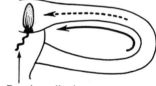

Resting discharge

When head stops rotating the endolymph tends to continue to rotate and the CUPULA is displaced in the opposite direction → HAIR CELLS are bent → Nerve fibres signal rotation of head to right → Individual feels for a moment as though he is rotating in opposite direction – when in fact he has ceased to rotate.

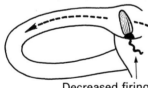

Decreased firing

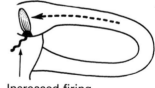

Increased firing

Rotating the head round a horizontal axis – i.e. tilting it backwards and forwards such as happens in the pitch and roll of a ship – stimulates the VERTICAL canals. This can lead to 'motion sickness'.

Stimulation of the semicircular canals also causes movements of the eyes to keep them fixed on the same point in the retina for as long as possible.

During rotation there is a slow movement of the eyes in the direction opposite to that of rotation, then a quick return to the normal position. This is **nystagmus** which can also be a pathological sign. It occurs continuously while rotating and continues for a short time after movement has ceased.

The semicircular canal mechanism predicts ahead of time that mal-equilibrium is going to occur. It allows equilibrium centres to make preventive adjustments.

VESTIBULAR PATHWAYS TO BRAIN

The vestibular end-organs in the **labyrinth** are linked through the **vestibular nuclei** with **receiving** and **integrating centres** in the **cerebellum**, and with **motor centres** in the **midbrain** and **spinal cord** through which they initiate reflex muscular movements of eyes, head and neck and trunk and limb muscles to adjust balance and posture.

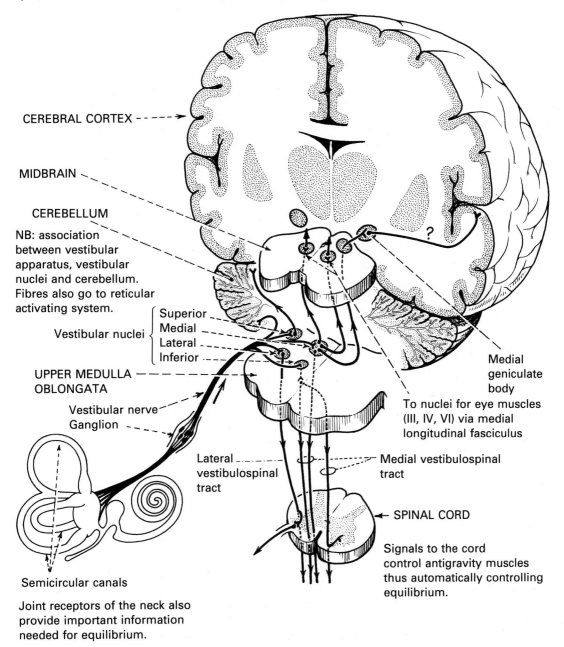

CEREBRAL CORTEX

MIDBRAIN

CEREBELLUM

NB: association between vestibular apparatus, vestibular nuclei and cerebellum. Fibres also go to reticular activating system.

Vestibular nuclei
{ Superior
  Medial
  Lateral
  Inferior

UPPER MEDULLA OBLONGATA

Vestibular nerve
Ganglion

Semicircular canals

Joint receptors of the neck also provide important information needed for equilibrium.

Lateral vestibulospinal tract

Medial geniculate body

To nuclei for eye muscles (III, IV, VI) via medial longitudinal fasciculus

Medial vestibulospinal tract

SPINAL CORD

Signals to the cord control antigravity muscles thus automatically controlling equilibrium.

287

CLASSIFICATION OF NERVE FIBRES

A **nerve fibre** is a dendrite of a neuron or it is a nerve axon and its sheath (p.21). A **nerve** e.g. sciatic or ulnar, consists of many nerve fibres. Usually, not all its fibres have the same function, e.g. there may be bundles of skeletal muscle motor fibres, efferent autonomic fibres, sensory afferents for skin sensation etc. The fibres of each of these bundles will have different diameters, some axons may be myelinated, others unmyelinated.

Large diameter fibres conduct action potentials at a faster rate than small fibres, thus, if a nerve is stimulated at one point and a recording is made of the arrival of the APs some distance from the stimulation point, APs in fast conducting fibres will arrive before APs in slower conducting fibres.

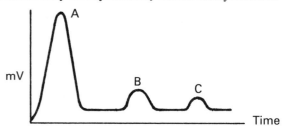

Erlanger and Glasser classified nerve fibres, mainly on this basis, into groups A, B and C. Later the A group, i.e. the fastest fibres, was subdivided into A-alpha(α), A-beta (β), A-gamma (γ) and A-delta (δ) since the A peak was found to have sub-peaks within it.

FIBRE TYPE	FUNCTION	FIBRE DIAM. (µm)	CONDUCTION VELOC. (m/s)	AFFERENT GROUP
Aα	Proprioception, somatic motor.	12–20	70–120	Ia,Ib
β	Touch, pressure, vibration.	5–12	30–70	II
γ	Motor to muscle spindles.	3–6	15–30	III
δ	Pain, cold, touch.	2–5	12–30	III
B	Preganglionic autonomic.	<3	3–15	
C	Postganglionic autonomic, pain, temperature, mechanoreception.	0.3–1.3	0.5–2.3	IV

This classification is unsatisfactory however, since the fastest conducting fibres in one nerve (classified as Aα) may have a different rate of conduction and size from those in another nerve. Consequently sensory physiologists have classified **afferent** fibres according to their diameters and origin and have numbered the groups Ia, Ib, II, III and IV.

NUMBER	ORIGIN	SIZE (µm)
Ia Ib	Muscle spindle, annulospiral. Golgi tendon organ.	12–20
II	Muscle spindle secondary ending, touch, pressure.	5–12
III	Pain and cold, some touch.	2–5
IV	Pain, temperature, mechanoreceptors.	0.1–0.3

There is thus a little confusion in nerve fibre classification. Some terms have been retained from the earlier classification, e.g. large motor fibres to skeletal muscle are alpha fibres, small motor fibres to muscle spindles are gamma fibres, and the term C fibre for small unmyelinated fibres is still commonly used.

The various classes in peripheral nerves vary in their sensitivity to pressure, hypoxia and local anaesthetics.

GENERAL PROPRIOCEPTORS

Proprioceptors are the sense organs stimulated by **movement** of the body itself. They make us aware of the movement or position of the body in space and the relative position of the various parts of the body to each other. They are important as ingoing afferent pathways in reflexes for adjusting posture and tone.

General proprioceptors are found in **skeletal muscles**, **tendons** and **joints**.

GOLGI ORGAN – in tendons – in series with muscle fibres – stimulated by tension forces which occur when muscle is STRETCHED passively and when it is CONTRACTED. Regulates muscle force by inhibiting nerves to muscle, in spinal cord.

BONE

MUSCLE SPINDLE
– in skeletal muscle in parallel to muscle fibres
– stimulated when muscle is actively or passively STRETCHED e.g. stretch reflex (p.258). They consist of specialized muscle fibres called intrafusal fibres to distinguish them from the true skeletal muscle fibres (extrafusal). They control muscle **stretch** by a feed back control system. See page 290.

PACINIAN CORPUSCLES (p.292)
similar to those in the skin are found in deep connective tissue and around joints. They are stimulated by *PRESSURE* of surrounding structures when joints are moved.

THE MUSCLE SPINDLE

The intrafusal muscle fibres that make up a **muscle spindle** (p. 289) consist of (a) two **nuclear bag** fibres (bag$_1$ and bag$_2$) with many nuclei in their distended middle third (**equatorial region**) and (b) four or more **nuclear chain** fibres with a single row of nuclei in the equatorial region. The ends of the bag fibres are attached to the connective tissue of the surrounding extrafusal fibres. Nuclear chain fibres, being shorter, are attached to the connective tissue of the nuclear bag fibres. Both fibre types have a motor and sensory innervation and their outer thirds (the **polar regions**) are striated and contractile.

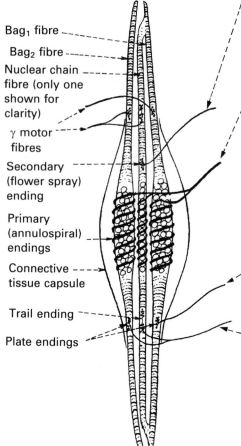

Bag$_1$ fibre

Bag$_2$ fibre

Nuclear chain fibre (only one shown for clarity)

γ motor fibres

Secondary (flower spray) ending

Primary (annulospiral) endings

Connective tissue capsule

Trail ending

Plate endings

Group II afferent nerves with **sensory**, or flower spray, endings are found on nuclear chain fibres next to the equatorial region. They generate action potentials at a rate which is proportional to the fibre's length. This is called the static or length-sensitive response.

Group Ia afferent nerves with **primary** or annulospiral endings which form a spiral round the centre of both types of fibre. One branch of the nerve goes to the bag$_1$ fibre, a second goes to the bag$_2$ fibre and the nuclear chain fibres. Rate of action potentials generated by the endings on the bag$_2$ and chain fibres is proportional to the amount of stretch (static response). The ending on the bag$_1$ fibre increases its rate of firing during stretching and reduces or stops firing during its release (dynamic or velocity-sensitive response).

Dynamic gamma (γ)-motor fibres: end with a plate-like ending on each pole of the bag$_1$ fibre. Activation of these fibres increases the spindle's sensitivity to dynamic responses.

Static gamma (γ)-motor fibres: end with multiple plate-like (trail) endings on nuclear chain fibres and usually single plates on bag$_2$ fibres. Activation of these fibres increases the spindle's sensitivity to static responses.

γ-motor stimulation causes contraction and hence **shortening** of the **poles** of the intrafusal fibres, thereby stretching the equatorial portion of the spindle thus generating impulses in the annulospiral endings. Stretch of the muscle spindle, as occurs in the stretch reflex, also causes generation of action potentials by the annulospiral endings.

Activation of α-motor neurons by descending fibres from the motor area of the cerebral cortex is accompanied by simultaneous activation of γ-motor neurons. This is **α-γ coactivation** and is very important for the accurate control of all muscle movements. See p. 308.

PROPRIOCEPTOR PATHWAYS TO BRAIN

General proprioceptive receptors are linked to centres especially in the **cerebellum**, but some also go to the **parietal lobe** of the **cerebral cortex** by a chain of 3 neurons.

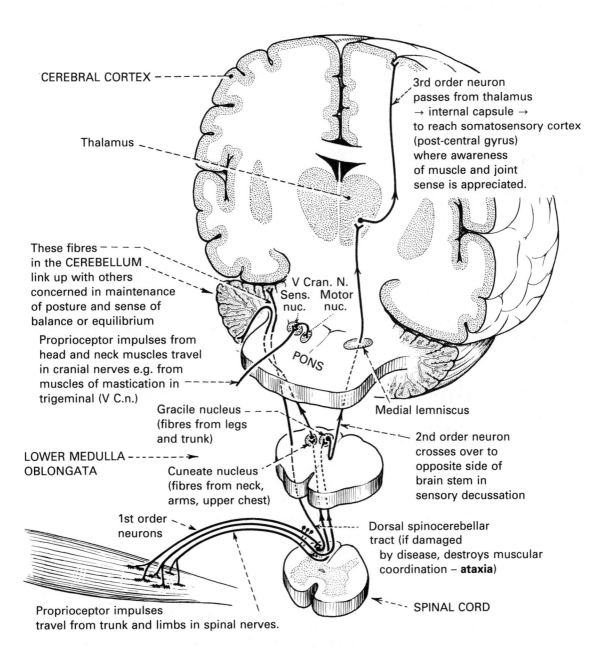

CEREBRAL CORTEX

3rd order neuron
passes from thalamus
→ internal capsule →
to reach somatosensory cortex
(post-central gyrus)
where awareness
of muscle and joint
sense is appreciated.

Thalamus

These fibres
in the CEREBELLUM
link up with others
concerned in maintenance
of posture and sense of
balance or equilibrium

V Cran. N.
Sens.   Motor
nuc.   nuc.

PONS

Proprioceptor impulses from
head and neck muscles travel
in cranial nerves e.g. from
muscles of mastication in
trigeminal (V C.n.)

Gracile nucleus
(fibres from legs
and trunk)

Medial lemniscus

LOWER MEDULLA
OBLONGATA

Cuneate nucleus
(fibres from neck,
arms, upper chest)

2nd order neuron
crosses over to
opposite side of
brain stem in
sensory decussation

1st order
neurons

Dorsal spinocerebellar
tract (if damaged
by disease, destroys muscular
coordination – **ataxia**)

SPINAL CORD

Proprioceptor impulses
travel from trunk and limbs in spinal nerves.

291

CUTANEOUS SENSATION

There are *five basic skin sensations* – **touch, pressure, pain, warmth,** and **cold**. There is much controversy as to how these are registered. In some areas they appear to be served by special nerve endings (sensory receptors or end-organs) in the skin. These receptors are not uniformly distributed over the whole body surface. (E.g. touch 'endings' are very numerous in hands and feet but are much less frequent in the skin of the back.)

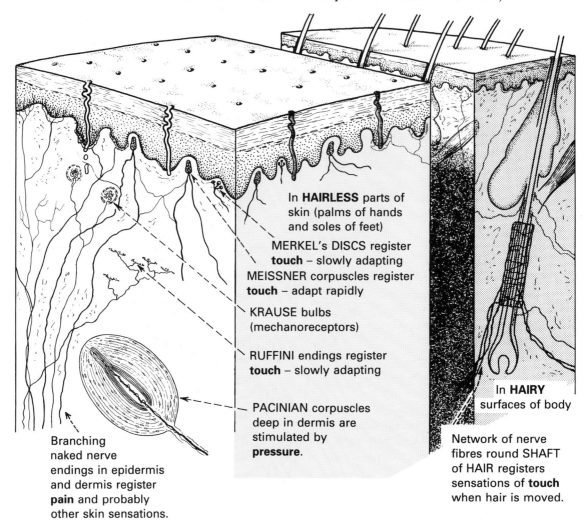

In **HAIRLESS** parts of skin (palms of hands and soles of feet)

MERKEL's DISCS register **touch** – slowly adapting
MEISSNER corpuscles register **touch** – adapt rapidly

KRAUSE bulbs (mechanoreceptors)

RUFFINI endings register **touch** – slowly adapting

PACINIAN corpuscles deep in dermis are stimulated by **pressure**.

Branching naked nerve endings in epidermis and dermis register **pain** and probably other skin sensations.

In **HAIRY** surfaces of body

Network of nerve fibres round SHAFT of HAIR registers sensations of **touch** when hair is moved.

Tickling, itching, softness, hardness, wetness are probably due to stimulation of two or more of these special endings and to a blending of the sensations in the brain.

Much has still to be discovered about skin receptors. Still to be explained, for example, is why in the cornea and the skin of the ear several types of sensation can be appreciated without the presence of specialized receptors.

PERIPHERAL PAIN

Pain is an important symptom which commonly causes a patient to consult a doctor. NB: pain is a **sensation** which is felt when **nociceptors** are stimulated by tissue damage. The terms pain and nociception are often used synonymously.

Nociceptors are free nerve endings which are stimulated by excessive heat, mechanical stimuli or chemicals, e.g. bradykinin released from γ-globulins as a result of cell damage.

Pain is either *fast* pain . . . . or . . . . *slow* pain
↓   ↓

Short, sharp, well localized, e.g. pin prick or knife cut. Conveyed by small myelinated fast Aδ or Group III fibres (12–30 m/sec).	Burning, aching, poorly localized, associated with tissue destruction. Conveyed by unmyelinated slower C or Group IV fibres (1 metre/s).

Nociceptive afferent fibres after synapsing in the dorsal horn ascend to the reticular formation, thalamus, sensory cortex and autonomic centres.

GATE CONTROL THEORY

In the dorsal horn of the spinal cord onward transmission of nerve impulses from nociceptive afferent fibres via **T** or **transmission cells** depends on the activity of large sensory afferent neurons from peripheral touch receptors. Impulses in these touch sensory afferents can block the pain pathway by stimulating an interneuron in the **substantia gelatinosa** which will presynaptically inhibit all input to the T-cell. If impulse traffic in the nociceptor afferents is greater than in the touch receptor afferents then afferent impulses will pass on and pain will be appreciated. This theory explains why rubbing your skin in a painful area can help to lessen the pain.

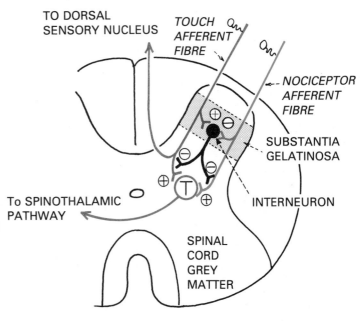

Impulses in nociceptor afferents can also be inhibited by descending fibres from the sensory cortex, the grey matter around the midbrain aqueduct and the brain stem reticular formation. These descending fibres terminate in the dorsal grey column of the spinal cord. They contain **opioid peptides** (encephalins, endorphins and dynorphins) which act as transmitters or neuromodulators.

293

POSTERIOR COLUMN – MEDIAL LEMNISCUS SENSORY PATHWAY

Receptors for proprioception, discriminative touch, stereognosis (recognize objects by feel), weight discrimination and vibratory sense are linked by a chain of 3 neurons with the sensory cortex. This is called the **posterior** (dorsal) **column—medial lemniscus pathway**.

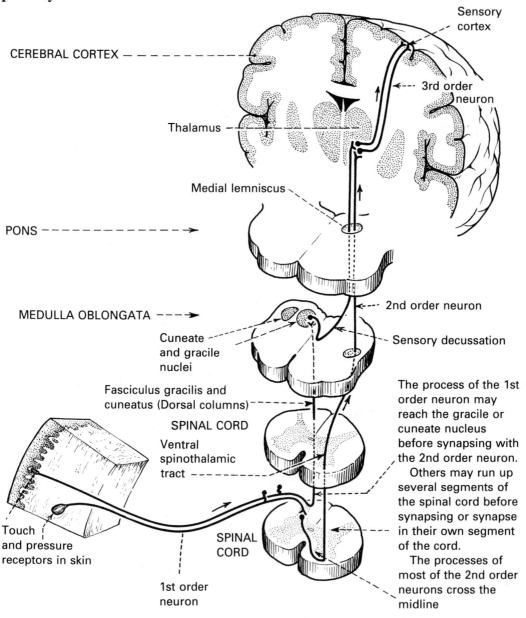

Sensory cortex

CEREBRAL CORTEX

3rd order neuron

Thalamus

Medial lemniscus

PONS

MEDULLA OBLONGATA

2nd order neuron

Cuneate and gracile nuclei

Sensory decussation

Fasciculus gracilis and cuneatus (Dorsal columns)

SPINAL CORD

Ventral spinothalamic tract

Touch and pressure receptors in skin

SPINAL CORD

1st order neuron

The process of the 1st order neuron may reach the gracile or cuneate nucleus before synapsing with the 2nd order neuron.

Others may run up several segments of the spinal cord before synapsing or synapse in their own segment of the cord.

The processes of most of the 2nd order neurons cross the midline

ANTEROLATERAL (SPINOTHALAMIC) SENSORY PATHWAY

Nerve pathways mainly for pain and temperature but also tickle, itch, poorly localized crude touch and pressure, are linked by a chain of 3 neurons with the somatosensory area in the postcentral gyrus of the **cerebral cortex**. It is called the **anterolateral** (spinothalamic) pathway. The lateral spinothalamic pathway conveys pain and temperature; the anterior, tickle, itch, crude touch and pressure, but they are now usually considered together as the anterolateral pathway.

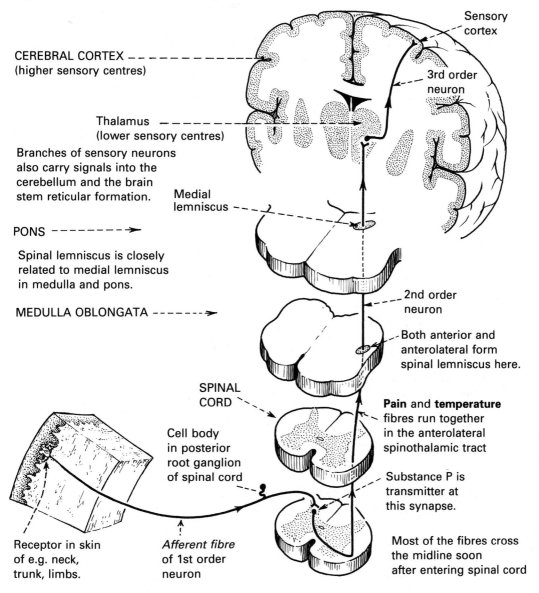

Sensory cortex

CEREBRAL CORTEX
(higher sensory centres)

3rd order neuron

Thalamus
(lower sensory centres)

Branches of sensory neurons also carry signals into the cerebellum and the brain stem reticular formation.

Medial lemniscus

PONS

Spinal lemniscus is closely related to medial lemniscus in medulla and pons.

MEDULLA OBLONGATA

2nd order neuron

Both anterior and anterolateral form spinal lemniscus here.

SPINAL CORD

Cell body in posterior root ganglion of spinal cord

Pain and **temperature** fibres run together in the anterolateral spinothalamic tract

Substance P is transmitter at this synapse.

Receptor in skin of e.g. neck, trunk, limbs.

Afferent fibre of 1st order neuron

Most of the fibres cross the midline soon after entering spinal cord

Pain *can* be perceived in the absence of the cerebral cortex. However the cortex is necessary to interpret the meaning of the pain and relate it to past experience.

SENSORY PATHWAYS FROM SKIN OF FACE

The receptors or nerve endings for **ordinary skin sensations** are linked by three neurons with receiving centres in the **sensory cortex**:

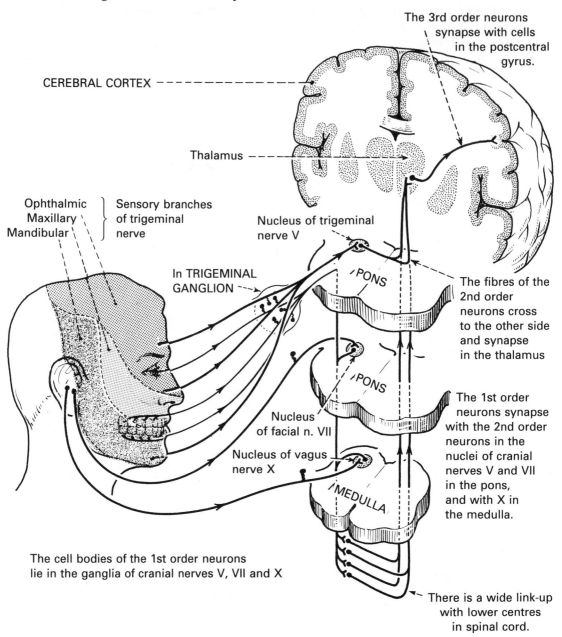

The 3rd order neurons synapse with cells in the postcentral gyrus.

CEREBRAL CORTEX

Thalamus

Ophthalmic
Maxillary
Mandibular

Sensory branches of trigeminal nerve

Nucleus of trigeminal nerve V

In TRIGEMINAL GANGLION

PONS

PONS

Nucleus of facial n. VII

Nucleus of vagus nerve X

MEDULLA

The fibres of the 2nd order neurons cross to the other side and synapse in the thalamus

The 1st order neurons synapse with the 2nd order neurons in the nuclei of cranial nerves V and VII in the pons, and with X in the medulla.

The cell bodies of the 1st order neurons lie in the ganglia of cranial nerves V, VII and X

There is a wide link-up with lower centres in spinal cord.

SENSORY CORTEX

The 3rd order neurons (conveying information from the *opposite side* of the body) synapse with cells in the somatosensory area of the **postcentral gyrus** of the **cerebral cortex**. The exact points on this gyrus at which impulses coming from the different regions of the skin surface terminate are indicated on this coronal view of the gyrus.

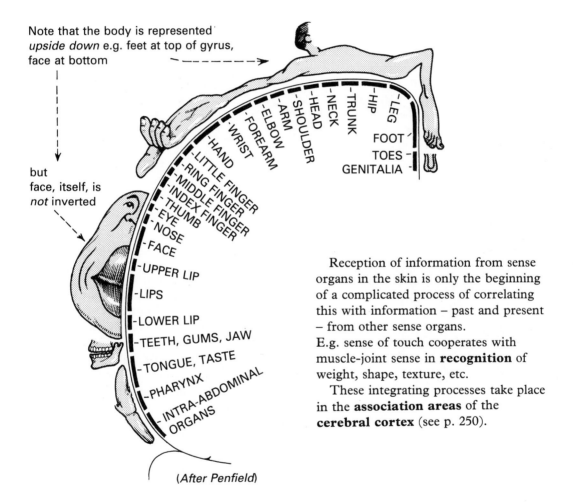

Note that the body is represented *upside down* e.g. feet at top of gyrus, face at bottom

but face, itself, is *not* inverted

LEG
HIP
TRUNK
NECK
HEAD
SHOULDER
ARM
ELBOW
FOREARM
WRIST
HAND
LITTLE FINGER
RING FINGER
MIDDLE FINGER
INDEX FINGER
THUMB
EYE
NOSE
FACE
UPPER LIP
LIPS
LOWER LIP
TEETH, GUMS, JAW
TONGUE, TASTE
PHARYNX
INTRA-ABDOMINAL ORGANS

FOOT
TOES
GENITALIA

(After Penfield)

Reception of information from sense organs in the skin is only the beginning of a complicated process of correlating this with information – past and present – from other sense organs.
E.g. sense of touch cooperates with muscle-joint sense in **recognition** of weight, shape, texture, etc.

These integrating processes take place in the **association areas** of the **cerebral cortex** (see p. 250).

The *sizes* of the receptive areas are directly proportional to the number of sensory receptors in each peripheral area of the body. Note the relatively large area devoted to **face** (especially lips) and to **hand** (especially thumb and index finger) while trunk representation is very small.

MOTOR CORTEX

The **motor nerve cells** which send out impulses to initiate **voluntary movement** of **skeletal muscles** lie in the **precentral gyrus** of each **frontal lobe** in the **cerebral cortex**.

Each cerebral hemisphere controls the muscles on the *opposite side* of the body.

The exact point in the **gyrus** where neurons controlling any one part of the body are situated is indicated in this coronal view of the gyrus.

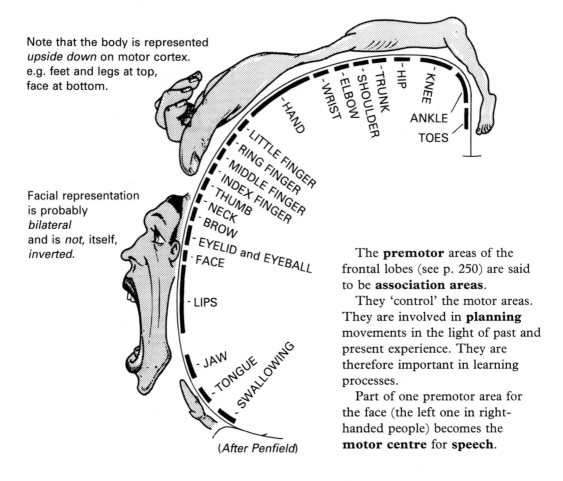

Note that the body is represented *upside down* on motor cortex. e.g. feet and legs at top, face at bottom.

Facial representation is probably *bilateral* and is *not*, itself, *inverted*.

(After Penfield)

The **premotor** areas of the frontal lobes (see p. 250) are said to be **association areas**.

They 'control' the motor areas. They are involved in **planning** movements in the light of past and present experience. They are therefore important in learning processes.

Part of one premotor area for the face (the left one in right-handed people) becomes the **motor centre** for **speech**.

The amount of motor cortex devoted to a particular part of the body is related, not to its relative size, but to the **precision** with which its movements can be controlled. Note the large area of the motor cortex (and therefore the very large number of neurons) devoted to the control of voluntary movements of the **hands**. This enables them to perform complicated movements and to acquire highly intricate skills: similarly with muscles of the mouth, lips, tongue and face which are used for talking.

MOTOR PATHWAYS TO HEAD AND NECK

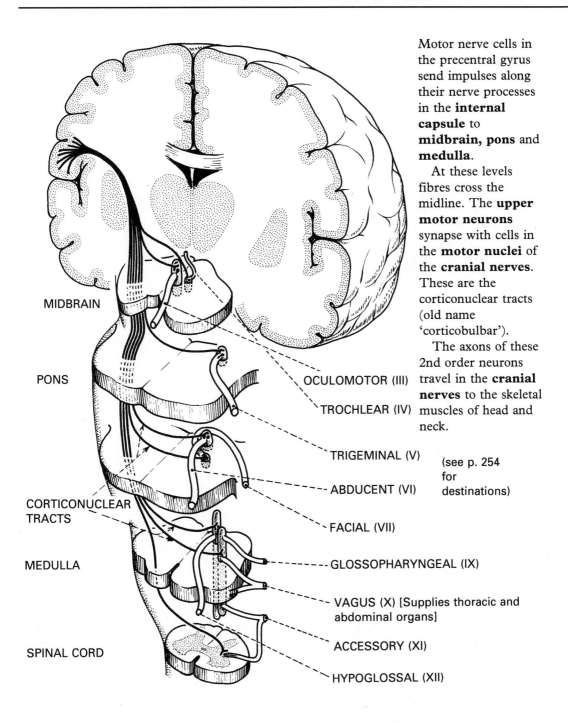

MIDBRAIN

PONS

CORTICONUCLEAR
TRACTS

MEDULLA

SPINAL CORD

OCULOMOTOR (III)

TROCHLEAR (IV)

TRIGEMINAL (V)

ABDUCENT (VI)

FACIAL (VII)

GLOSSOPHARYNGEAL (IX)

VAGUS (X) [Supplies thoracic and
abdominal organs]

ACCESSORY (XI)

HYPOGLOSSAL (XII)

Motor nerve cells in
the precentral gyrus
send impulses along
their nerve processes
in the **internal
capsule** to
midbrain, pons and
medulla.

At these levels
fibres cross the
midline. The **upper
motor neurons**
synapse with cells in
the **motor nuclei** of
the **cranial nerves**.
These are the
corticonuclear tracts
(old name
'corticobulbar').

The axons of these
2nd order neurons
travel in the **cranial
nerves** to the skeletal
muscles of head and
neck.

(see p. 254
for
destinations)

DIRECT (PYRAMIDAL) MOTOR PATHWAYS TO EXTREMITIES

Nerve impulses from the **motor cortex** to the **skeletal muscles** of the extremities can take a direct or indirect route. The controlling centres in the **motor cortex** are sometimes linked by only 2 neurons (upper and lower motor neurons) with the voluntary muscles. These routes form the **direct** or **pyramidal** pathways.

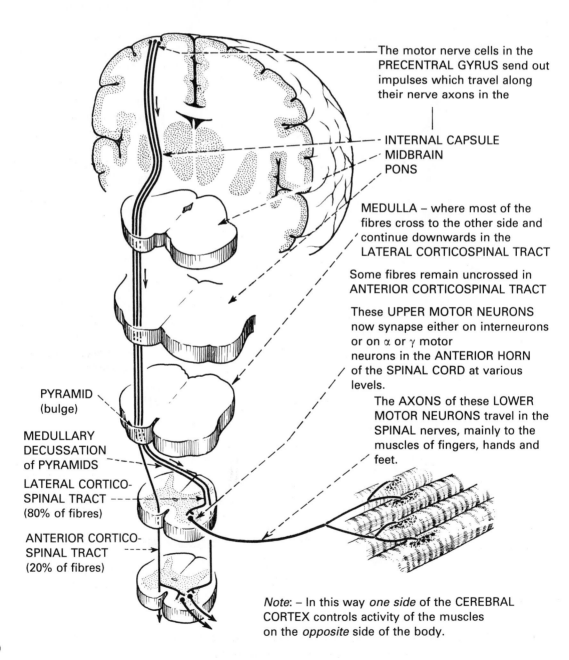

The motor nerve cells in the PRECENTRAL GYRUS send out impulses which travel along their nerve axons in the

INTERNAL CAPSULE
MIDBRAIN
PONS

MEDULLA – where most of the fibres cross to the other side and continue downwards in the LATERAL CORTICOSPINAL TRACT

Some fibres remain uncrossed in ANTERIOR CORTICOSPINAL TRACT

These UPPER MOTOR NEURONS now synapse either on interneurons or on α or γ motor neurons in the ANTERIOR HORN of the SPINAL CORD at various levels.

The AXONS of these LOWER MOTOR NEURONS travel in the SPINAL nerves, mainly to the muscles of fingers, hands and feet.

PYRAMID (bulge)

MEDULLARY DECUSSATION of PYRAMIDS

LATERAL CORTICO-SPINAL TRACT (80% of fibres)

ANTERIOR CORTICO-SPINAL TRACT (20% of fibres)

Note: – In this way *one side* of the CEREBRAL CORTEX controls activity of the muscles on the *opposite* side of the body.

INDIRECT (EXTRAPYRAMIDAL) PATHWAYS

The indirect (extrapyramidal) pathways include all descending motor tracts apart from the corticospinal and corticonuclear tracts.

The actual performance of a **voluntary movement** – initiated in the **cortex** – involves planning and programming by **motor centres** in the **basal ganglia** and **brain stem**.

Fibres from the direct and indirect pathways converge on the motor neurons in the anterior horns and cranial nerves.

Controls coordinated movements involving many muscles.

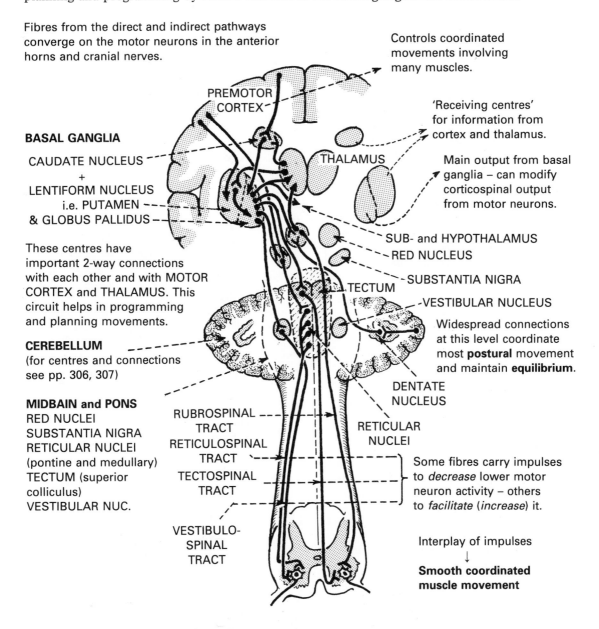

PREMOTOR CORTEX

THALAMUS

'Receiving centres' for information from cortex and thalamus.

Main output from basal ganglia – can modify corticospinal output from motor neurons.

BASAL GANGLIA

CAUDATE NUCLEUS
+
LENTIFORM NUCLEUS
i.e. PUTAMEN
& GLOBUS PALLIDUS

SUB- and HYPOTHALAMUS
RED NUCLEUS
SUBSTANTIA NIGRA
TECTUM
VESTIBULAR NUCLEUS

These centres have important 2-way connections with each other and with MOTOR CORTEX and THALAMUS. This circuit helps in programming and planning movements.

Widespread connections at this level coordinate most **postural** movement and maintain **equilibrium**.

CEREBELLUM
(for centres and connections see pp. 306, 307)

DENTATE NUCLEUS

MIDBAIN and PONS
RED NUCLEI
SUBSTANTIA NIGRA
RETICULAR NUCLEI
(pontine and medullary)
TECTUM (superior colliculus)
VESTIBULAR NUC.

RUBROSPINAL TRACT
RETICULOSPINAL TRACT
TECTOSPINAL TRACT

RETICULAR NUCLEI

Some fibres carry impulses to *decrease* lower motor neuron activity – others to *facilitate* (*increase*) it.

VESTIBULO-SPINAL TRACT

Interplay of impulses
↓
Smooth coordinated muscle movement

If part of this system, especially the basal ganglia, is damaged by disease, varying types of rigidity, tremor and uncoordinated muscle movement result.

FINAL COMMON PATHWAY

Each **motor neuron** in the **anterior horns** of the **spinal cord** serves as the **pathway** for motor impulses initiated in:

THE CEREBRUM (*of opposite side*)

and travelling in –

1 CORTICO-SPINAL TRACT

The motor neuron also serves as the **pathway** for coordinating corrective (restraining or facilitating) impulses discharged by – NUCLEI in the BRAIN STEM (*of same or opposite side*) and travelling in –

2 RUBROSPINAL TRACT
from red nucleus (*opposite side*)

3 DORSAL VESTIBULOSPINAL TRACT
from dorsal vestibular nucleus (*same side*)

4 OLIVOSPINAL TRACT
from olivary nucleus (*same side*)

5 RETICULOSPINAL TRACT
from reticular nuclei (*same side*)

6 VENTRAL VESTIBULOSPINAL TRACT
from vestibular nuclei (*opposite side*)

7 TECTOSPINAL TRACT
from tectum (*opposite side*)

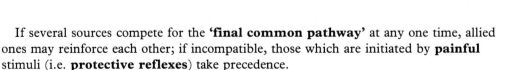

'Final common pathway'

Skeletal muscle fibres

The motor neuron also receives relays of afferent impulses from other reflex centres in –

spinal cord

8 For REFLEXES of *same* segment of cord and from *same* side of cord.

9 For REFLEXES of *same* segment but *other* side of cord and body.

10 For REFLEXES from *other* segments of cord but *same* side of cord.

11 For REFLEXES from *other* segments and *other* side of cord.

If several sources compete for the **'final common pathway'** at any one time, allied ones may reinforce each other; if incompatible, those which are initiated by **painful** stimuli (i.e. **protective reflexes**) take precedence.

PATHWAYS CONTROLLING MOTOR ACTIVITY

Many **sensory receptors**, **cerebral nuclei** and **integrating centres** are involved in the control of **motor activity**.

Sensory input comes from **skin**, **joints**, **muscle** and the **special senses** of **vision**, **hearing** and **balance**

The **cerebellum** constantly monitors movement and regulates the range, rate and force of contraction.

The **basal ganglia** and **brain stem nuclei** are all involved in integrating the control of **motor output**.

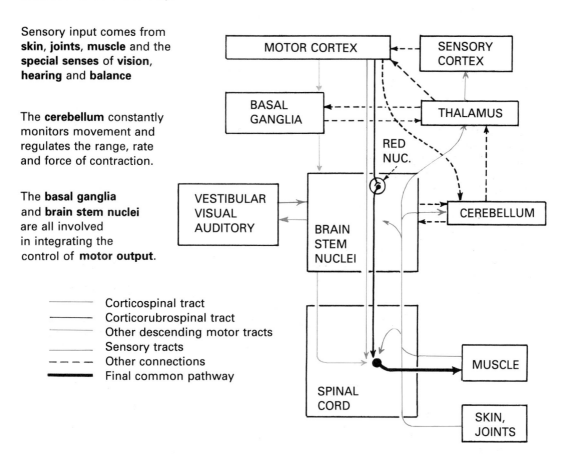

- ———— Corticospinal tract
- ———— Corticorubrospinal tract
- ———— Other descending motor tracts
- ———— Sensory tracts
- – – – – Other connections
- ━━━━ Final common pathway

The **corticospinal pathway** was formerly called the **pyramidal** tract since it runs through the **medullary pyramids**. All other descending pathways except the cerebellar were called the **extrapyramidal system**. The concept of two independent systems controlling movement is incorrect and most authors regard the terms as redundant. However the terms may persist for some time.

A more recent classification is based on the position of **termination** of the descending fibres in the grey matter of the spinal cord. The **lateral motor system** includes the **corticospinal** tracts and the **corticorubrospinal** pathway. It controls fine movements, particularly of the fingers and hands. The **medial motor system** includes the other descending tracts which originate primarily in the **brain stem**. It controls the muscles of the trunk and proximal parts of the limbs, thus it controls posture and equilibrium.

MOTOR UNIT

The **axon** of the **lower motor neuron** divides into many branches. Each branch ends at the **motor end-plate** of a single muscle fibre.

A **motor nerve** with the group of **muscle fibres** it supplies is known as a **motor unit**.

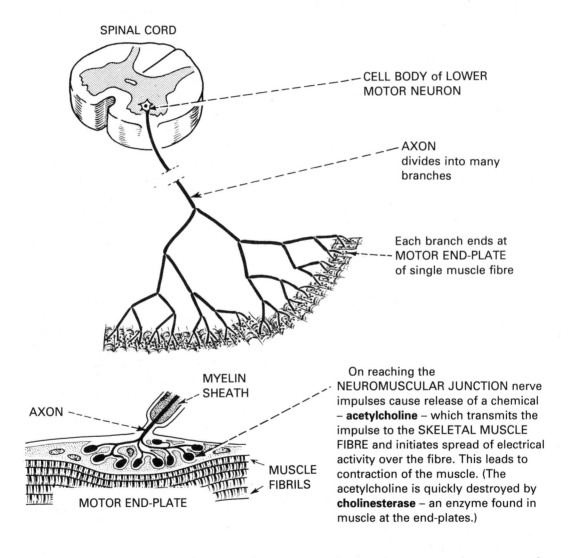

SPINAL CORD

CELL BODY of LOWER MOTOR NEURON

AXON
divides into many branches

Each branch ends at MOTOR END-PLATE of single muscle fibre

MYELIN SHEATH

AXON

MUSCLE FIBRILS

MOTOR END-PLATE

On reaching the NEUROMUSCULAR JUNCTION nerve impulses cause release of a chemical – **acetylcholine** – which transmits the impulse to the SKELETAL MUSCLE FIBRE and initiates spread of electrical activity over the fibre. This leads to contraction of the muscle. (The acetylcholine is quickly destroyed by **cholinesterase** – an enzyme found in muscle at the end-plates.)

In muscles requiring very fine control, e.g. extraocular muscles, *one* axon innervates only about *ten* muscle fibres. In muscles requiring less precise control *one* axon may innervate about 2000 muscle fibres.

CEREBELLUM

The cerebellum is important in the control of posture and movement and for learning patterns of movement. It has 2 hemispheres each with 3 **lobes, anterior, posterior** and **flocculonodular**. Functionally, the anterior and posterior lobes are organized into 3 longitudinal zones, lateral, intermediate and vermis.

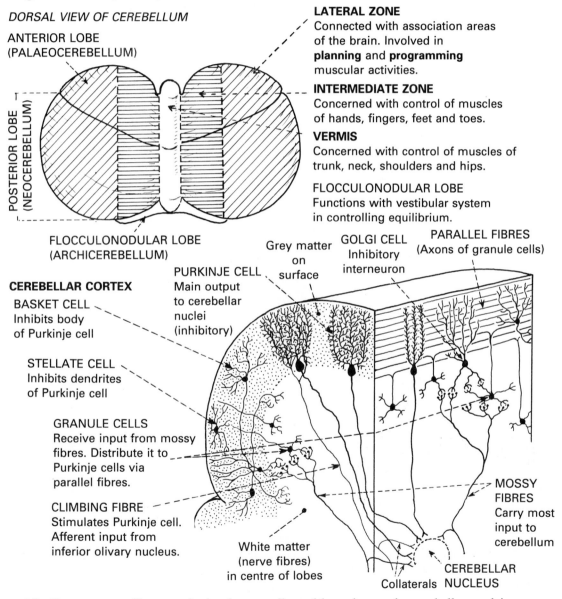

DORSAL VIEW OF CEREBELLUM

ANTERIOR LOBE
(PALAEOCEREBELLUM)

POSTERIOR LOBE
(NEOCEREBELLUM)

FLOCCULONODULAR LOBE
(ARCHICEREBELLUM)

LATERAL ZONE
Connected with association areas
of the brain. Involved in
planning and **programming**
muscular activities.

INTERMEDIATE ZONE
Concerned with control of muscles
of hands, fingers, feet and toes.

VERMIS
Concerned with control of muscles of
trunk, neck, shoulders and hips.

FLOCCULONODULAR LOBE
Functions with vestibular system
in controlling equilibrium.

CEREBELLAR CORTEX

BASKET CELL
Inhibits body
of Purkinje cell

STELLATE CELL
Inhibits dendrites
of Purkinje cell

GRANULE CELLS
Receive input from mossy
fibres. Distribute it to
Purkinje cells via
parallel fibres.

CLIMBING FIBRE
Stimulates Purkinje cell.
Afferent input from
inferior olivary nucleus.

PURKINJE CELL
Main output
to cerebellar
nuclei
(inhibitory)

Grey matter
on
surface

GOLGI CELL
Inhibitory
interneuron

PARALLEL FIBRES
(Axons of granule cells)

White matter
(nerve fibres)
in centre of lobes

Collaterals

MOSSY
FIBRES
Carry most
input to
cerebellum

CEREBELLAR
NUCLEUS

All afferent mossy fibres send stimulatory collateral branches to the cerebellar nuclei. Output from these nuclei is modulated by the inhibition from Purkinje cells (GABA is transmitter) which in turn is modulated by the effects of granule cells, Golgi cells, basket cells and stellate cells.

CEREBELLUM

INGOING PATHWAYS
The cerebellum
receives information . . .

. . . from SPINAL CORD
(Ventral spinocerebellar tract)
– information about the arrival
and strength of motor signals in
spinal cord.

. . . from EYES and EARS
(Tectocerebellar tracts
from colliculi)

. . . from CEREBRAL CORTEX
(Corticopontocerebellar
tract) – information
about muscle movements
'planned' by cortex. Largest
source of **mossy fibres**

. . . from OLIVARY NUCLEUS
(Olivocerebellar tract)
Receives proprioceptive and
cutaneous information from spinal
cord. Also connections from
motor cortex, basal ganglia
and reticular formation.
Sole source of **climbing fibres**.

Three bundles of nerve fibres – the superior, middle and
inferior **peduncles** – link the cerebellum with the
midbrain, pons and medulla respectively.

All sensory ingoing fibres to cerebellum send
collateral branches to deep cerebellar nuclei.

SUPERIOR
PEDUNCLE

MIDLINE

NUCLEI
PONTIS

MIDDLE
PEDUNCLE

INFERIOR
PEDUNCLE

MIDLINE

OLIVARY
NUCLEUS

CUNEATE
NUCLEUS

. . . from GENERAL PROPRIOCEPTORS (Dorsal
spinocerebellar tract) in sacral, lumbar and
thoracic regions – information about tension and
contraction of muscle, joint position, forces acting
on body surface.

. . . from SPECIAL PROPRIOCEPTORS (Vestibulocerebellar tract)
Semicircular canals – information about **movement** of head in space.

Utricle }
Saccule } – information about **position** of head in
space

. . . from CUNEATE NUCLEUS
(Cuneocerebellar tract)
– same information as
dorsal spinocerebellar
tract but from neck and
upper limbs.

The synaptic activity of cerebellar neurons is
modulated by afferent monoaminergic neurons from the
brain stem.

The cerebellum continuously receives information
about the exact position of all parts of the body in space
and what movements are 'planned'. Since the
information is received below the level of consciousness
it gives no sensation.

CEREBELLUM

OUTGOING PATHWAYS
Originate in VERMIS.
LATERAL and INTERMEDIATE
ZONES and FLOCCULONODULAR LOBE

The **intermediate zone** sends signals to GLOBOSE and EMBOLIFORM nuclei. Thence to RED NUCLEUS of opposite side to influence activity of rubrospinal motor pathway controlling proximal muscles of limbs – lateral motor system.

The **vermis** sends impulses direct to vestibular nucleus. Also via FASTIGIAL NUCLEUS to pontine and medullary reticular formation. Helps to control posture.

The **flocculonodular lobe** sends signals direct and via fastigial nucleus to VESTIBULAR NUCLEUS. Thence to vestibulospinal tract to coordinate movements and position of head with postural tone of limb muscles.

The **lateral zone** sends impulses to DENTATE nucleus, thence to CEREBRAL CORTEX via THALAMUS. Coordinates corticospinal motor activities. Also a small projection to RED NUCLEUS of opposite side to influence activity of the rubrospinal motor pathway.

White matter lies below the grey matter of the cerebellar cortex and in it are buried the deep **cerebellar nuclei – dentate, emboliform, globose** and **fastigial**.

The cerebral cortex probably initiates purposeful movements. During such movements proprioceptors are continually supplying information to the cerebellum about the changing positions of muscles and joints. The cerebellum compares intended movement with what is actually happening and can, if necessary, send feedback signals to the motor cortex to adjust the activity of the skeletal muscles to attain that intention. It smooths and coordinates complex sequences of skilled movements and regulates posture and balance.

307

CONTROL OF MUSCLE MOVEMENT

The muscle spindle is the key structure in the complex self-regulating mechanism for the control of movement of skeletal muscle.

In **voluntary movement** a muscle can be made to contract by impulses reaching it by one of *two routes*:-

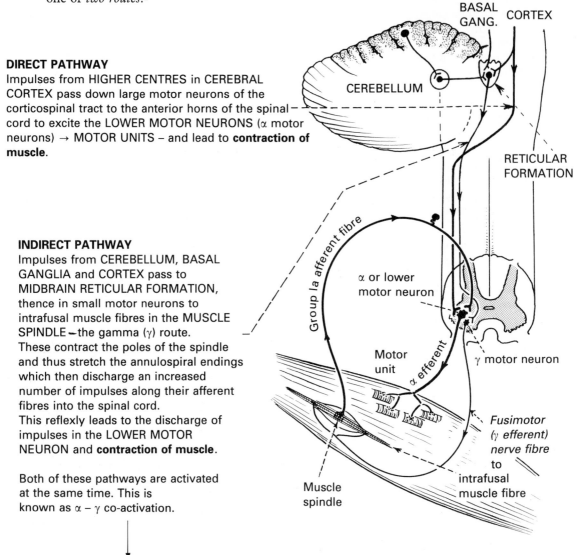

DIRECT PATHWAY
Impulses from HIGHER CENTRES in CEREBRAL CORTEX pass down large motor neurons of the corticospinal tract to the anterior horns of the spinal cord to excite the LOWER MOTOR NEURONS (α motor neurons) → MOTOR UNITS – and lead to **contraction of muscle**.

INDIRECT PATHWAY
Impulses from CEREBELLUM, BASAL GANGLIA and CORTEX pass to MIDBRAIN RETICULAR FORMATION, thence in small motor neurons to intrafusal muscle fibres in the MUSCLE SPINDLE – the gamma (γ) route.
These contract the poles of the spindle and thus stretch the annulospiral endings which then discharge an increased number of impulses along their afferent fibres into the spinal cord.
This reflexly leads to the discharge of impulses in the LOWER MOTOR NEURON and **contraction of muscle**.

Both of these pathways are activated at the same time. This is known as α – γ co-activation.

The length of the spindle thus alters at the same time as the length of the extrafusal fibres. The spindle therefore remains constantly capable of responding to stretch throughout the period of contraction and to change, if necessary, the α motor discharge to its muscle, and hence its contraction force, and therefore control muscle movement very accurately.

SKELETAL SYSTEM

BONES and MUSCLES – concerned with **movement** of the body.

SKELETON —— RIGID FRAMEWORK gives **shape** and **support** to body.
is JOINTED to permit **movement**.

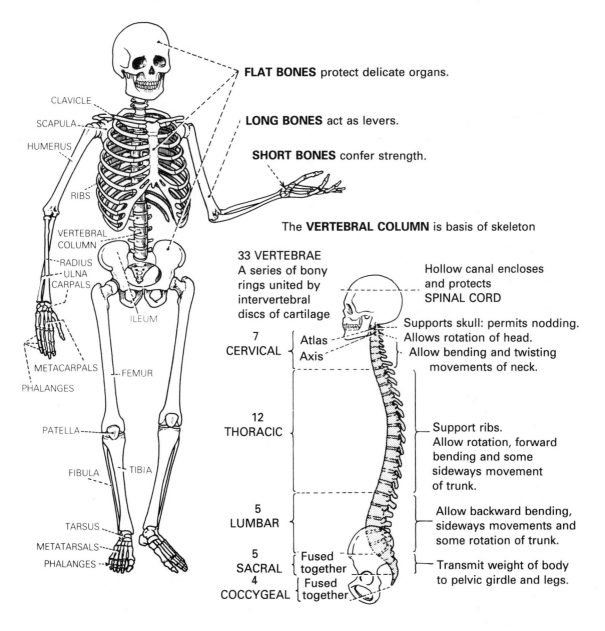

CLAVICLE
SCAPULA
HUMERUS
RIBS
VERTEBRAL COLUMN
RADIUS
ULNA
CARPALS
ILEUM
METACARPALS
PHALANGES
FEMUR
PATELLA
FIBULA
TIBIA
TARSUS
METATARSALS
PHALANGES

FLAT BONES protect delicate organs.

LONG BONES act as levers.

SHORT BONES confer strength.

The **VERTEBRAL COLUMN** is basis of skeleton

33 VERTEBRAE
A series of bony
rings united by
intervertebral
discs of cartilage

Hollow canal encloses
and protects
SPINAL CORD

7
CERVICAL

Atlas
Axis

Supports skull: permits nodding.
Allows rotation of head.
Allow bending and twisting
movements of neck.

12
THORACIC

Support ribs.
Allow rotation, forward
bending and some
sideways movement
of trunk.

5
LUMBAR

Allow backward bending,
sideways movements and
some rotation of trunk.

5
SACRAL

Fused
together

4
COCCYGEAL

Fused
together

Transmit weight of body
to pelvic girdle and legs.

All bones give attachment to muscles.

SKELETAL MUSCLES

Bones are moved at joints by the *contraction* and *relaxation* of **muscles** attached to them.

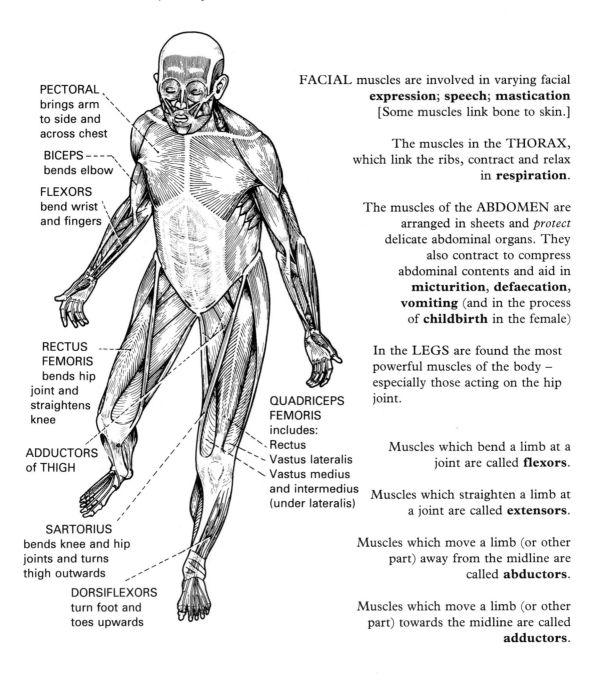

PECTORAL
brings arm
to side and
across chest

BICEPS
bends elbow

FLEXORS
bend wrist
and fingers

RECTUS
FEMORIS
bends hip
joint and
straightens
knee

ADDUCTORS
of THIGH

SARTORIUS
bends knee and hip
joints and turns
thigh outwards

DORSIFLEXORS
turn foot and
toes upwards

QUADRICEPS
FEMORIS
includes:
Rectus
Vastus lateralis
Vastus medius
and intermedius
(under lateralis)

FACIAL muscles are involved in varying facial **expression; speech; mastication** [Some muscles link bone to skin.]

The muscles in the THORAX, which link the ribs, contract and relax in **respiration**.

The muscles of the ABDOMEN are arranged in sheets and *protect* delicate abdominal organs. They also contract to compress abdominal contents and aid in **micturition, defaecation, vomiting** (and in the process of **childbirth** in the female)

In the LEGS are found the most powerful muscles of the body – especially those acting on the hip joint.

Muscles which bend a limb at a joint are called **flexors**.

Muscles which straighten a limb at a joint are called **extensors**.

Muscles which move a limb (or other part) away from the midline are called **abductors**.

Muscles which move a limb (or other part) towards the midline are called **adductors**.

310

SKELETAL MUSCLES

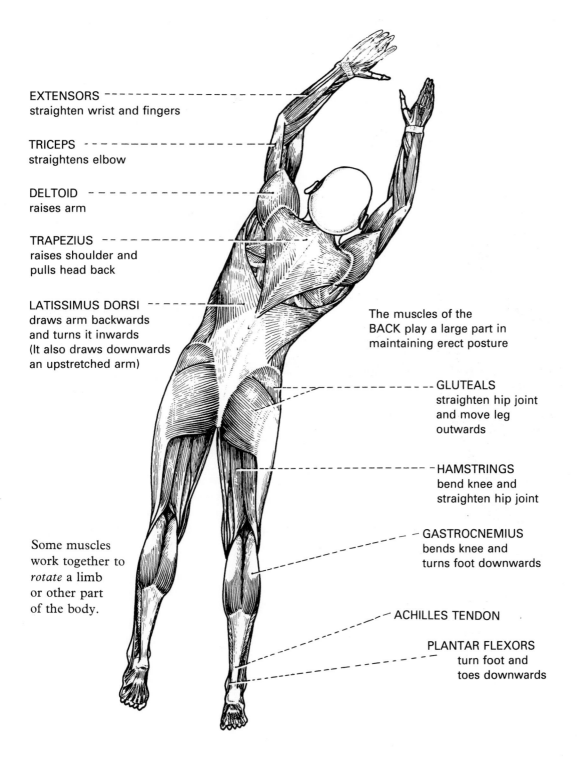

EXTENSORS
straighten wrist and fingers

TRICEPS
straightens elbow

DELTOID
raises arm

TRAPEZIUS
raises shoulder and
pulls head back

LATISSIMUS DORSI
draws arm backwards
and turns it inwards
(It also draws downwards
an upstretched arm)

The muscles of the
BACK play a large part in
maintaining erect posture

Some muscles
work together to
rotate a limb
or other part
of the body.

GLUTEALS
straighten hip joint
and move leg
outwards

HAMSTRINGS
bend knee and
straighten hip joint

GASTROCNEMIUS
bends knee and
turns foot downwards

ACHILLES TENDON

PLANTAR FLEXORS
turn foot and
toes downwards

311

MUSCULAR MOVEMENTS

The long bones particularly form a light framework of **levers**.
The skeletal muscles attached to them contract to operate these levers.

When a muscle contracts it shortens.

This brings its two ends closer together.

Since the two ends are attached to different bones by **tendons** one or other of the bones must move.

Two bones meet or articulate at a **joint**.

Joint surfaces are covered with a layer of smooth **cartilage**.

To avoid friction when the two surfaces move on one another a **synovial membrane** secretes a **lubricating fluid**.

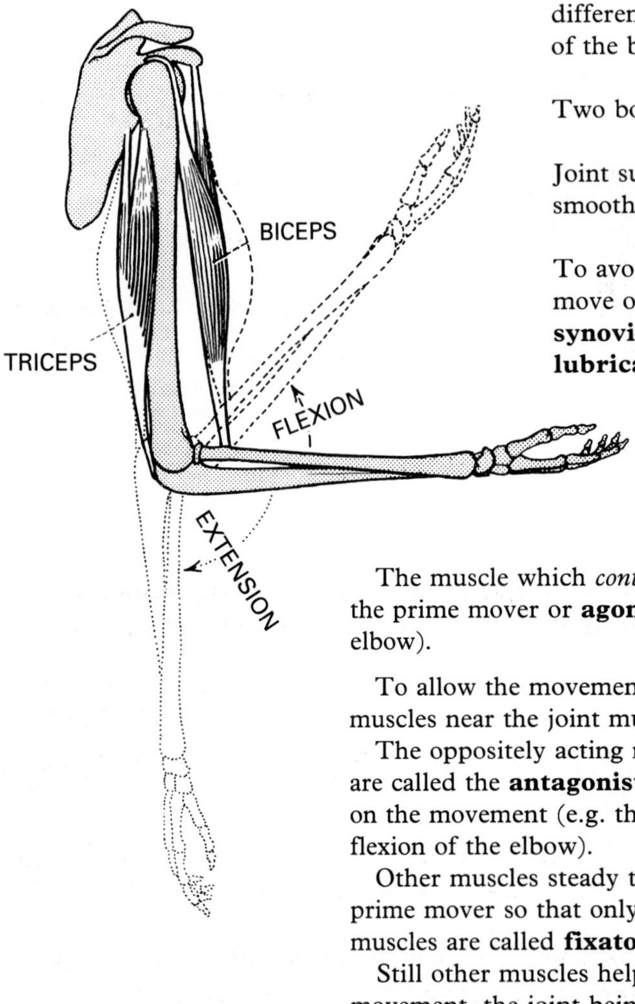

BICEPS

TRICEPS

FLEXION

EXTENSION

The muscle which *contracts* to move the joint is called the prime mover or **agonist** (the biceps in flexion of elbow).

To allow the movement to take place, however, other muscles near the joint must cooperate:-
The oppositely acting muscles gradually *relax* – these are called the **antagonists** and exercise a 'braking' control on the movement (e.g. the extensors – chiefly triceps – in flexion of the elbow).
Other muscles steady the bone giving 'origin' to the prime mover so that only the 'insertion' will move – these muscles are called **fixators**.
Still other muscles help to steady, for most efficient movement, the joint being moved – called **synergists**.

When the elbow is straightened the reverse occurs:-
Triceps, the prime mover, *contracts*; biceps, the antagonist, *relaxes*.

RECIPROCAL INNERVATION

The coordinated group action of muscles is made possible by the many synaptic connections between interneurons of the *ingoing* or **proprioceptive neurons** of one muscle group and the *outgoing* or **motor neurons** of the functionally opposite group of muscles.

This is shown diagrammatically for the reciprocal contraction and relaxation of the extensors and flexors during the **stretch reflex**. See also page 258.

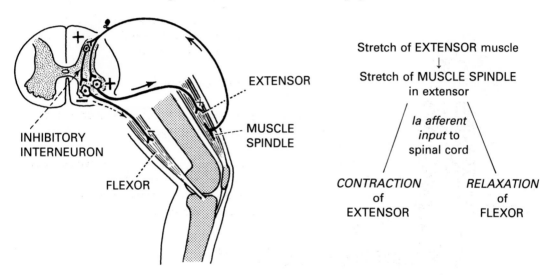

Stretch of EXTENSOR muscle
↓
Stretch of MUSCLE SPINDLE
in extensor

*la afferent
input* to
spinal cord

CONTRACTION
of
EXTENSOR

RELAXATION
of
FLEXOR

Reciprocal innervation is due to an **inhibitory** interneuron (within the spinal cord) interposed between the sensory nerve fibre and the α-motor neuron of the **flexor** muscle.

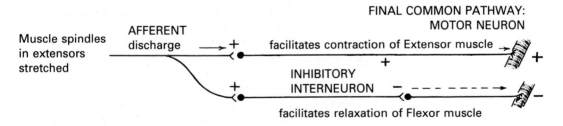

Reciprocal **inhibition** of the flexor muscle is mediated by a **disynaptic** (two synapses) pathway. Contraction of the **extensor** muscle is mediated by a **monosynaptic** pathway.

SKELETAL MUSCLE AND THE MECHANISM OF CONTRACTION

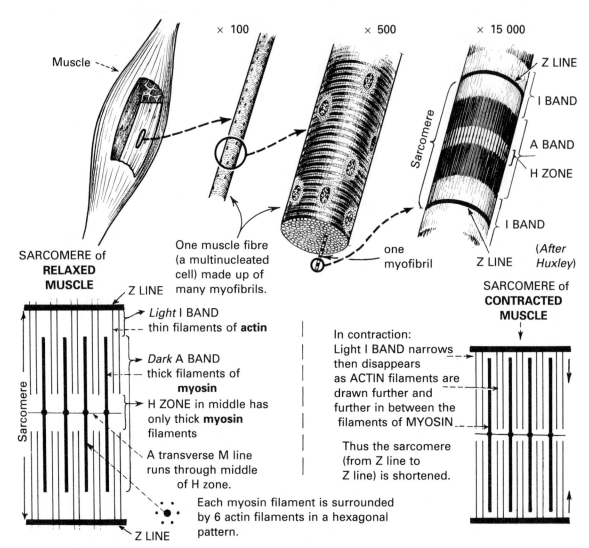

× 100   × 500   × 15 000

Muscle

Z LINE

I BAND

A BAND

H ZONE

I BAND

Sarcomere

(After Huxley)

SARCOMERE of **RELAXED MUSCLE**

Z LINE

One muscle fibre (a multinucleated cell) made up of many myofibrils.

one myofibril

Z LINE

SARCOMERE of **CONTRACTED MUSCLE**

Light I BAND — thin filaments of **actin**

Dark A BAND — thick filaments of **myosin**

H ZONE in middle has only thick **myosin** filaments

A transverse M line runs through middle of H zone.

In contraction: Light I BAND narrows then disappears as ACTIN filaments are drawn further and further in between the filaments of MYOSIN

Thus the sarcomere (from Z line to Z line) is shortened.

Each myosin filament is surrounded by 6 actin filaments in a hexagonal pattern.

Z LINE

Sarcomere

Energy for contraction is derived from glucose and fat in the mitochondria (page 12). The energy is transported in ATP from the mitochondria to the contractile filaments. ATP splits readily into ADP and phosphate, releasing its trapped energy where needed (page 49).

There are 3 types of skeletal muscle fibre based on the **speed** of contraction and **fatigue** resistance. **Type I** are slow twitch and fatigue resistant; have **many** blood vessels and mitochondria and much myoglobin. Its myosin molecules split ATP **slowly**. **Type IIA** are fast twitch and fatigue resistant; also have **many** blood vessels and mitochondria and much myoglobin. Its myosin molecules split ATP **rapidly**. **Type IIB** are fast twitch and fatiguable; have **few** blood vessels and mitochondria and little myoglobin. Its myosin molecules split ATP **rapidly**.

SKELETAL MUSCLE – MOLECULAR BASIS OF CONTRACTION

Actin and **myosin** filaments *slide* past each other during *contraction* of skeletal muscle.

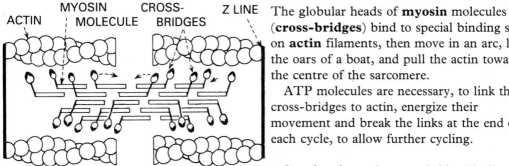

SARCOMERE

ACTIN — MYOSIN MOLECULE — CROSS-BRIDGES — Z LINE

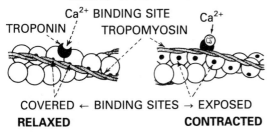

CHAINS OF ACTIN MOLECULES

TROPONIN — Ca^{2+} BINDING SITE — TROPOMYOSIN — Ca^{2+}

COVERED ← BINDING SITES → EXPOSED
RELAXED   **CONTRACTED**

The globular heads of **myosin** molecules (**cross-bridges**) bind to special binding sites on **actin** filaments, then move in an arc, like the oars of a boat, and pull the actin towards the centre of the sarcomere.

ATP molecules are necessary, to link the cross-bridges to actin, energize their movement and break the links at the end of each cycle, to allow further cycling.

In *relaxed* muscle, cross-bridge binding is inhibited by regulatory proteins, **troponin** and **tropomyosin**. Tropomyosin *covers* the actin binding sites. Troponin *holds* the tropomyosin in this blocking position. To initiate cross-bridge cycling Ca^{2+} attaches to troponin and changes its *shape*. This change moves tropomyosin away from and thus exposes the binding sites, allowing cross-bridge cycling and contraction to proceed. Removal of Ca^{2+} *reverses* the process and the muscle *relaxes*.

To initiate *contraction* Ca^{2+} is released from the **lateral sacs** of the **sarcoplasmic reticulum**, segments of which are wrapped round the myofibrils covering each A and I band. Between each segment a **transverse** or **T-tubule** system which is continuous with the plasma membrane forms a grid perforated by the myofibrils. Its lumen is continuous with the extracellular fluid. Action potentials travelling along the muscle membrane pass down into the **T-tubules** and cause release of Ca^{2+} from the sarcoplasmic reticulum to initiate contraction. At the end of contraction Ca^{2+} is pumped back into the sacroplasmic reticulum, removing it from the troponin and thus *relaxation* occurs.

T. TUBULE — SARCOPLASMIC RETICULUM — PLASMA MEMBRANE

MYOFIBRILS — LATERAL SACS — Z LINE — ← A BAND → — I BAND

CHAPTER 11

AUTONOMIC NERVOUS SYSTEM AND CHEMICAL TRANSMISSION AT NERVE ENDINGS

THE AUTONOMIC NERVOUS SYSTEM

The **autonomic nervous system** (ANS) consists of **efferent nerves** from the central nervous system (CNS) which innervate cardiac muscle, smooth muscle and some gland cells (effector cells). The ANS has 2 divisions: (1) the **parasympathetic** or craniosacral system and (2) the **sympathetic** or thoraco-lumbar system. The parasympathetic system consists of outflows in **cranial nerves** III, VII, IX and X and outflows from the **sacral** part of the spinal cord (S2, 3 and 4). The sympathetic system consists of outflows from the **thoraco-lumbar** part of the spinal cord (T1-L3).

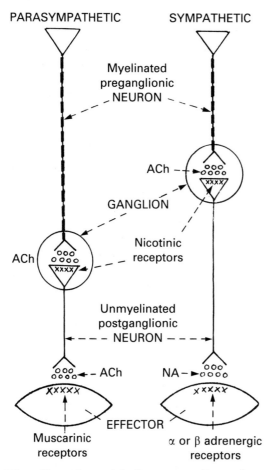

A nerve impulse in the ANS has to travel along **2 neurons in series** to get from the CNS to an effector cell. The first neuron has its cell body in the CNS; it is myelinated and called the **preganglionic neuron**. The second is unmyelinated and called the **postganglionic neuron**.

The nerve impulse is transmitted from the pre- to the postganglionic neuron by the chemical transmitter **acetylcholine** (ACh). Where this occurs, the nerve cell body forms a swelling or **ganglion**. Collections of nerve cell bodies in the peripheral nervous system are called ganglia (singular, a ganglion). NB: Collections of nerve cell bodies in the CNS are called **nuclei**.

In the parasympathetic system the nerve impulse is transmitted from the postganglionic neuron to the effector cell by **acetylcholine**; in the sympathetic system it is *normally* by **noradrenaline** (NA). In a few exceptional cases post-ganglionic sympathetic neurons release acetylcholine e.g. in sweat glands and in vasodilator fibres in skeletal muscle blood vessels.

The effect of acetylcholine at ganglion cells can be mimicked by the drug nicotine, so acetylcholine receptors on postganglionic neurons are classified as **nicotinic** receptors. Similarly, acetylcholine effects at parasympathetic postganglionic junction can be mimicked by the drug muscarine, so acetylcholine receptors on the effector cells are classified as **muscarinic** receptors. Compare this with **somatic motor nerves** which are cholinergic and the receptors on skeletal muscle are **nicotinic** receptors (see p. 323).

Noradrenergic receptors are classified as α_1, α_2, β_1 and β_2. The different receptors result in different effects on the **second messenger system** (pp. 69, 70) in the effector cell.

AUTONOMIC GANGLIA

The nerve cell bodies of preganglionic sympathetic nerves lie in the **lateral horns** of the grey matter of thoracic 1 to lumbar 3 spinal cord segments (T1–L3). The preganglionic fibres leave in the anterior nerve root and synapse in **paravertebral** or **prevertebral** ganglia.

The paravertebral ganglia consist of 22 pairs of ganglia linked by nerve fibres which form the **sympathetic trunks** (or chains). These trunks run from the base of the skull down through the neck, then through the inside of the thoracic and abdominal cavities on either side of the vertebral column to the coccyx. In the neck (cervical region) there are only 3 ganglia, the **superior, middle** and **inferior cervical** ganglia.

The **prevertebral** ganglia are situated at the origin of the main arteries which come off the abdominal aorta and take their names from these arteries: the **coeliac, superior mesenteric** and **inferior mesenteric** ganglia. Postganglionic fibres accompany the blood vessels from there to the abdominal viscera.

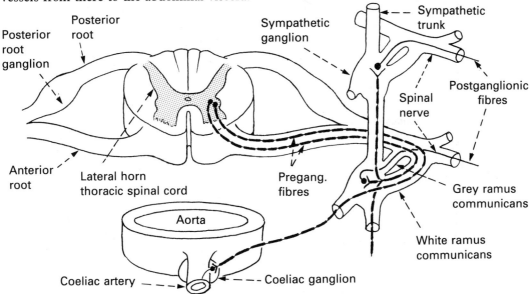

The preganglionic sympathetic fibres which leave the spinal nerve to run to the sympathetic trunk, because they are myelinated, are white and form a **white ramus communicans** (plural, rami communicantes). The postganglionic fibres which run from the sympathetic trunk back to the spinal nerve are unmyelinated, appear grey and form a **grey ramus communicans**.

A single preganglionic fibre may run up or down in the trunk and synapse with 20 or more postganglionic fibres. **Sympathetic** responses are thus **widespread**.

The preganglionic parasympathetic fibres are long. Their nerve cell bodies are in the nuclei of the cranial nerves III, VII, IX and X; those of the sacral outflow are in the lateral horns of the grey matter of sacral segments 2, 3 and 4 (S2, 3 and 4) of the spinal cord. The parasympathetic ganglia are in or very near the organ which they innervate and are called **terminal** (or intramural) ganglia. One preganglionic parasympathetic fibre usually synapses with only 4 or 5 postganglionic neurons which are short. **Parasympathetic** effects are thus more **localized**.

PARASYMPATHETIC OUTFLOWS

The functions of the autonomic system are normally reflexly controlled and are carried out below the level of consciousness.

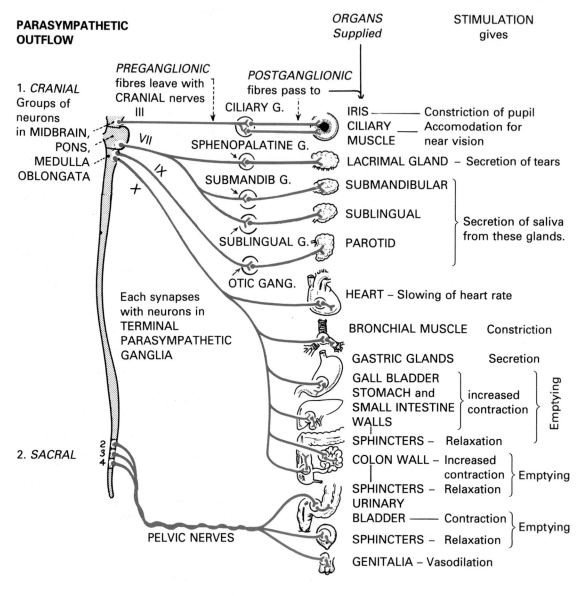

PARASYMPATHETIC OUTFLOW

PREGANGLIONIC fibres leave with CRANIAL nerves

POSTGANGLIONIC fibres pass to

ORGANS Supplied

STIMULATION gives

1. *CRANIAL* Groups of neurons in MIDBRAIN, PONS, MEDULLA OBLONGATA

III — CILIARY G.

VII — SPHENOPALATINE G.

IX — SUBMANDIB G.

SUBLINGUAL G.

OTIC GANG.

IRIS — Constriction of pupil
CILIARY MUSCLE — Accomodation for near vision

LACRIMAL GLAND – Secretion of tears

SUBMANDIBULAR
SUBLINGUAL
PAROTID
} Secretion of saliva from these glands.

Each synapses with neurons in TERMINAL PARASYMPATHETIC GANGLIA

HEART – Slowing of heart rate

BRONCHIAL MUSCLE — Constriction

GASTRIC GLANDS — Secretion

GALL BLADDER
STOMACH and
SMALL INTESTINE WALLS
} increased contraction } Emptying

SPHINCTERS – Relaxation

2. *SACRAL*
2
3
4

COLON WALL – Increased contraction } Emptying

SPHINCTERS – Relaxation

URINARY BLADDER — Contraction } Emptying

SPHINCTERS – Relaxation

GENITALIA – Vasodilation

PELVIC NERVES

The parasympathetic system is concerned mainly with the production and conservation of energy, e.g. it promotes reabsorption from the gut, slows the heart, etc.

SYMPATHETIC OUTFLOWS

The parasympathetic and sympathetic systems usually act in balanced reciprocal fashion. The activity of an organ at any one time is the result of the two opposing influences. However this is not *always* true, e.g. most blood vessels have only a sympathetic innervation.

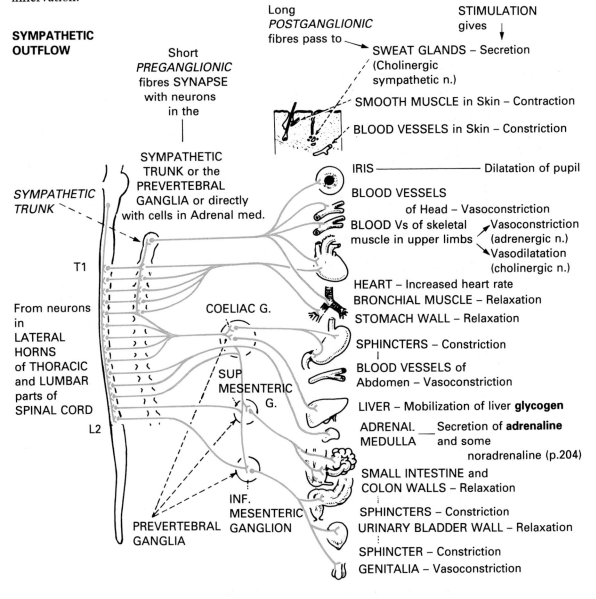

SYMPATHETIC OUTFLOW

Short *PREGANGLIONIC* fibres SYNAPSE with neurons in the

SYMPATHETIC TRUNK or the PREVERTEBRAL GANGLIA or directly with cells in Adrenal med.

SYMPATHETIC TRUNK

T1

From neurons in LATERAL HORNS of THORACIC and LUMBAR parts of SPINAL CORD

L2

PREVERTEBRAL GANGLIA

COELIAC G.

SUP. MESENTERIC G.

INF. MESENTERIC GANGLION

Long *POSTGANGLIONIC* fibres pass to

STIMULATION gives

SWEAT GLANDS – Secretion (Cholinergic sympathetic n.)

SMOOTH MUSCLE in Skin – Contraction

BLOOD VESSELS in Skin – Constriction

IRIS ——————— Dilatation of pupil

BLOOD VESSELS of Head – Vasoconstriction

BLOOD Vs of skeletal muscle in upper limbs — Vasoconstriction (adrenergic n.) / Vasodilatation (cholinergic n.)

HEART – Increased heart rate

BRONCHIAL MUSCLE – Relaxation

STOMACH WALL – Relaxation

SPHINCTERS – Constriction

BLOOD VESSELS of Abdomen – Vasoconstriction

LIVER – Mobilization of liver **glycogen**

ADRENAL MEDULLA — Secretion of **adrenaline** and some noradrenaline (p.204)

SMALL INTESTINE and COLON WALLS – Relaxation

SPHINCTERS – Constriction

URINARY BLADDER WALL – Relaxation

SPHINCTER – Constriction

GENITALIA – Vasoconstriction

The sympathetic system is regarded as preparing the animal for 'fight' or 'flight'.

321

AUTONOMIC REFLEX

Autonomic centres in the **brain** and **spinal cord** receive *sensory inflows* from the **viscera**. (Less is known about their exact pathways than about *motor outflows*.) Some of the *sensory neurons* convey information about events in the viscera to **higher autonomic centres** which send impulses to modify the activity of

Both *visceral* and *somatic afferents* serve as *afferent pathways* for **autonomic reflexes** by means of which much of the nervous regulation of vegetative functions is carried out below the level of consciousness.

E.g. the simplest autonomic reflex arc:–

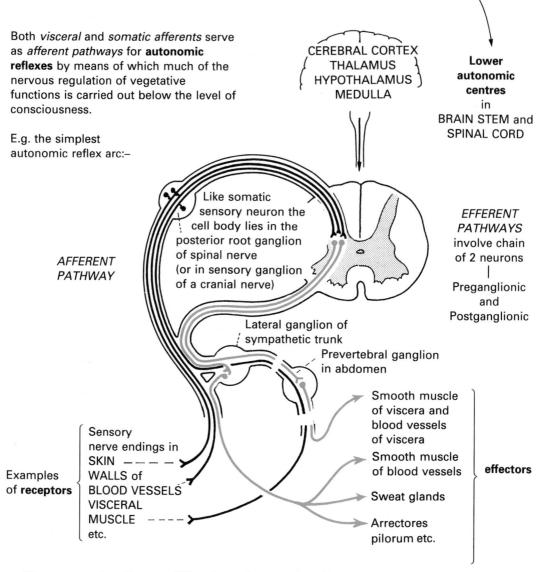

CEREBRAL CORTEX
THALAMUS
HYPOTHALAMUS
MEDULLA

Lower autonomic centres in BRAIN STEM and SPINAL CORD

AFFERENT PATHWAY

Like somatic sensory neuron the cell body lies in the posterior root ganglion of spinal nerve (or in sensory ganglion of a cranial nerve)

EFFERENT PATHWAYS involve chain of 2 neurons

Preganglionic and Postganglionic

Lateral ganglion of sympathetic trunk

Prevertebral ganglion in abdomen

Examples of **receptors**

Sensory nerve endings in
SKIN
WALLS of
BLOOD VESSELS
VISCERAL
MUSCLE
etc.

Smooth muscle of viscera and blood vessels of viscera

Smooth muscle of blood vessels

Sweat glands

Arrectores pilorum etc.

effectors

The autonomic reflex arc differs from the somatic reflex arc mainly in that it has *two efferent neurons*. Transmission of impulse from *afferent* to *efferent* probably involves one or more interneurons.

Reflex control of blood pressure is a more complex and an important example of an autonomic reflex (see pp. 124, 125).

322

CHEMICAL TRANSMISSION AT NERVE ENDINGS

When an **action potential** reaches the endings of a nerve, a **neurotransmitter** is liberated. It diffuses across the gap between the nerve endings and the next neuron or effector cell and attaches itself to **receptors** on the membrane of the cell. This attachment alters the permeability of the post-synaptic membrane to Na^+ ions and results in onward spread of the action potential over the post-synaptic cell. Some transmitters can **inhibit** the post-synaptic membrane by altering its permeability to Cl^- or K^+.

Some nerves when stimulated liberate acetylcholine. These are called *cholinergic* nerves. Others liberate noradrenaline. These are called *adrenergic* nerves.

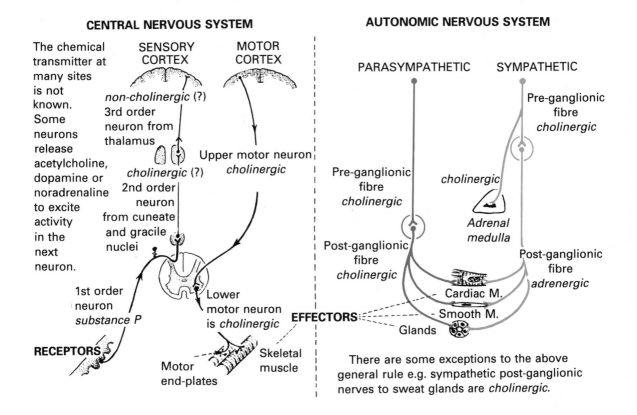

Acetylcholine, adrenaline, noradrenaline, dopamine and the amino acids glutamate, glycine and gamma aminobutyric acid (GABA) are important neurotransmitters in the CNS. GABA and glycine are **inhibitory** transmitters; glutamate is an important **excitatory** transmitter, it can kill cells by overstimulating them.

Possibly all neurons contain more than one transmitter; i.e. they contain cotransmitters e.g. neuropeptide Y is released with noradrenaline and potentiates its action. VIP is secreted with and potentiates the action of acetylcholine.

323